IAC-IARC-WHO Cytopathology Reporting Systems • 1st Edition

WHO Reporting System for Pancreaticobiliary Cytopathology

International Academy of Cytology – International Agency for Research on Cancer – World Health Organization
Joint Editorial Board

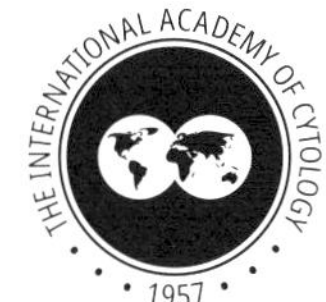

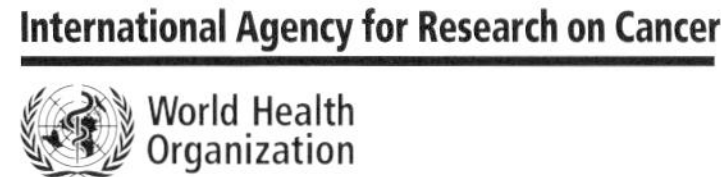

Suggested citation

International Academy of Cytology – International Agency for Research on Cancer – World Health Organization Joint Editorial Board. WHO Reporting System for Pancreaticobiliary Cytopathology. Lyon (France): International Agency for Research on Cancer; 2022. (IAC-IARC-WHO cytopathology reporting systems series, 1st ed.; vol. 2). https://publications.iarc.fr/621.

Sales, rights, and permissions

Print copies are distributed by WHO Press, World Health Organization, 20 Avenue Appia, 1211 Geneva 27, Switzerland
Tel.: +41 22 791 3264; Fax: +41 22 791 4857; email: bookorders@who.int; website: https://whobluebooks.iarc.fr

To purchase IARC publications in electronic format, see the IARC Publications website (https://publications.iarc.fr).

Third-party materials

General disclaimers

First print run (2500 copies)

Updated corrigenda can be found at https://publications.iarc.fr

IARC Library Cataloguing-in-Publication Data

Names: International Academy of Cytology – International Agency for Research on Cancer – World Health Organization Joint Editorial Board.
Title: WHO reporting system for pancreaticobiliary cytopathology / edited by International Academy of Cytology – International Agency for Research on Cancer – World Health Organization Joint Editorial Board.
Description: First edition. | Lyon: International Agency for Research on Cancer, 2022. | Series: IAC-IARC-WHO cytopathology reporting systems. | Includes bibliographical references and index.
Identifiers: ISBN 9789283245186 (pbk.) | ISBN 9789283245193 (ebook)
Subjects: MESH: Pancreas--pathology. | Biliary Tract--pathology. | Pancreatic Diseases--diagnosis. | Biliary Tract Diseases--diagnosis. | Cytodiagnosis--classification.
Classification: NLW WI 750

The WHO Reporting System for Pancreaticobiliary Cytopathology presented in this book reflects the views of the International Academy of Cytology (IAC) – International Agency for Research on Cancer (IARC) – World Health Organization (WHO) Joint Editorial Board that convened via video conference 27–29 April 2021.

The IAC-IARC-WHO Joint Editorial Board

Expert members: Pancreaticobiliary cytopathology

Standing members

* Standing members marked with an asterisk also served as expert members for this volume.

For the complete list of all contributors and their affiliations, see pages 181–182.

WHO Reporting System for Pancreaticobiliary Cytopathology

Edited by	The IAC-IARC-WHO Joint Editorial Board
IAC-IARC Pathology Editors	Martha Bishop Pitman Andrew S. Field Ian A. Cree
Additional IARC Editing	Gabrielle Goldman-Lévy
Project Assistant	Asiedua Asante
Assistants	Anne-Sophie Bres Laura Brispot Nandini Deleu Nicole Suty
Production Editor	Jessica Cox
Copy Editing	Julia Slone-Murphy
Principal Information Assistant	Alberto Machado
Information Assistant	Catarina Marques
Layout	Catarina Marques
Printed by	Omnibook 74370 Argonay, France
Publisher	International Agency for Research on Cancer (IARC) 150 Cours Albert Thomas 69372 Lyon Cedex 08, France

Contents

List of abbreviations

2D	two-dimensional
3D	three-dimensional
ACR	American College of Radiology
AR	androgen receptor
BDB	bile duct brushing
CEP	chromosome enumeration probe
CI	confidence interval
CNB	core needle biopsy
CT	computed tomography
CXR	chest X-ray
DNA	deoxyribonucleic acid
EBV	Epstein–Barr virus
ER	estrogen receptor
ERCP	endoscopic retrograde cholangiopancreatography
EUS	endoscopic ultrasound, endoscopic ultrasonography
EUS-FNAB	endoscopic ultrasound–guided fine-needle aspiration biopsy
FISH	fluorescence in situ hybridization
FNAB	fine-needle aspiration biopsy
H&E	haematoxylin and eosin stain
HGA	high-grade atypia
HGEA	high-grade epithelial atypia
IAC	International Academy of Cytology
IARC	International Agency for Research on Cancer
ICC	immunocytochemistry
ICDC	international consensus diagnostic criteria
LGEA	low-grade epithelial atypia
MRI	magnetic resonance imaging
MSI	microsatellite instability
NGS	next-generation sequencing
NOS	not otherwise specified
NSE	neuron-specific enolase
OGC	osteoclast-like giant cell
Pap	Papanicolaou stain
PAS	periodic acid–Schiff
PASD	periodic acid–Schiff with diastase
PCR	polymerase chain reaction
PET	positron emission tomography
PET-CT	positron emission tomography–computed tomography
PR	progesterone receptor
PSC	Papanicolaou Society of Cytopathology
RNA	ribonucleic acid
ROM	risk of malignancy
ROSE	rapid onsite evaluation
SNV	single-nucleotide variant

Foreword

The classification of tumours can be viewed from many perspectives. To a histopathologist it is all about the histological patterns, to a molecular pathologist or geneticist it is all about which genes are affected, and to an epidemiologist it is about the tumours' incidence. The WHO Classification of Tumours series started in the 1960s as a result of the histopathologist's need to make diagnoses by grouping tumours according to their microscopic appearance. The programme now includes contributions from many specialties, including, of course, cytopathology. However, the cytopathologist looks at tumours slightly differently than other specialists do, and although the main classification is helpful, it has become clear that reporting systems based on the key diagnostic cytopathological features are needed, tailored to the diagnostic categories in widespread use. There is also a need for these reporting systems to be truly international, serving the needs of patients worldwide.

The International Academy of Cytology (IAC), a scientific, non-profit organization with members from 49 other cytopathology-affiliated societies, therefore approached the International Agency for Research on Cancer (IARC) – home to the WHO Classification of Tumours Programme – to see whether it would be possible to produce a complementary series of WHO Reporting Systems, particularly for the areas of diagnostic cytopathology that did not already have agreed systems published by others. The two organizations signed a memorandum of understanding in early 2020 and, despite the problems of the COVID-19 pandemic, have produced the first WHO Reporting System for Lung Cytopathology and now the series' second volume – the WHO Reporting System for Pancreaticobiliary Cytopathology. Reporting systems for lymph node and soft tissue cytopathology are reaching completion, and further systems are planned.

Cytopathology plays a critical role in the diagnosis of many pancreaticobiliary conditions, including tumours. With recent developments in sampling technology, there now remain only a few lesions that cannot be sampled for cytopathological examination. Endoscopic ultrasound–guided fine-needle aspiration biopsy (EUS-FNAB) has emerged as the standard of care for the diagnosis of solid pancreatic lesions by cytopathology. Imaging detection of ever-smaller lesions, combined with the ability to obtain tissue from all but a few, facilitates cytopathological diagnosis in addition to, or in some instances instead of, histopathological diagnosis. Endoscopic examination of bile ducts is used to produce washings for cytological examination. Ancillary methods such as immunocytochemistry and in situ hybridization are applicable to smears and cell blocks, which also provide material for next-generation sequencing. The avoidance of formalin in cytopathological preparations allows molecular methods to be applied, whether simple PCR or next-generation sequencing, for diagnosis and predictive testing.

Just as the WHO Classification of Tumours series (also known as the WHO Blue Books), published in print volumes and as a website (https://tumourclassification.iarc.who.int), is an essential tool for standardizing diagnostic practice worldwide and serves as a vehicle for the translation of cancer research into practice, we hope that these first-edition WHO Reporting Systems will fulfil the same role for cytopathology. The key diagnostic cytopathological features listed for each tumour type under the diagnostic categories represent the first international consensus and are described in precise, uniform language. These diagnostic criteria are underpinned by evidence that has been evaluated and debated by experts in the field. Each lesion-specific section includes a dedicated subsection discussing the differential diagnosis of the lesion's cytopathological features that can be used worldwide, including in low-resources settings, followed by a subsection describing the current best-practice application of ancillary testing (including next-generation sequencing) on cytopathology material. About 70 authors and editors participated in the production of this volume, and gave their time freely to this task. We are very grateful for their help; it is a remarkable team effort.

This volume, like those of the WHO Classification of Tumours series, has been led by an editorial board composed of standing and expert members. The standing members include the chair of the WHO Classification of Tumours Editorial Board and others nominated by the IAC. The expert members, selected on the basis of informed bibliometric analysis and advice from the standing members, represent a broad international expertise, as does the authorship group. The diagnostic process is increasingly multidisciplinary, and we are delighted that several radiology and clinical experts have joined us to address specific needs.

In addition to using the International System of Units (SI) for all measurements, we have standardized the genomic nomenclature by using Human Genome Variation Society (HGVS) notation. We have also further standardized our use of units of length, adopting the convention used by the International Collaboration on Cancer Reporting (https://www.iccr-cancer.org) and the UK Royal College of Pathologists (https://www.rcpath.org/), so that the size of tumours is now given exclusively in millimetres (mm) rather than centimetres (cm). This is clearer, in our view, and avoids the use of decimal points – a common source of medical errors.

We hope this is the start of a long-term solution to meeting the needs of the cytopathology community. Like the WHO Classification of Tumours, the WHO Reporting Systems (books and website) are published on a non-profit basis, with proceeds ploughed directly back into the series to support the costs involved, including production, printing, and distribution. There are substantial discounts available for residents of low- and middle-income countries and trainees. It is of vital importance that cancers continue to be classified and diagnosed according to the same standards internationally so that patients can benefit from multicentre clinical trials and studies, as well as from the results of local research conducted on different continents.

Ian A. Cree, Fernando Schmitt, Martha Bishop Pitman, Ravi Mehrotra, Andrew S. Field

International Agency for Research on Cancer
International Academy of Cytology

December 2022

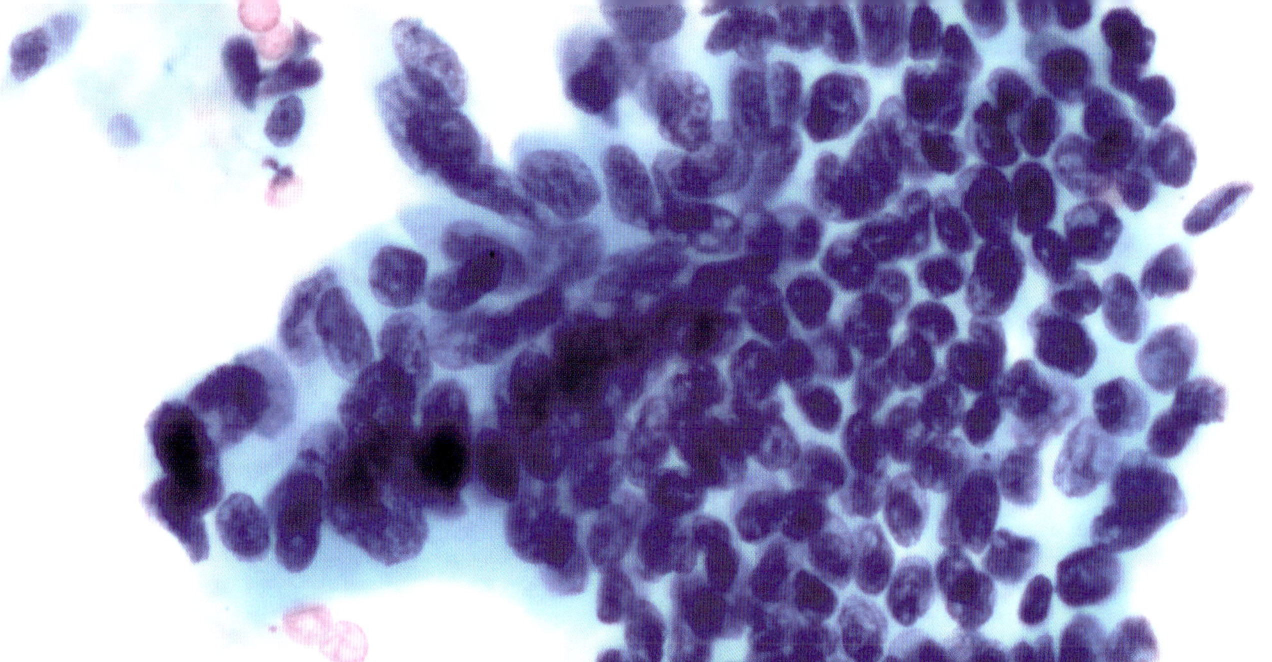

1

Introduction to the WHO Reporting System for Pancreaticobiliary Cytopathology

Edited by: Field AS, Mehrotra R, Pitman MB

Background

Stelow EB
Centeno BA
Field AS
Fukushima N
Layfield LJ
Lozano MD
Perez-Machado MA
Saieg M
Schmitt F
Siddiqui MT
Weynand B

Pancreaticobiliary pathology, mostly neoplasia, affects millions of people worldwide. It is estimated that each year nearly half a million people are diagnosed with pancreatic cancer {553}. The incidence rate of cholangiocarcinoma varies greatly throughout the world, and although in most places it is less than that of pancreatic cancer, some populous areas of the world, particularly regions of eastern Asia, have incidence rates that are actually higher than those of pancreatic cancer {690}.

Our understanding of pancreaticobiliary pathology has increased tremendously over the past 20 years. This is especially true with regard to neoplasia. Large multi-institutional studies, replete with extensive molecular analysis, have improved our understanding of pancreaticobiliary neoplasia and have allowed for the development of a more reproducible and meaningful classification system that is contained within the fifth-edition WHO classification of tumours of the digestive system {910}. We also have a better understanding of non-neoplastic disease. For example, our understanding of tumefactive inflammatory processes, such as autoimmune pancreatitis, has allowed us to recognize and treat some patients with apparent mass lesions without surgery {516}.

Obtaining diagnostic tissue in a minimally invasive way is the goal for optimal patient care. The pancreas is a deeply situated organ, making biopsy of pancreatic masses and nodules difficult and often associated with significant patient morbidity and mortality. FNAB of the pancreas was essentially ignored by early investigators including Martin and Ellis {526} and Stewart {818}. The first FNAB directed by imaging of the pancreas utilized selective angiographic guidance. Oscarson et al. {617} and Tylen et al. {861} demonstrated the successful use of selective angiographic guidance for the diagnosis of pancreatic carcinoma. It was not until the early 1970s that reliable imaging techniques including CT and ultrasound allowed more accurate needle placement into lesions of the pancreas. This allowed pancreatic core needle biopsy and FNAB to be performed for the diagnosis of pancreatic nodules and masses. A number of investigators in the USA, Scandinavia, and Japan have documented the usefulness of percutaneous techniques for the cytopathological diagnosis of pancreatic neoplasms {249,250,406,666,795,213,266,274}. Because ultrasound allowed real-time needle placement and was less expensive than CT guidance techniques, it became the predominant technique for percutaneous FNAB of the pancreas. Diagnostic accuracy of the percutaneous method was good, but percutaneous FNAB was associated with a small number of adverse events and a lower than desired diagnostic sensitivity {609}.

EUS was introduced in 1982, and the technique allowed detailed imaging of the oesophagus and gastric wall, as well as adjacent structures including lymph nodes, bile ducts, and the pancreas. With increasing experience, EUS-FNAB became the standard method for the investigation of abnormalities of the pancreas {490}. Further progress occurred with the development of the linear array echoendoscope, which made it possible to perform EUS-FNAB of mural and extramural lesions {914,881,115}. Diagnostic sensitivity and specificity for pancreatic lesions was excellent {622,438, 200,299}. EUS instruments also allowed the development of brushing and washing techniques for the investigation of biliary tract and pancreatic duct lesions. Endoscopic retrograde cholangiopancreatography improved the diagnosis and tissue sampling of abnormalities involving the bile ducts and pancreas. Currently, the combination of FNAB guided by linear array endoscopy with brushing techniques guided by endoscopic retrograde cholangiopancreatography allows accurate, sensitive, and specific cytopathological sampling of abnormalities of the pancreas, biliary tract, and neighbouring structures.

These advances in imaging techniques have facilitated the improved identification and characterization of lesions of the pancreaticobiliary system. A larger number of smaller (and thus earlier) lesions of the intrahepatic and extrahepatic biliary system and pancreas are recognized by imaging every year, often before they cause symptoms. For example, with modern imaging techniques, the majority of people aged > 70 years are found to have early cystic neoplasia of the pancreas {871}. Our understanding of the premalignant nature of mucinous cysts has changed the management and workup of patients with pancreatic cysts. Preoperative assessment of the cyst type and its risk of malignancy are paramount for the early detection of pancreatic cancer {839,472}.

Better, earlier, and more sensitive detection techniques, coupled with better treatments based on our increasing understanding of disease states, have led to a great demand for correct and precise tissue diagnostics. Now more than ever, anatomical pathologists must provide specific and reproducible diagnoses for pancreaticobiliary samples. For example, the advent of neoadjuvant chemoradiation treatment for patients with ductal adenocarcinoma makes a definitive preoperative diagnosis an absolute requirement {45,664}.

Finally, advances in surgical care, radiation therapy, and pharmacology have led to better outcomes for patients with pancreaticobiliary disease. Our understanding of the various diseases has allowed more directed treatments, often specific for the disease state that is present {553}.

The comprehensive diagnostic reporting system presented in this volume is a revision of the Papanicolaou System for Reporting Pancreaticobiliary Cytology {650}. The WHO Reporting System fully acknowledges the role of the previous authors and system, and is a product of the collaborative project between WHO, the International Agency for Research on Cancer (IARC), and the International Academy of Cytology (IAC) to produce international reporting systems in cytopathology. This WHO Reporting System has been developed, written, and produced by an international expert editorial board with the support of IARC.

This WHO Reporting System is intended to assist and guide pathologists with the interpretation and reporting of cytopathological samples from the pancreaticobiliary system in line with the WHO classification of tumours of the pancreas {910}. The aim is to provide clear information to clinicians to better guide them in the diagnostic approach to pancreaticobiliary disease, and ultimately to improve patient care.

The role of pancreaticobiliary cytopathology

Stelow EB
Pitman MB

The pancreas and extrahepatic biliary system are located deep within the retroperitoneum and are difficult to sample with conventional imaging and sonographic techniques. Previously, transabdominal FNAB and core biopsy sampling of the pancreas were most commonly performed using either CT or ultrasound {415}. However, over the past 20 years, endoscopic visualization and sampling have greatly improved the diagnosis of pancreaticobiliary cancer, and have, for many cytopathology laboratories, led to a marked increase in the number of pancreaticobiliary samples {813}. Direct access of the extrahepatic biliary tract and pancreas can be gained through endoscopic retrograde cholangiopancreatography (ERCP) {343}. The pancreas, extrahepatic biliary system, and adjacent structures can all be visualized and sampled by EUS, through either the gastric wall or the duodenal wall {553,800}. Both ERCP and EUS can gather cytopathological samples through either brushing or FNAB, and both can also garner small tissue fragments. Newer needle designs, such as the fork-tipped needle, have allowed for large tissue fragments and intact cores that can be used both for smears for rapid onsite evaluation (ROSE) and for histological processing with fewer passes {220,366,799}.

ERCP and EUS currently afford the two easiest methods for the sampling of the pancreas and extrahepatic biliary system. Indeed, because sampling via other methods is so difficult and because surgery is contraindicated in most pancreaticobiliary disease, ERCP and EUS often provide the only sample of a patient's pancreaticobiliary disease {734}. Therefore, pathologists are called to render meaningful diagnoses from the cytopathological and small biopsy specimens obtained by these procedures with as much precision as possible.

Integration of clinical, radiological, and key FNAB cytopathological features with ancillary testing in a diagnostic approach

Pitman MB
Centeno BA

The management of patients with pancreatic masses is best decided within a multidisciplinary team. Integrating the clinical, radiological, cytopathological, histopathological, and ancillary testing parameters in the final diagnosis greatly improves diagnostic accuracy and, ultimately, patient care {364,787,651,270, 700,646}. Before obtaining a tissue sample, the clinical team has often established a differential diagnosis based on the clinical and imaging findings. The task of the pathologist is to incorporate the cytopathological and histopathological features and ancillary testing results with those clinical and imaging findings into a final pathological diagnosis.

Clinical characteristics that may be relevant include patient age, sex, social factors, and family history of cancer or familial syndromes. Social factors, such as smoking, diet, and alcohol use, may predispose the patient to pancreatitis and pancreatic cancer. Patients with germline mutations and familial syndromes may be at risk for neoplasms and ductal malignancy. Laboratory values, particularly serum tumour markers, also provide essential information to assist the diagnostic process {910}.

The imaging appearance determines the differential diagnosis and algorithmic approach to biopsy evaluation. Not only is knowledge of the imaging findings a critical piece of information to have before assessing the biopsy sample, but this information also provides context for recognizing potential gastrointestinal contamination. A transduodenal approach is used to access lesions in the pancreatic head, and a transgastric approach is used for lesions in the body and tail of the gland.

Lesions of the pancreas are broadly divided into solid lesions, cystic lesions, and mixed solid and cystic lesions. Solid masses can be divided into ductal and non-ductal lesions. Ductal lesions represent most masses with a primary differential diagnosis of ductal adenocarcinoma and chronic pancreatitis. Mixed solid and cystic lesions represent either secondarily cystic solid tumours or primary cysts with complex architecture usually representing progressed disease. Imaging features are the key parameter by which patients with pancreatic cysts are managed {838,839}. The differential diagnosis for cystic lesions includes pseudocysts, lymphoepithelial cysts, developmental cysts, and cystic neoplasms. The two main clinical questions directing management of patients with a pancreatic cyst include whether the cyst is mucinous or non-mucinous, and whether the cyst is low-risk or high-risk for malignancy, and it is the combination of cytopathology, biochemical testing, and molecular analysis that best answers these questions {364,140}.

Ancillary testing results are not always available, leaving cytopathology and histopathology as the sole means of diagnosis. Cytomorphological analysis of solid lesions often provides a definite diagnosis, but ancillary studies are beneficial for the FNAB that is indeterminate for malignancy and for the diagnosis of non-ductal neoplasms {549}. Ancillary studies are critical in the evaluation of pancreatic cysts, which are often paucicellular {364,787,651,270,700,646}. Without ancillary studies, pancreatic cyst fluid FNABs are often non-diagnostic or indeterminate.

A recommended algorithmic approach to diagnosis is presented (see Fig. 1.01). The details of the clinical, imaging, cytomorphological, and ancillary studies are covered in detail in the corresponding sections for specific entities.

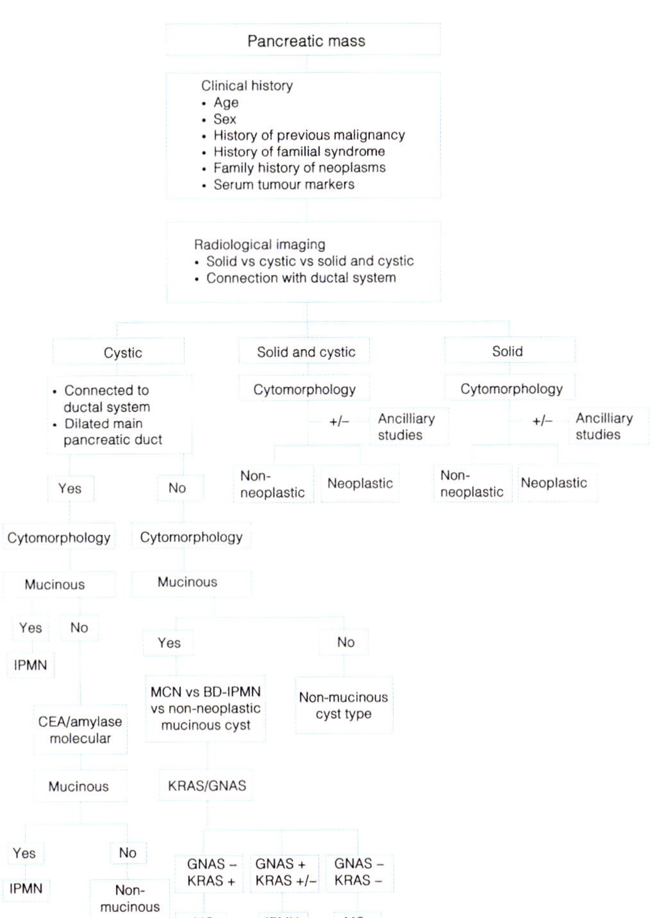

Fig. 1.01 Algorithm for the integration of cytomorphology with ancillary testing for the diagnosis of pancreatic FNABs. BD-IPMN, branch duct intraductal papillary mucinous neoplasm; IPMN, intraductal papillary mucinous neoplasm; MC, mucinous cyst; MCN, mucinous cystic neoplasm.

Diagnostic categories and report structure

Pitman MB
Saieg M

A standardized interpretation scheme for reporting pancreaticobiliary cytopathology provides a framework to be used by pathologists, so that pancreaticobiliary lesions are consistently categorized in the same manner in cytopathology reports that relate clear and consistent diagnostic information, with language uniformly understood by pathologists and clinicians all around the world. This proposed WHO Reporting System for Pancreaticobiliary Cytopathology is a revision of the Papanicolaou Society of Cytopathology (PSC) System for Reporting Pancreaticobiliary Cytology {643}.

The PSC system was developed by a multidisciplinary group of experts with input and feedback from practising pathologists from all over the globe. It uses a six-tiered system with the following categorizations: "Non-diagnostic", "Negative (for malignancy)", "Atypical", "Neoplastic: benign", "Neoplastic: other", "Suspicious (for malignancy)", and "Positive or malignant". The "Neoplastic" category is separated into clearly benign tumours (mainly composed of serous cystadenoma) and other tumours, which include premalignant tumours and low-grade malignant tumours. It advocates close correlation with imaging and encourages incorporation of ancillary testing into the final diagnosis, including biochemical tests for CEA and amylase and molecular testing of pancreatic cyst fluid {643}. One of the clear benefits of incorporating radiological information and ancillary testing is the decrease in the number of "Atypical" and "Non-diagnostic" reports in addition to an increase in both sensitivity and specificity for the detection of neoplasia, which has helped to refine the risk of malignancy (ROM) in the diagnostic categories {643,535,633,502,824,924,712,792,848,21}.

Controversial issues related to the PSC system have primarily revolved around the inclusion of low-grade malignant tumours (i.e. well-differentiated pancreatic neuroendocrine tumours [PanNETs] and solid pseudopapillary neoplasms) in the "Neoplastic: other" category, a non-malignant diagnostic category. The rationale for this was to provide maximum flexibility for patient management, which has become increasingly conservative, especially for small, grade 1 PanNETs. The "Positive or malignant" category was reserved for high-grade and/or aggressive malignancies.

The WHO Reporting System for Pancreaticobiliary Cytopathology presented here changes this categorization of tumours so as to align the categorization with the WHO classification of digestive system tumours {910}, with a refined ROM based on recent publications. Incorporation of ancillary studies will continue to be emphasized, but with the understanding that this information may not be available in all laboratories worldwide.

The WHO Reporting System for Pancreaticobiliary Cytopathology has seven diagnostic categories (listed in Box 1.01). Each of the categories is associated with a ROM that is directly linked to a recommendation for further diagnostic testing aimed at achieving a specific diagnosis or refining a differential diagnosis. The WHO Reporting System uses categories to assist in the communication of ROM, but a specific diagnosis or differential diagnosis further refined by ancillary testing is the aim of all cytopathology reporting and paramount in the report. Currently there are limited publications defining the ROM for the "PaN-low" and "PaN-high" categories, and there is a need for further research using the WHO Reporting System to more clearly define the ROM.

The principal differences between this system and the PSC system revolve around the classification of neoplasia. In the PSC system, there is a category for neoplastic lesions not diagnostic of adenocarcinoma or other aggressive malignancies that includes two groups, one for benign neoplasms, primarily serous cystadenoma, and one named "Other", which encompasses a broad range of premalignant and low-grade malignant neoplasms including intraductal papillary mucinous neoplasm, mucinous cystic neoplasm, well-differentiated PanNET, solid pseudopapillary neoplasm, and (rarely) low-grade spindle lesions. With such a diverse amalgam of neoplasia, it has been difficult to determine a meaningful ROM for the neoplastic category as a whole and even for the "Other" group, because the "Other" category includes a range of low-grade dysplastic lesions with a low ROM and high-grade dysplastic intraductal lesions with a much higher ROM {307,824}.

In the present WHO Reporting System, benign neoplasms with no ROM are included in the "Benign / Negative for malignancy" category, and low-grade malignancies including PanNET and solid pseudopapillary neoplasm are included in the "Malignant" category, as per the WHO classification of digestive system tumours {910}. This leaves in the pancreatic neoplasm categories primarily those non-invasive premalignant lesions of the ductal system. Because these lesions can be divided by the cytomorphological grade of the epithelium into low-grade and high-grade, with distinctly different ROMs, the "Neoplastic: other" category of the PSC system is converted to two distinct categories in the WHO Reporting System: "Pancreaticobiliary neoplasm, low-risk/grade (PaN-low)" and "Pancreaticobiliary neoplasm, high-risk/grade (PaN-high)".

An individual cytopathologist and a department with more than one cytopathologist should choose one term from "Insufficient", "Inadequate", and "Non-diagnostic" for cases where there is no material for assessment or where there are technical problems preventing the assessment and diagnosis of the material on the slides. If FNAB specimens have adequate benign material in the

Box 1.01 The seven categories of the WHO Reporting System for Pancreaticobiliary Cytopathology

1. Insufficient/Inadequate/Non-diagnostic
2. Benign / Negative for malignancy
3. Atypical
4. Pancreaticobiliary neoplasm, low-risk/grade (PaN-low)
5. Pancreaticobiliary neoplasm, high-risk/grade (PaN-high)
6. Suspicious for malignancy
7. Malignant

setting of a clearly defined targeted lesion, then this can either be reported as "Non-diagnostic", because it does not explain the mass lesion, or it can be reported as "Benign", with a mandatory caveat in the report that the material "does not explain the lesion seen on imaging and further diagnostic workup is recommended". The argument for using "Non-diagnostic" instead of "Benign" for these very likely false negative FNAB specimens is to maintain a low ROM in the "Benign" category, but further research is required to confirm any impact on the ROM.

The "Benign" category includes normal pancreas components, inflammatory processes, and benign tumours (e.g. serous cystadenoma). If the features are benign but a precise diagnosis cannot be made, the features should be described and a differential diagnosis provided if possible. As with all categories, correlation with clinical and imaging is mandatory, and, as above, if the "Benign" category is used to classify benign tissue in the setting of a targeted lesion, then this should be stated in a caveat in the conclusion.

The "Atypical" category is expected to have a relatively low to intermediate ROM and allows for a high negative predictive value for a benign diagnosis, whereas the "Suspicious for malignancy" category is expected to have a high ROM and provide for a high positive predictive value for a malignant diagnosis. The categories stratify the ROM and allow for the development of management recommendations. The "Atypical" category will include cases where there is scant or poorly prepared but atypical material, as well as cases where mainly benign cytopathological features are present, but there are some features (e.g. nuclear atypia, presence of mucin, or limited necrosis) that may raise the possibility of malignancy. If any atypical features are seen in a case showing otherwise insufficient material, the case is regarded as "Atypical" and not "Insufficient" or "Non-diagnostic".

The "Pancreaticobiliary neoplasm, low-risk/grade (PaN-low)" category is expected to have a low ROM, whereas the "Pancreaticobiliary neoplasm, high-risk/grade (PaN-high)" category is estimated to have a much higher ROM {306}.

The "Suspicious for malignancy" category includes cases where there is scant, poorly smeared, or poorly prepared and stained material suggestive of malignancy, and cases where there is considerable material, some of which suggests a "Malignant" categorization but in which not all features of a particular malignancy are present or there may be discrepant features.

The "Malignant" category is reserved for those cases in which there are unequivocal features of malignancy without any discrepant findings. All cytopathology specimen types are a sampling technique and it is not always possible to make a precise diagnosis of a specific carcinoma or other malignancy, even with ancillary testing. The precise diagnosis of carcinoma subtypes may require assessment of the entire resected tumour.

The presentation of tumours in this reporting system follows the order found in the fifth-edition WHO classification of digestive system tumours, but not all tumours are included because they have not been described in the cytopathology literature.

Structured reporting

Each cytopathology report from an FNAB or a bile duct brushing should have a structured format, with a heading of a specific diagnostic category using the WHO Reporting System standardized descriptive terminology and a diagnosis. Structured reporting improves the quality, clarity, and reproducibility of reports within individual pathology departments and between countries, and it will improve patient management and facilitate research and quality assurance measures. Standard guidelines for cell block preparation, immunocytochemistry, in situ hybridization, and other molecular tests of prognostic and predictive markers improve diagnostic accuracy, reduce cost, and improve patient care. The establishment of key diagnostic cytopathological findings for each lesion, which will act as a checklist for the reporting cytopathologist, will also improve reporting.

There are essential or core components in a cytopathology report presented here. It is not intended to make any particular format mandatory, but some components are required: the diagnostic category, using the defined terminology of the WHO Reporting System (not the category number), and a diagnosis, which may be specific or descriptive with a differential diagnosis. A comment or note outlining ancillary tests (when used) and their results is also required. A microscopic description of the key diagnostic features may be informative when a specific diagnosis is not made and when a differential diagnosis is rendered, but it may not be necessary when a specific diagnosis is made. A quality indicator (e.g. "limited by scant cellularity") may also be helpful, particularly when an indeterminate diagnosis is made. A diagnostic summary or conclusion may also be helpful if there are multiple parts to a single biopsy procedure.

A number should not be used in place of the diagnostic category terminology or a specific diagnosis. A category number can be included in the body of the report for audit and research purposes, but not in the conclusion. Reducing a cytopathology report to a number reduces the information that can be given to the clinician and management team and increases the risk of error.

When used, the microscopic description should provide a clear, concise cytopathological description, which can include the degree of cellularity but should focus on the presence or absence of key cytopathological diagnostic features.

The aim of cytopathology is to provide as specific a diagnosis as possible in the vast majority of cases, and this remains the priority. The indeterminate categories of "Atypical" and "Suspicious for malignancy" establish a ROM and subsequent diagnostic management recommendations as part of an algorithm to aid communication with the clinician about a particular biopsy and any further management of the patient.

The ancillary tests should always be part of the final cytopathology report, and if cyst biochemical results, in situ hybridization, or molecular pathology reports are issued by a different laboratory, then it is recommended that they should be referred to in the report.

The WHO Reporting Systems are based on cytomorphology for the initial categorization and reporting of the lesion, which can be applied in any well-resourced or low- and middle-income country setting, but they also incorporate the application of appropriate ancillary testing as current best practice. Subsequent ancillary testing may well change the final diagnostic category and provide a specific diagnosis of a particular case.

The standardized cytopathology report

Demographic information

- Patient's name, date of birth, address, patient identifiers / patient episode, date of request, and laboratory accession number
- Referring doctor and contact details

Type of specimen

- FNAB (EUS, transabdominal), biliary duct brushing

Clinical and imaging information

- Provided by the interventional physician: site, size (mm), imaging (ultrasound, CXR, tomogram, CT, MRI) features

Quality indicator

- Optional

Diagnostic summary

Category

- Using the terminology of the WHO Reporting System

Diagnosis

- Specific diagnosis or differential diagnosis

Comment/note (optional)

- Includes details of ancillary studies, microscopic description (optional)

Other information included in the report

Macroscopic description

- Number of air-dried slides, number of alcohol-fixed slides
- Type (saline, RPMI medium, formalin, only specimen without diluent) and volume of fluid received, with description of fluid (colour, presence of blood, viscosity, presence of particulate matter), including any other specimens received and specifically designated for cyst fluid biochemistry, microbiology, cell block

Details of rapid onsite evaluation (ROSE) (if conducted)

- Number of passes, gauge of needle used, imaging modality used
- Names of those performing the clinical and diagnostic procedures, including the cytology biomedical scientist, pathology trainee, or cytopathologist attending ROSE
- Number of slides processed and stained at ROSE, air-dried and alcohol-fixed, and other specimen types prepared
- The specific ROSE report provided verbatim and documented, and the name of the cytopathologist or cytotechnologist issuing ROSE, with further noting of any subsequent ROSE

Microscopic description

- This is optional if a specific diagnosis of a lesion or tumour is made, but in cases where the diagnosis is not specific and involves a differential diagnosis and discussion, a description of the features present is required; this includes cases that are categorized as "Atypical" or "Suspicious for malignancy"

Sample report

Specimen adequacy: Satisfactory for evaluation.
Category: Pancreaticobiliary neoplasm, low-risk/grade (PaN-low).
Diagnosis: Mucinous cyst with low-grade atypia (low/intermediate-grade dysplasia). See comment.
Comment: A mucinous etiology is established by the presence of mucinous epithelium with mild to moderate atypia and thick extracellular mucin. Cyst fluid CEA is also elevated to 541 ng/mL. Amylase is 12 431 U/L. These findings, in the context of imaging showing multiple cysts along the pancreatic duct and communication with the pancreatic duct, support the diagnosis of a branch duct intraductal papillary mucinous neoplasm. Molecular studies are pending and will be reported separately.

Risk of malignancy and management recommendations

Hoda RS
Klapman J
Layfield LJ
Schmitt F

The risk of malignancy (ROM) for the diagnostic categories of the WHO Reporting System for Pancreaticobiliary Cytopathology is extrapolated from the Papanicolaou Society of Cytopathology (PSC) system published in 2014 {650}. Since its publication, several large academic institutions have published their experience with the PSC system {461,792,124,307,824,244}. The WHO Reporting System for Pancreaticobiliary Cytopathology follows the fifth-edition of the WHO classification of tumours of the digestive system {910} and thus modifies terminology of the PSC system as well as the classification of tumours among the categories. For example, the "Neoplastic: other" category, which includes both low- and high-grade/risk lesions, is now split into two separate categories: "Pancreaticobiliary neoplasm, low-risk/grade (PaN-low)" and "Pancreaticobiliary neoplasm, high-risk/grade (PaN-high)". Well-differentiated pancreatic neuroendocrine tumour (PanNET) and solid pseudopapillary neoplasm are now in the "Malignant" category.

Few prior studies provide data on associated ROM that translate well into this new categorization system {792,307,824,244, 306}. The estimated ROMs associated with the diagnostic categories, as well as diagnostic management recommendations, are shown in Table 1.01. The estimated ROMs for pancreatic lesions are 0–15% for the "Benign / Negative for malignancy" category and 99–100% for the "Malignant" category. For the new categories of "PaN-low" and "PaN-high", estimated ROMs are 5–20% and 60–95%, respectively {306}. Prior studies reporting ROM for pancreatic FNAB vary in their cohort size, study nature (retrospective or prospective), inclusion of cystic and/or solid lesions, and length of clinical follow-up. Despite these differences in study design, the ROMs for the "Suspicious for malignancy" and "Malignant" categories across multiple studies were consistently close to 100%, and "Benign / Negative for malignancy" ROMs were very low (< 15%). With the redistribution of certain tumours within the categories from the PSC system to this current WHO Reporting System, the associated ROM for the "PaN-low" and "PaN-high" categories probably lie within their estimated ranges, particularly given that both PanNET and solid pseudopapillary neoplasm are now categorized as "Malignant" {306}. In the current oncological environment, where many patients get neoadjuvant chemotherapy and radiation therapy for pancreatic cancer regardless of resectability, obtaining a definitive diagnosis to initiate treatment is of paramount importance. FNAB results in the "Atypical" and "Suspicious for malignancy" categories are not considered diagnostic for malignancy, and repeat FNAB is recommended to confirm a diagnosis of malignancy.

The ROM for bile duct brushing (BDB) specimens is higher per diagnostic category than for FNAB of pancreatic masses. Because criteria are lacking for the diagnosis of specific premalignant intraductal bile duct neoplasms, most cytopathological interpretations fall in the "Benign / Negative for malignancy", "Malignant", or conventional indeterminate categories of "Atypical" and "Suspicious for malignancy", and not into the "PaN-low" or "PaN-high" categories. Using these conventional categories, an estimated ROM is shown in Table 1.02 {875,111,192,952,658, 468,595}. There is a high threshold for a "Malignant" interpretation in BDB specimens because of the significant overlap in reactive/reparative changes and carcinoma, which can be caused from stones, indwelling stents, instrumentation, and underlying inflammatory processes such as in primary sclerosing cholangitis. In one study of cytomorphological features of BDB specimens, > 50% of cases considered not malignant demonstrated genetic mutations of neoplasia, and over half of these cases were late mutations indicating a high-risk stricture {699}. For this reason, the ROM is as high as 55% in the "Benign / Negative for malignancy" category, 77% in the "Atypical" category, and

Table 1.01 The WHO Reporting System for Pancreaticobiliary Cytopathology on pancreas FNAB: implied risk of malignancy (ROM) and clinical management options by diagnostic category

Diagnostic category	Estimated ROM[a]	Clinical management options[b]
Insufficient/Inadequate/Non-diagnostic	5–25%	Repeat FNAB
Benign / Negative for malignancy	0–15%	Correlate clinically
Atypical	30–40%	Repeat FNAB
Pancreaticobiliary neoplasm, low-risk/grade (PaN-low)	5–20%	Correlate clinically
Pancreaticobiliary neoplasm, high-risk/grade (PaN-high)	60–95%	Surgical resection in surgically fit patients; conservative management optional
Suspicious for malignancy	80–100%	If patient to be surgically managed, treat as positive; if patient requires preoperative therapy, repeat FNAB
Malignant	99–100%	Per clinical stage

[a]Estimated ROMs are based on retrospective and prospective studies with risk analysis based on pancreatic neoplasia with low-grade and high-grade cytopathological atypia {792, 307,824,306}. [b]Management options for patients with pancreatic lesions may depend on a variety of factors, including clinical and imaging characteristics and the overall functional status of the patient. Some clinical management suggestions are outlined above.

Table 1.02 The WHO Reporting System for Pancreaticobiliary Cytopathology on bile duct brushing specimens: implied risk of malignancy (ROM) and clinical management options by diagnostic category

Diagnostic category	Estimated ROM[a]	Clinical management options[b]
Insufficient/Inadequate/Non-diagnostic	28–69%	Repeat ERCP with cholangioscopy, brushing, and biopsies
Benign / Negative for malignancy	26–55%	Correlate clinically
Atypical	25–77%	Repeat ERCP with cholangioscopy, brushing, and biopsies; consider ancillary testing with FISH and/or NGS
Pancreaticobiliary neoplasm, low-risk/grade (PaN-low)	n/a[c]	n/a
Pancreaticobiliary neoplasm, high-risk/grade (PaN-high)	n/a[c]	n/a
Suspicious for malignancy	74–100%	Repeat sampling with ancillary testing (FISH and/or NGS) or, if other factors support malignancy, surgical intervention; for neoadjuvant therapy, repeat ERCP with cholangioscopy / brushings / biopsies / ancillary studies
Malignant	96–100%	Per clinical stage

ERCP, endoscopic retrograde cholangiopancreatography; n/a, not available / not applicable; NGS, next-generation sequencing.
[a]Estimated ROMs are based on retrospective and prospective studies with risk analysis based on pancreatic neoplasia with low-grade and high-grade cytological atypia {875,111, 192,952,658,468,595}. [b]Management options for patients with bile duct strictures may depend on a variety of factors, including clinical and imaging characteristics and the overall functional status of the patient. Some clinical management suggestions are outlined above. [c]Cytological criteria for premalignant neoplasms of the bile duct are lacking, so there are no data on bile duct categorization in the "PaN-low" and "PaN-high" categories.

as high as 100% for the "Suspicious for malignancy" category. A definitive diagnosis of malignancy is rarely incorrect, with a ROM of 96–100%. This correlates with the high specificity and low sensitivity associated with BDB cytopathology.

Management of patients with a bile duct stricture is continued surveillance regardless of a "Benign" interpretation, with increasing concern for surgical intervention with each diagnostic category. In patients with primary sclerosing cholangitis, there is a 5–10% lifetime risk of developing cholangiocarcinoma, which is a contraindication for liver transplant for most patients, so the detection of bile duct dysplasia is the goal of surveillance {877,85}. To further improve the diagnostic yield of BDB, ancillary techniques have been developed over the past 10–20 years, initially with FISH and more recently with next-generation sequencing. Both tests have shown that when positive and used in combination with BDB cytomorphology, the sensitivity for a high-risk stricture with at least high-grade dysplasia increases without decreasing the high specificity of the results {386,483,192,788}. The clinical diagnostic management for each diagnostic category for BDB is shown in Table 1.02. Patients with a "Benign" interpretation are generally followed clinically, depending on the clinical concern for malignancy. Repeat endoscopic retrograde cholangiopancreatography with cholangioscopy, brushing, and biopsies are warranted when malignancy is clinically suspected. The addition of ancillary testing with FISH and/or next-generation sequencing can provide supportive evidence for a benign or malignant diagnosis, if these tests are available. Detection of a *KRAS* mutation supports neoplasia over reactive changes, and the detection of high-risk mutations, including *TP53* mutation, or *SMAD4* or *CDKN2A* (*P16*) deletion, support a high-risk stricture, warranting consideration of surgical intervention {788,192,699,733}.

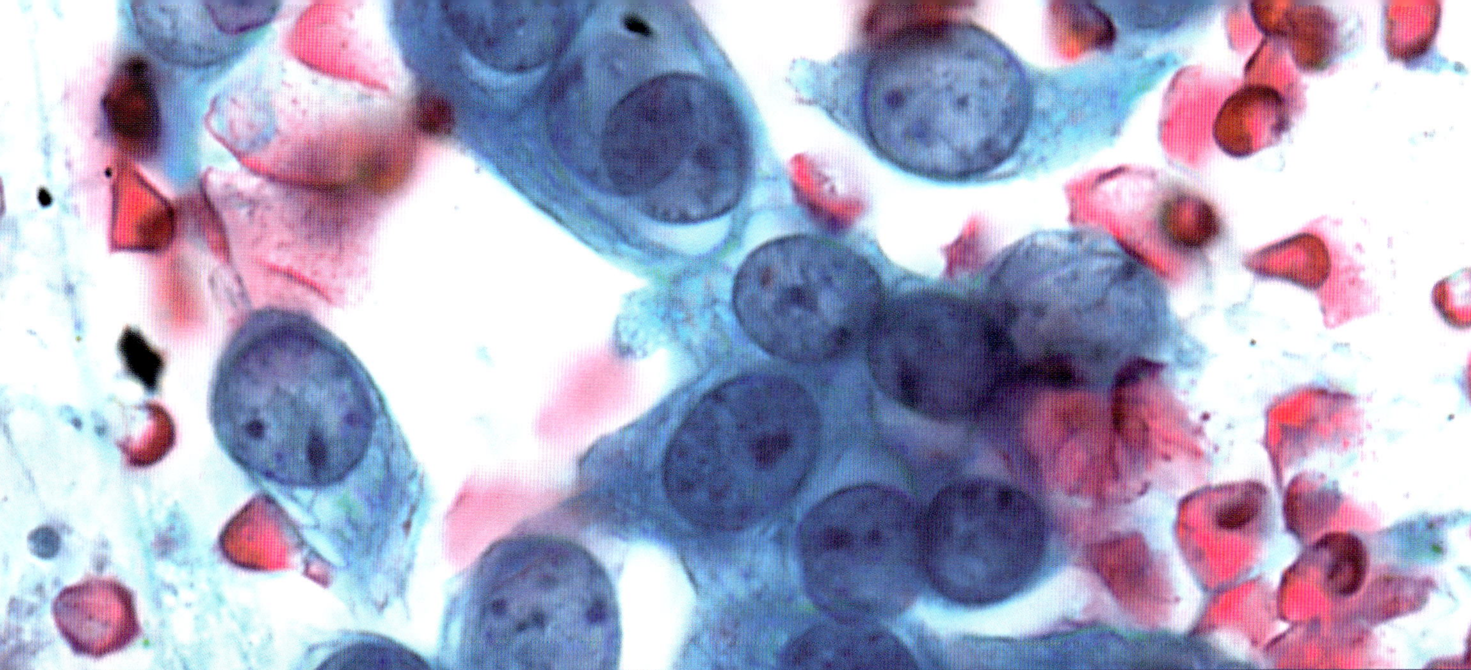

2

Pancreaticobiliary cytopathology techniques

Edited by: Cree IA, Layfield LJ, Mehrotra R, Perez-Machado MA, Pitman MB, Schmitt F, Siddiqui MT

FNAB techniques and specimen management for solid pancreatic masses

Krishnan K
Itoi T
Klapman J
Policarpio Nicolas ML

EUS-guided tissue acquisition has emerged as the standard of care for the diagnosis of solid pancreatic lesions. In a meta-analysis of 41 studies, which assessed 4766 cases, the pooled sensitivity and specificity of EUS-FNAB for the diagnosis of a solid pancreatic mass were 86.8% (95% CI: 85.5–87.9) and 95.8% (95% CI: 94.6–96.7), respectively {660}. Over the past decade, there has been considerable interest in improving the diagnostic yield of EUS-FNAB. This has occurred through enhanced technology advances and improvement in tissue procurement via EUS. Tissue triage using rapid onsite evaluation (ROSE) has also played a critical role in improving diagnostic yield.

The three main techniques of EUS-FNAB include dry suction, stylet slow-pull, and wet suction {42,475,657}.

The dry-suction technique is reported to increase sample cellularity, diagnostic sensitivity, and accuracy {657,48}. However, there have been concerns in regard to the damage and crushing of the cellular structure of the tissue sample and blood contamination of the specimen {901}. Several studies have evaluated the effect of the stylet slow-pull technique for pancreatic solid lesions and found comparable diagnostic quality to standard suction methods {99,183,731}. The wet capillary suction technique has also been reported {42,880}. Some authors prefer the stylet slow-pull technique when using a fine core needle to limit blood within the specimen and prevent tissue fragmentation.

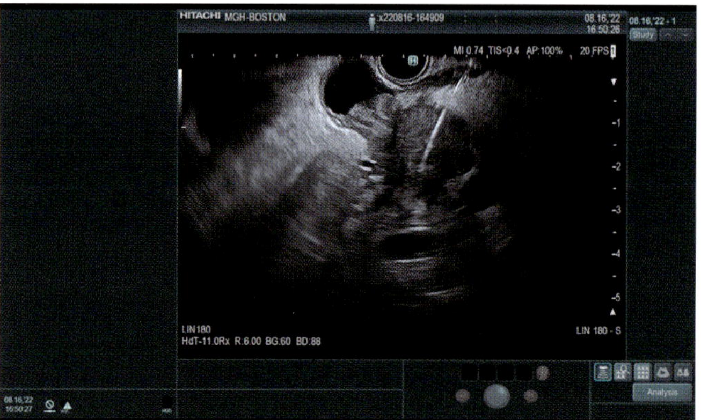

Fig. 2.01 EUS-FNAB of ductal adenocarcinoma. EUS shows the biopsy needle in a large, irregular, solid mass in the head of the pancreas.

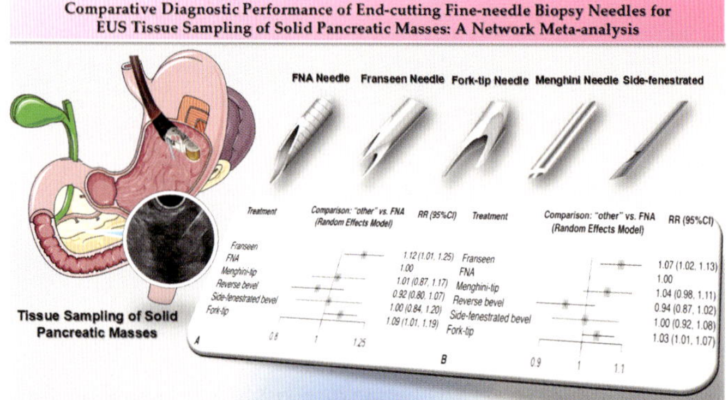

Fig. 2.02 Comparative diagnostic performance of end-cutting fine-needle biopsy needles for EUS tissue sampling of solid pancreatic masses. RR, risk ratio {246A}.

Puncturing the target lesion with a mounted stylet from the needle lumen is routinely practised by endosonographers, because it is believed to prevent the contamination of the sample from the gastrointestinal tract {657}. However, some studies have shown no added advantage of the stylet with regard to diagnostic accuracy, adequacy, quality, cellularity, or blood contamination {402, 452,902,945}. The effect of stylet use with fork-tip and other larger bore needles has not been evaluated.

EUS needles are available in three sizes: 19, 22, and 25 gauge. There appears to be no difference in the diagnostic accuracy between these various needle gauges, but some studies recommend using the 25 gauge needle, for easier manipulation during the biopsy procedure {48,474}.

Despite the yield of EUS-guided FNAB, the interest in tissue architecture and molecular analysis has resulted in substantial interest in procuring core needle biopsy (CNB) tissue specimens from pancreatic lesions. As a result, small core needles have been developed to procure core biopsy specimens, also known as fine-needle biopsy or fine CNB. Comparative studies of FNAB and fine CNB have demonstrated similar diagnostic accuracy; however, fewer passes and shorter procedure times were noted with fine CNB compared with FNAB {799,830}.

FNAB techniques and specimen management for pancreatic cysts

Itoi T
Pereira SP
Yoon WJ
Zhang ML

EUS features of pancreatic cysts are defined as follows: (1) macrocystic and/or microcystic septations; (2) solid component (nodule); (3) thickened wall; (4) suspected mucin; (5) communication with a pancreatic duct; (6) dilatation of the main pancreatic duct; (7) a mucous plug in the papilla; and (8) hypervascularity {260}. EUS provides high-resolution morphological imaging of pancreatic cysts and allows detection of lesions as small as a few millimetres in diameter, whereas septa, mural nodules, mucin balls, and thickened cysts cannot be detected on CT or MRI. In addition, EUS has the important role of tissue sampling using FNAB or fine CNB techniques.

EUS-FNAB of pancreatic cysts is performed using linear echoendoscopes. Lesions in the head or uncinate process of the pancreas are accessed via a transduodenal approach, whereas those in the body or the tail of the pancreas are accessed via a transgastric approach {960}. When performing the FNAB and passing the fine needle into the lesion, Doppler imaging is used to identify and avoid blood vessels {915}. After puncturing the cyst, it is important to aspirate all the fluid with one needle pass using suction {90}. Any solid component should be separately biopsied and identified as a solid component or mural nodule. Prophylactic antibiotics are used to minimize the risk of infection {657,38}. However, a recent randomized trial demonstrated that the incidence of infections did not differ with or without antibiotic prophylaxis {143}. A microforceps biopsy needle can be used to sample the cyst wall. This biopsy device is threaded through a 19 gauge needle and should be used before draining the cyst. The small tissue sample often improves the specificity of diagnosis {982,56}.

Rapid onsite evaluation (ROSE) is not recommended for pancreatic cysts because it does not aid in patient management and risks wasting the (often scant) fluid needed for ancillary testing. Instead, all drained cyst fluid should be saved and triaged for cytopathology, CEA/amylase analysis, and molecular testing (see Fig. 2.03 for workflow) {640,112,139}. Fresh, unfixed, and undiluted pancreatic cyst fluid is required for accurate evaluation and analysis. Fixing and/or diluting cyst fluid in saline or liquid-based preservatives precludes the ability to perform accurate biochemical analysis. If the cyst fluid is very thick, a direct smear should be made, because the viscous nature of the cyst fluid already indicates that the cyst is mucinous, and further ancillary testing does not contribute additional information. Either an aliquot of fresh, homogenized fluid or an aliquot of supernatant fluid can be submitted for molecular testing if available. The residual fluid is spun down for cytology and the supernatant is sent for biochemical testing with CEA prioritized over amylase. Each ancillary test requires at least 0.3 mL.

Recently, shear-wave elastography, contrast agents, and needle-based confocal laser endomicrography have been developed to evaluate tissue hardness, vascularity, and histopathology without tissue sampling, respectively, and offers the potential to enhance EUS imaging to aid in the diagnostic yield of the pancreatic cyst lining {476}.

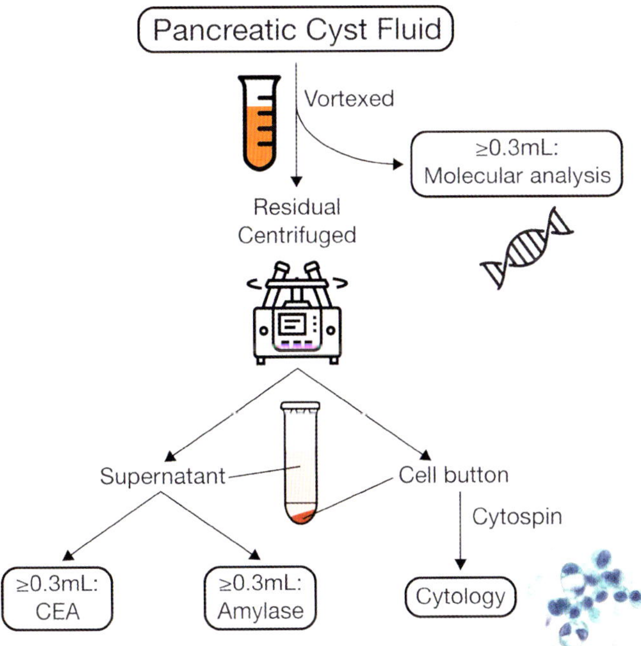

Fig. 2.03 Pancreatic cyst fluid triage.

FNAB techniques and specimen management for bile duct brushings

Eltoum IA
Pitman MB
Yoon WJ

As many as 30% of bile duct lesions may be benign {860}, and close to 20% may remain indeterminate after exhaustive diagnostic workup {83}. The decision to obtain tissue for diagnosis depends on clinical features, imaging findings, and the availability of resources, including technical expertise for procurement of specimens, for interpreting the pathological findings, and for providing surgical and/or palliative management {193, 929,222,578,576}. For instance, according to the National Comprehensive Cancer Network (NCCN), if a neoplasm is highly suspected, tissue acquisition before surgery may not be required {587}. Likewise, if liver transplant is contemplated, a transperitoneal procedure such as FNAB or fine core needle biopsy (CNB) may carry a risk of seeding the peritoneal cavity and is not recommended {294}. Finally, expertise in cytopathology and CNB interpretation may not be available in all health care settings across the world. Once a decision is made to obtain a specimen before surgical or palliative intervention, the choices are either FNAB, CNB, forceps biopsy, or ductal brushing. Again, which procedure is used depends on the location of the lesion along the bile duct, where it can be close to the liver hilum, close to the ampulla (i.e. distal), or in between, and the lesion's relationship to the bile duct wall, where it can be luminal, intramural, or periductal. The decision also depends on whether or not there is a mass, especially in the hilar region where MRI/CT-guided FNAB/CNB may be the last resort (see Table 2.01 and Box 2.01).

FNAB

The European Society of Gastrointestinal Endoscopy (ESGE) and the Papanicolaou Society of Cytopathology (PSC) have published clear guidelines on some of the best practices regarding EUS-FNAB, but worldwide practice varies substantially from one region to another {657,649,872}. Generally, a 25 or 22 gauge needle is thrust into the lesion under EUS visualization, with or without a stylet, with a jabbing and/or fanning technique with or without aspiration to obtain cellular material. If rapid onsite evaluation (ROSE) is not available, three to four passes are recommended {657}. Albeit less commonly than EUS-FNAB, CT/MRI-guided FNAB can be performed percutaneously for hilar ductal masses. The sensitivity of EUS-FNAB is modestly higher than that of endoscopic retrograde cholangiopancreatography (ERCP)-procured tissue, and the combined procedure is better than either alone {170}.

Fine CNB and forceps biopsy

Obtaining a bile duct biopsy via CNB or forceps biopsy is as technically difficult as FNAB. Tissue can be acquired using forceps during ERCP; during cholangioscopy; during percutaneous, transhepatic, spyglass cholangiopancreatoscopy; with EUS guidance; or by using a 19 or 22 gauge needle to procure tiny cores of tissue {657,649,589,588,614,632,947}. A tissue biopsy, even if small, generally preserves architecture and may allow differentiation between an intraductal lesion and invasive carcinoma. However, CNB and forceps biopsy are frequently small, fragmented, superficial, and/or crushed rendering them inadequate for a definitive diagnosis. ERCP-directed forceps biopsy and brush cytopathology are comparable in their diagnostic performance {589}.

Bile duct brushing

Brushing strictures of the bile ducts is usually performed during ERCP by passing a brush through the endoscope under fluoroscopy. The brush, with its catheter sheath, is inserted into the bile duct and positioned just distal to the stricture. The brush is advanced from the catheter to the point proximal to the stricture and moved across the stricture in a to-and-fro fashion approximately 10 times. The brush is retracted into the catheter, and the brush and catheter are withdrawn as a unit from the endoscope

Table 2.01 Imaging modality and tissue acquisition

Imaging modality	Notes on tissue acquisition
Percutaneous ultrasound	First-line diagnostic imaging; generally, no tissue obtained unless there is a reachable mass
MRCP	Better than ultrasound in localization, staging, and diagnostic features; no tissue
CT	Good for staging; lower sensitivity for malignant diagnosis than MRCP; CT-guided FNAB when there is a mass
EUS without FNAB	Useful in diagnosing strictures with no mass and in staging
EUS-FNAB	Used for obtaining both FNAB and core needle biopsy
ERCP	Has diagnostic and therapeutic advantage; brush cytology and forceps biopsy; more invasive than EUS-FNAB
Percutaneous transhepatic cholangioscopy	Has diagnostic and therapeutic advantage; direct visualization with both brush cytology and forceps biopsy
Peroral cholangioscopy	Direct visualization; higher sensitivity than biopsy obtained under conventional ERCP
Spyglass peroral cholangiopancreatoscopy	More advanced direct visualization and biopsy (SpyBite), with reported high sensitivity
Intraductal ultrasound	Used in conjunction with ERCP; excellent for localization and staging; no tissue

ERCP, endoscopic retrograde cholangiopancreatography; MRCP, magnetic resonance cholangiopancreatography.

{165}. Brushing a pancreatic duct stricture is done in a similar manner {938}; however, pancreatic duct brushing may be technically difficult, and cannulation may not be possible in as many as 25% of cases {165}.

Box 2.01 Variables to be considered when performing FNAB of the bile duct

- Lesion size and site
- Endoscope location/distance in relation to the lesion (for EUS-FNAB)
- Transgastric or transduodenal approach (for EUS-FNAB)
- Needle size (22 or 25 gauge)
- Number of passes
- Number of slides per pass
- Needle movement (fanning vs to-and-fro)
- Application of suction
- Air vs saline flushing of material
- Presence of cytologist for rapid onsite evaluation (ROSE)
- Who prepared the smear
- Whether it was an air-dried or alcohol-fixed smear
- Whether liquid-based cytology was used

Tissue triage

Bile duct brushings can be smeared directly onto glass slides; for this, it is imperative that for alcohol-fixed Pap-stained material the slides are placed immediately (i.e. within seconds) into alcohol. Air-dried Giemsa-stained smears can also be prepared. Alternatively, the brush can be placed immediately into preservative solutions and gently rotated for liquid-based processing. The latter offers better cellular preservation and less mechanical artefact changes in the cells, which already have instrumentation effect from the procedure alone. Rapidly well-smeared material offers advantages in showing the pattern of material on the slide and less rounding up of tissue fragments. Tissue in a liquid medium provides cells for cell block preparation and/or ancillary studies such as FISH and next-generation sequencing. Molecular analysis of the cells from bile duct brushings are an important factor in improving the sensitivity of the test {192, 788,603,979,411}. ROSE is not needed, because the interpretation does not affect the procedure or patient management.

Tissue obtained from CNB or forceps biopsy should be placed directly into formalin for routine histopathological processing.

Percutaneous FNAB and specimen management

Kalra N
Pitman MB

Percutaneous pancreaticobiliary FNAB is a method of obtaining material for cytopathological diagnosis from a tumour of the pancreas or biliary tree by accurate localization and targeted placement of a fine needle through the abdominal wall using image guidance. Percutaneous FNAB of the pancreas was first described in 1974 {794}. Pancreaticobiliary cancers are often small and incite a desmoplastic reaction, making diagnostic yield challenging. Biliary cancers may only cause a stricture. Gallbladder cancers may present as a mass replacing the gallbladder, as a polypoid lesion extending into the gallbladder lumen, or as an asymmetrical mural thickening. Advances in imaging techniques have improved the sensitivity of image-guided percutaneous FNAB. The combined use of sonographic and fluoroscopic guidance has been shown to improve the sensitivity of FNAB both for pancreatic cancers (66.7–77.5%) and for biliary cancers (40–60%) {271}.

Ultrasound, CT, or MRI may be used for image guidance after local anaesthesia at the site of skin entry. The platelet count should be > 50 000/mL and international normalized ratio (INR) < 1.5. Ultrasound guidance may be done freehand or with the use of a lateral probe-mounted guiding kit. Ultrasound has the advantage of real-time guidance. It is inexpensive and easily available. Use of colour Doppler delineates the vessels in relation to the tumour, as well as showing the vascularity of the tumour. CT is relatively expensive and has the disadvantage of involving ionizing radiation. MRI is not widely available and there is less expertise for using this technique. Fusion image guidance, combining ultrasound and CT/PET-CT or combining ultrasound and MRI, has limited availability.

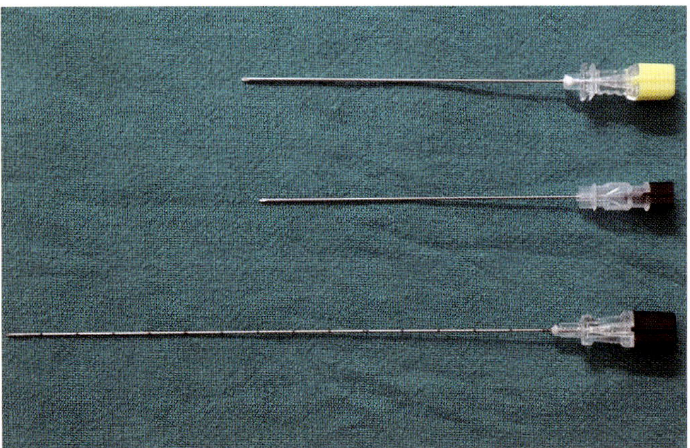

Fig. 2.04 Needles for percutaneous FNAB. From top to bottom: 20 gauge spinal needle, 22 gauge spinal needle, 22 gauge Chiba needle.

The needle used for percutaneous FNAB can be a 20–22 gauge needle, a spinal needle, or a 20–21 gauge Chiba needle. A coaxial system using a stationary guiding needle makes multiple passes easier. The suction/aspiration method combined with passing the fine needle into the lesion with a to-and-fro motion is preferred over the capillary action method (which does not include aspiration) because of an increased yield {316}. The presence of rapid onsite evaluation (ROSE) improves diagnostic yield {188}.

The sensitivity of percutaneous pancreatic FNAB ranges from 62% to 100%, with specificity ranging from 82% to 100% {970, 188}. CT-guided pancreatic biopsies had lower accuracy than ultrasound-guided biopsies in one series {86}. The accuracy of FNAB has been reported to be as low as 60% for pancreatic cysts {806}. A randomized control trial comparing EUS-FNAB and CT- or ultrasound-guided FNAB found no statistically significant difference between these different modalities {318}. The diagnostic accuracy for adequate FNAB of a gallbladder mass has been reported to be 95.3% {442}. In a series of gallbladder FNABs from 791 patients, 10.2% samples were non-diagnostic {443}. False negative results on FNAB may be a sampling error due to small tumour size, tumour necrosis, fibrosis, or vascularity. Repeat FNAB should be performed to obtain a conclusive diagnosis. The reported rate for false negative pancreatic FNAB is 5.4% {188}. The incidence of false negative gallbladder FNAB varies from 11% to 41% {769}.

Complications are very uncommon (0–4.9%) for pancreatic FNAB and include abdominal pain, pancreatitis, and ascites. There is a risk of needle tract seeding or peritoneal spread, and this has been reported to be more common with pancreatic cysts, although it is difficult to prove because peritoneal nodules on follow-up could also represent disease progression {303,958}.

Rapid onsite evaluation

Layfield LJ
Weynand B

Rapid onsite evaluation (ROSE) has been used for two decades, with the goals of increasing specimen adequacy, reducing the number of passes necessary for adequate sampling, and allowing appropriate triage of material for ancillary testing. ROSE has been shown to increase overall diagnostic yield by 10–30% {115,336}, and this is especially true for solid pancreatic lesions. Despite this, the method's utility and benefit–cost ratio remain controversial {430,739,740,460}.

ROSE is not recommended for pancreatic cysts. Cysts should be drained as much as possible, with all of the fresh, undiluted cyst fluid submitted to the cytology laboratory for processing {139,112,221,640}. ROSE on cyst fluid wastes the typically scant cyst fluid, which is better used for ancillary tests. If available, either an aliquot of fresh, homogenized fluid or an aliquot of supernatant fluid can be submitted for molecular testing. The residual fluid is spun down for cytology and the supernatant is send for biochemical testing, with CEA prioritized over amylase. Each test generally requires ≥ 0.3 mL.

ROSE is an interpretive service generally provided by cytopathologists, but in certain circumstances experienced cytotechnologists will provide immediate evaluation of specimen adequacy. An aliquot of FNAB material is immediately smeared and stained, either with an alcohol-based stain or with an air-dried Giemsa-type stain. The material is examined microscopically, and an evaluation of adequacy is provided, although a cytopathologist may provide a provisional diagnosis. Repeat passes are performed until adequate or diagnostic tissue is obtained or the endoscopist decides to terminate the procedure. When preliminary evaluation discloses an adequate specimen, additional tissue may be requested for ancillary testing such as flow cytometry, cell culture, or molecular testing.

In some studies, ROSE has been shown to reduce the number of passes necessary to obtain a diagnosis and reduce the incidence of repeat biopsy procedures {740,943,145,434}. Not all studies have demonstrated this beneficial impact, with the degree of improvement resulting from ROSE depending on the adequacy rate for non-ROSE procedures {739,740}. In cases where the adequacy rate is high in non-ROSE procedures, the improvement provided by ROSE is modest {739,740}. With next-generation fine core needle biopsy needles, diagnostic yield rates were similar with and without ROSE. Of note, many of these centres were high-volume experienced centres {35,168}. ROSE may be most beneficial when EUS-FNAB is performed by less experienced endoscopists {434}. Multivariate analyses have not shown a consistent improvement in EUS-FNAB adequacy {430}. Overall, these studies indicate that ROSE plays a critical role in improving diagnostic yield when performing standard FNAB, in situations where institutional yield rates are low and when performing fine core needle biopsy in lesions with a prior "Inadequate" or "Non-diagnostic" outcome.

One important issue relating to the utility of ROSE is the availability of trained staff. The availability of ROSE services varies by geographical area. ROSE is available in only 48% of European centres, but it is available in a significant majority of centres located in the USA {872}. This issue of limited staff availability may potentially be addressed by telecytopathology or by training endoscopists to perform ROSE {943}.

Introduction: The role of ancillary testing

Centeno BA
Stelow EB

Immunocytochemistry (ICC) and molecular-based testing have improved the diagnostic accuracy of cytopathology and small biopsy samples derived from pancreaticobiliary lesions. Ancillary tests available include special stains; ICC; biochemical analysis of cyst fluid; FISH; flow cytometry for suspected lymphomas; and molecular analysis for mutations, fusions, and other genetic abnormalities {459,462,549}.

The use of special stains has been mostly supplanted by an extensive menu of ICC antibodies. ICC panels are used to resolve a number of diagnostic dilemmas, including the distinction of benign from malignant ductal lesions in the pancreaticobiliary tract {109,549}, the diagnosis of non-ductal neoplasms of the pancreas {182,549}, and the workup of possible metastatic neoplasms {549,104}. ICC is also used to assess the grade of neuroendocrine tumours (NETs) {531,677} and biomarkers predictive of tumoural response to therapy.

The selection of ancillary tests is based on the site sampled and the nature of the lesion. All of the indications listed above apply to FNAB samples from solid pancreatic or bile duct masses or biliary tract strictures sampled by bile duct brushing. The differential diagnosis of pancreatic cysts includes a unique set of entities, such as non-neoplastic pseudocysts, developmental cysts that include enteric cysts and lymphoepithelial cysts, and intraductal and secondarily cystic neoplasms. Ancillary studies in pancreatic cysts are indicated to differentiate non-mucinous from mucinous cysts and to identify cysts at risk of progression to invasive carcinoma. The addition of ancillary studies is crucial to the evaluation of pancreatic cyst fluids. In this scenario, the usual ICC panels are often of limited utility because of the scant amount of representative cellular material. In addition to cytopathology, the most accurate diagnosis of cyst fluid includes testing the fluid for the biochemical markers CEA and amylase {651,549}. Analysis of molecular alterations is increasingly becoming an important part of the diagnostic workup, and although the results are typically not available at the time of sign-out, they can be added to an integrated final cytopathology report and will inform management by the patient care team {364,700}. For example, cyst fluid with a single *KRAS* mutation supports a neoplastic mucinous cyst, whereas the addition of a *GNAS* mutation supports the diagnosis of an intraductal papillary mucinous neoplasm, and the detection of late mutations in the adenoma-to-carcinoma progression (such as *SMAD4* or *CDKN2A* [*P16*] deletion or mutations in *TP53*) supports a high-risk cyst or bile duct stricture warranting surgical resection {787}.

Immunocytochemistry

Centeno BA
Sigel C

Introduction

Immunocytochemistry (ICC) is primarily used for the workup of solid pancreaticobiliary masses but may also be used in pancreaticobiliary brushings of strictures and pancreatic cysts. Indications include the identification of cellular lines of differentiation, site of origin for metastases, confirmation of malignancy, and biomarkers for therapeutic intervention and prognostication.

Technical requirements

Successful ICC, whether performed manually or using automated equipment, is dependent on having well-fixed and well-preserved tissue and a robust, optimized, and reproducible staining regime that uses high-quality and specific reagents {545}. Antigen retrieval is one of the first required steps and in theory can be performed using a protease step or heat-induced epitope retrieval, although heat-induced epitope retrieval is the only form of antigen retrieval recommended for direct smears, because protease treatment will cause the cells to fall off the slides.

The primary antibody needs to be optimized for each specimen type. Using antibody concentrations optimized for formalin-fixed, paraffin-embedded tissues may give a false positive result when applied to smears.

Management of types of cytopathological specimens

ICC may be performed on formalin-fixed, paraffin-embedded cell blocks; smears; cytospins; and liquid-based cytopathology preparations. Formalin-fixed, paraffin-embedded cell blocks are preferred, because these use the same controls and technical processes as routine histopathology specimens. The technique used to prepare the cell block should be considered, because different preparation techniques can impact the reliability of the ICC {121}. ICC may be performed on destained Pap slides or unstained alcohol-fixed or air-dried smears {159,4}. If a sample is limited, cell transfer techniques may be used to increase the amount of material available for staining with different antibodies {545}. When preparing smears, non-adhesive slides have been advocated in case slide transfer is needed, but cells may be lost when staining if a non-adhesive slide is used for initial staining {545,121}. Liquid-based cytopathology slides may be used, but caution is indicated, because the methanol fixative may lead to aberrant cytoplasmic and nuclear staining {158,252}.

Fixation

The preferred fixative is formalin, and the preferred sample is a good-quality formalin-fixed, paraffin-embedded cell block. For non–cell block cytopathology, most fixatives can be used after validation. The following results have been reported: both immediate fixation in alcohol or postfixation in normal saline provide good antigen presentation but may produce high background staining {826}; air-dried smears fixed in 0.1% normal saline and postfixed in 100% ethanol produced the best and most consistent results; acetone gave inconsistent results; and saline-rehydrated air-dried smears fixed in 95% alcohol plus 5% acetic acid were unsatisfactory {214,479,766}. Air-dried smears fixed in 4–10% formalin are well suited for nuclear antigens. Certain antigens (e.g. S100, ER, BAP1, and MTAP) are leached in alcohol fixative.

Controls

Positive and negative controls are required. The purpose of the positive control is to demonstrate that the ICC protocol is able to detect the antigen of interest (qualitative positive control) and is sensitive at the level of clinical relevance (calibrated positive controls, low and high expressers). Positive controls include samples that have previously been tested for the marker in question, or samples that are known to express the marker at levels within the desired range for the intended use after sample preparation, including fixation and retrieval variables {545}. For cell blocks, formalin-fixed, paraffin-embedded controls are preferred. For cytopathology samples, controls similar to the test specimen should be prepared using scrapes from surgical specimens, cell lines, or effusions.

Procedures

ICC can be performed either manually or using automated immunostainers. Most laboratories employ either the ABC method or a polymer-based antibody–antigen detection system. The majority of cytoplasmic and membranous antigens do not require antigen retrieval in alcohol-fixed preparations {172,252,337}. A short period of heat-induced antigen retrieval is recommended for uncovering epitope reactivity for most nuclear and some membranous antigens in alcohol-fixed preparations, for all formalin-fixed preparations, and for selected antigens in liquid-based cytopathology {172,173}. Protease should be avoided {277,172,225}.

Diagnostic applications

The following is a summary of the antibodies commonly used in pancreaticobiliary cytopathology.

Diagnostic markers

Cytokeratins

All normal epithelial cells of the pancreas, including acinar, islet, and ductal, express CK8 and CK18. Ductal cells also express CK7 and CK19 {24,745}. Cytokeratin cocktails are used in diagnostic practice to identify a neoplasm as epithelial. AE1/AE3 recognizes CK1–8, CK10, CK14–16, and CK19, and it will recognize both non-ductal and ductal epithelium. CAM5.2 recognizes CK7 and CK8. CK17 is rarely expressed in normal ductal cells, but its expression is upregulated during pancreatic carcinogenesis and it therefore serves as a marker of malignancy {671,261}. CK20 is also expressed only by ductal carcinoma and not by benign ducts.

Table 2.02 Immunocytochemistry (ICC) useful in the diagnosis of pancreatic FNABs

ICC stain	Target	Diagnostic utility	Limitations
SMAD4	Loss of nuclear staining	Adenocarcinoma	Strong staining in non-tumour disorders and other tumours; lost in ~50% of adenocarcinomas
p53	Positive nuclear staining	Adenocarcinoma	Also mutated in high-grade intraepithelial neoplasia
Mesothelin	Positive cytoplasmic staining	Adenocarcinoma	Focal staining in pancreatitis
IMP3	Strong cytoplasmic staining	Adenocarcinoma	Focal staining in pancreatitis
S100P	Strong cytoplasmic and nuclear staining	Adenocarcinoma	Strong staining of gastric epithelium
Monoclonal CEA	Strong cytoplasmic staining	Adenocarcinoma	
CA125 (MUC16)	Strong cytoplasmic staining	Adenocarcinoma	
VHL protein	Loss of membranous and cytoplasmic staining	Adenocarcinoma	Membranous and cytoplasmic expression in normal biliary and pancreatic ductal cells; loss in AIP
Synaptophysin	Strong, diffuse cytoplasmic staining	Neuroendocrine neoplasms	Focal staining in other tumours and normal islet cells
Chromogranin A	Strong to patchy cytoplasmic staining	Neuroendocrine neoplasms	Patchy staining, sometimes weak
INSM1	Strong, diffuse nuclear staining	Neuroendocrine neoplasms	Focal staining in other tumours
Trypsin	Strong cytoplasmic granular staining	Acinar cell carcinoma and other acinar proliferations	High background staining; focal staining in other tumours
Chymotrypsin	Strong cytoplasmic granular staining	Acinar cell carcinoma and other acinar proliferations	High background staining; focal staining in other tumours
BCL10	Cytoplasmic staining	Acinar cell carcinoma and other acinar proliferations	
CD99	Perinuclear dot-like pattern	Solid pseudopapillary neoplasm	Specific
β-Catenin	Strong nuclear staining	Solid pseudopapillary neoplasm	Nuclear staining in other tumours, but usually much more high-grade (acinar cell carcinoma)
E-cadherin	Membranous staining	PanNET vs solid pseudopapillary neoplasm	Loss in solid pseudopapillary neoplasm, depends on epitope
AR	Nuclear staining	Solid pseudopapillary neoplasm	High specificity, lacks sensitivity
SOX11	Nuclear staining	Solid pseudopapillary neoplasm	High sensitivity and specificity
MUC6	Cytoplasmic staining	Serous cystadenoma; oncocytic differentiation	Pyloric glands
α-Inhibin	Cytoplasmic staining	Serous cystadenoma	Focal staining in NETs

AIP, autoimmune pancreatitis; AR, androgen receptor; NET, neuroendocrine tumour; PanNET, pancreatic neuroendocrine tumour.

Vimentin

Vimentin is expressed by mesenchymal cells, such as fibroblasts and endothelial cells. It is expressed in undifferentiated carcinomas and is the only intermediate filament consistently expressed by solid pseudopapillary neoplasm (SPN).

Oncofetal antigens

Antibodies to oncofetal antigens routinely used in the pathological assessment of pancreaticobiliary specimens include CA19-9, CA125, and CEA. CA19-9 is a marker of pancreaticobiliary differentiation but is also expressed by other gastrointestinal carcinomas. CA19-9 is expressed both by reactive ductal cells and by pancreatic ductal adenocarcinoma (PDAC), and therefore, alone, it is not useful as a marker to differentiate benign from malignant disease {517,747}. CA125 is also known as MUC16 and is encoded by the *MUC16* gene {954}. Approximately 50% of PDACs may express this antigen, and coexpression of CA125 with CA19-9 is considered indicative of pancreatic ductal differentiation. CA125 (MUC16) is not expressed in benign ductal epithelium and could be useful as a marker to differentiate benign from malignant glands {507}. Intensity and quantity decrease with increasing grade {507}. Monoclonal CEA is not expressed by benign pancreatic ducts, but it is expressed by PDAC, making it a useful antibody for distinguishing benign pancreatic ducts from PDAC on FNAB and small biopsy samples {64}.

Markers of malignancy in ductal epithelium

Loss of ICC staining for SMAD4, the protein product of *SMAD4* (*DPC4*), is a good surrogate marker for mutations in this gene. Somatic inactivation of the *SMAD4* (*DPC4*) gene occurs in approximately half of PDACs, resulting in a loss of nuclear staining in PDAC, compared with the retained staining in benign ductal cells and gastrointestinal contamination. *SMAD4* loss occurs late in pancreatic carcinogenesis, in high-grade pancreatic intraepithelial neoplasia (HG-PanIN) and intraductal papillary mucinous neoplasm with high-grade dysplasia. *SMAD4*

Table 2.03 MUC protein immunoprofiles in pancreaticobiliary benign and neoplastic epithelium and gastrointestinal epithelium

Tissue	EMA (MUC1)	MUC2	MUC4	MUC5AC	MUC6
Gastric epithelium	+ (luminal)	Goblet cells in intestinal metaplasia	–	+	+ (pyloric glands) (– in foveolar glands)
Duodenal epithelium	– (luminal) (+ in crypts)	Goblet cells	–	–	Brunner glands
Intercalated ducts	+	–	–	–	
Intralobular ducts	+	–	–	–	
Interlobular ducts	+	–	–	–	
Main pancreatic duct	–	–	–	–	–
Periductal glands, pancreas	–	–	–	–	+
Benign biliary epithelium	+ (weak)	–	–	–	+
Serous cystadenoma	–	–	–	–	+
Mucinous cystic neoplasm	+ (invasive)	Goblet cells	+ (invasive)	+	–
LG-PanIN	+ (membranous)	–	–	+	+
HG-PanIN	+ (cytoplasmic)	–	–	+	+
IPMN and IPNB, gastric	–/+ (luminal)	–	–	+	–/+
IPMN, intestinal	–	+ (cytoplasmic)	+	+	–
IPMN and IPNB, pancreaticobiliary	+	–	–	+	+
IPMN and IPNB, oncocytic	+/–	–	–	+	+
PDAC, tubular	+	–/+	+	+	–/+
PDAC, colloid	–	+	+	+	–

HG-PanIN, high-grade pancreatic intraepithelial neoplasia; IPMN, intraductal papillary mucinous neoplasm; IPNB, intraductal papillary neoplasm of the bile duct; LG-PanIN, low-grade pancreatic intraepithelial neoplasia; PDAC, pancreatic ductal adenocarcinoma.

loss also occurs late in distal extrahepatic bile duct carcinogenesis {580,136,843}. Therefore, malignant-appearing epithelial groups with loss of expression are not necessarily representative of invasive carcinoma. *SMAD4* loss has been reported in pancreatoblastoma {7} and (rarely) in high-grade neuroendocrine carcinoma (NEC) of the pancreas {933}.

The von Hippel–Lindau syndrome tumour suppressor protein (VHL protein), localized to the cell membrane and cytoplasm, is the protein product of the gene *VHL*. Loss of VHL protein expression serves as a surrogate marker for mutations in *VHL* and is associated with extrahepatic cholangiocarcinoma and PDAC, but not with intrahepatic cholangiocarcinoma {492,495, 482,738,763,499}. Loss of VHL protein has been identified in ducts of autoimmune pancreatitis, which may present a pitfall in interpretation {292}. The use of a panel of antibodies including the ones described in this section is recommended to avoid false positive and false negative interpretations.

ICC for p53 reflects an accumulation of the protein in the nucleus, either due to mutation of the *TP53* gene or due to stabilization by other mechanisms {932}. Like SMAD4 (DPC4), this marker is not specific for invasion because it also occurs in non-invasive ductal lesions, mostly high-grade pancreatic intraepithelial neoplasia (HG-PanIN). Two patterns of staining are noted with mutation: strong, diffuse nuclear staining, which is most common; and no staining at all, i.e. the null pattern. This is in contrast to the wildtype pattern, indicating no mutation, where there is pale, patchy nuclear staining.

Other markers of malignancy include the oncofetal protein IMP3, as well as S100P and mesothelin. A cell is considered to show positive staining for S100 when there is strong nuclear and cytoplasmic staining. Gastric epithelium is positive for S100, limiting its utility in EUS-FNAB {495}.

Markers useful for the assessment of differentiation

SMARCA4 (BRG1), SMARCA2 (BRM), and SMARCB1 (INI1/BAF47)

Inactivating mutations in the genes *SMARCA4*, *SMARCA2*, and *SMARCB1* are implicated in tumorigenesis at various anatomical sites, including the pancreas, where tumours may show rhabdoid or undifferentiated morphology. Abnormalities in these genes are detected by ICC staining for loss of nuclear expression of the related proteins, SMARCA4 (BRG1), SMARCA2 (BRM), and SMARCB1 (INI1).

Differential diagnosis of non-ductal neoplasms

Markers useful in the differential diagnosis of non-ductal neoplasms of the pancreas are outlined in Table 2.02.

Acinar differentiation

BCL10 (monoclonal antibody 331.3) is a highly sensitive (80–100%) and highly specific (near 100%) marker of acinar differentiation {451,321}. Labelling of adenosquamous carcinoma has been reported {321}. The combination of trypsin and BCL10 is currently the most useful panel for identifying acinar differentiation, and BCL10 may be positive in trypsin-negative acinar neoplasms.

Trypsin is highly sensitive (95%) and specific. Although it is the best marker to use for the confirmation of acinar differentiation, it is commonly paired with another enzyme marker such as chymotrypsin or BCL10 to enhance sensitivity {315,419}.

Chymotrypsin has a lower sensitivity (38%) than trypsin and BCL10 for detecting acinar cell carcinoma. The staining pattern tends to be more focal than that of trypsin {419}, but it remains a useful marker, because tumours can be positive for chymotrypsin while being negative for trypsin.

Neuroendocrine differentiation

ICC is recommended for the cytopathological diagnosis of most cases of neuroendocrine tumours (NETs). Labelling for synaptophysin, chromogranin A, and/or INSM1 provides support for neuroendocrine differentiation {497}. CD56 (NCAM) and CD57 (LEU7) have insufficient specificity for clinical utility {536,420}. Staining for specific peptide hormones is not usually indicated, because functioning NETs are defined clinically {420}.

Grading of pancreatic NETs

Ki-67

The Ki-67 antigen is a marker of proliferation expressed in dividing cells. The Ki-67 proliferation index (i.e. the number of positively stained tumour cells divided by the total counted tumour cells) forms the basis of grading NET, as detailed in *Neuroendocrine tumour* (p. 142) {773,82,209}.

Markers to distinguish well-differentiated NETs from poorly differentiated NECs

DAXX and ATRX

Loss of expression of either DAXX or ATRX occurs in as many as 40% of well-differentiated NETs and is not seen in NEC {403, 291,873}.

RB1

RB1 expression can be lost in NEC but is maintained in most untreated well-differentiated NETs. RB1 loss can also be seen in PDAC, acinar cell carcinoma, and pancreatoblastoma. SPN does not label for RB1 {850}.

Markers of pancreatic origin for NETs

Several transcription factors key to pancreatic development have been studied for their utility to support the site of NET origin, but only a few have performance characteristics supporting their practical utility {810,772,488}.

ISL1

Insulin gene enhancer protein ISL1 (islet-1) is expressed in NET of the pancreas and rectum, but not NEC of the pancreas. The sensitivity is approximately 70% for pancreatic origin {772}. A staining pattern of positive for ISL1 and negative for CDX2 and thyroid transcription factor 1 (TTF1) has moderate to high sensitivity and high specificity for determining that a NET is of pancreatic or rectal origin {949}.

PDX1

PDX1 is a transcription factor essential for pancreatic differentiation and beta-cell function. The performance in detecting NET is highly variable, with < 30% sensitivity and 89% specificity, because it also labels acinar cell carcinoma and PDAC {114,810,627}.

NESP55

NESP55 is a marker of primary pancreatic origin for NET with 32% sensitivity and 97% specificity {810}.

Markers commonly used in the diagnosis of solid pseudopapillary neoplasm

Mutated *CTNNB1* in SPN leads to a loss of surface β-catenin expression and intense, diffuse nuclear labelling. β-Catenin is widely considered to be one of the most useful markers for SPN diagnosis because the sensitivity is > 90%, but it is often combined with other markers such as E-cadherin and CD99 because the specificity is limited, specifically because of staining in acinar cell carcinoma and pancreatoblastoma {93,607}. A paranuclear dot-like labelling pattern with CD99 has almost 100% sensitivity for SPN {264}. Stains for other WNT pathway proteins, including LEF1, TFE3, PR, CD56, and cyclin D1, also support a diagnosis of SPN {534,785,850,478,359}.

Mucin apomucins

Mucins are heavily glycosylated proteins that constitute the major components of mucus covering the surface of epithelial tissues. EMA (MUC1), MUC2, MUC5AC, and MUC6 are the most commonly used in diagnostic pancreaticobiliary pathology. Mucin proteins are expressed in normal tissues of the gastrointestinal and pancreaticobiliary tracts, and expression in the pancreas changes with intraductal and invasive ductal neoplasia {801,92,255}. Normal biliary ductal epithelium expresses MUC3A, MUC5B, and MUC6 {339} (see Table 2.03, p. 21).

EMA (MUC1) exists in various forms, from a fully glycosylated form to a poorly glycosylated form and a sialylated form. Tissue expression is dependent on the antibody epitope used {575}. EMA (MUC1) is expressed in benign pancreatic ducts and on the surface membranes of low-grade pancreatic intraepithelial neoplasia (LG-PanIN). HG-PanIN and intraductal papillary mucinous neoplasm with high-grade dysplasia overexpress EMA (MUC1) in the cytoplasm, as does PDAC. MUC2 is known as the intestinal-type mucin. It is expressed in goblet cells, but not in normal gastric epithelium or normal pancreaticobiliary ducts. Expression of MUC2 in a pancreaticobiliary neoplasm indicates intestinal differentiation. MUC5AC is the gastric-type mucin and is expressed by gastric foveolar epithelium. It is not expressed in normal pancreaticobiliary ducts, but it is expressed in all types of intraductal papillary mucinous neoplasm, bile duct intraductal papillary neoplasia, mucinous cystic neoplasm, and PDAC. MUC6 is expressed in periductal glands and benign ducts and by neoplasms with oncocytic and pancreaticobiliary differentiation {404,61}.

In situ hybridization

Lozano MD
Clayton A
Gómez-Román JJ
Savic Prince S
Troncone G

Introduction

FISH is a well-established method for visualizing and diagnosing numerical and structural abnormalities in chromosomal DNA. It is widely used to identify aneuploidy, deletions, amplifications, and rearrangements of selected chromosomes and genes {730,529}. The advantages of FISH include the fact that only a small number of cells are required for analysis and that alterations within cells of interest can be detected directly on the cytopathological specimen. Because chromosomal alterations are a hallmark of malignant cells, FISH can improve the accuracy of pancreaticobiliary cytopathology and may select patients for targeted therapies {463,489,43,311,946}.

Technical requirements

FISH analysis requires a fluorescence microscope with appropriate filters, ideally equipped with an automated stage and coupled with relocation software. Recording the location of photodocumented target cells on the Pap-stained cytopathology specimen enables rapid identification of these cells after hybridization and greatly facilitates FISH evaluation {730,885}. The use of adhesive slides with electrostatic positive charge is recommended to prevent cell loss during pretreatment and DNA denaturation {730,503}.

FISH scoring is ideally supervised by an experienced cytotechnologist or cytopathologist, in order to correlate FISH findings with cytomorphology. Scoring FISH signals can be done directly at the fluorescence microscope or at the computer screen after high-quality z-stack scanning, which facilitates signal evaluation and allows for the documentation of FISH findings {730}.

Management of types of cytopathological specimens

Most cytopathological preparations are suitable for FISH analysis, including Pap- or Giemsa-stained smears; unstained smears; cytospins; liquid-based preparations (liquid-based cytopathology); specimens after ICC; and unstained tissue in formalin-fixed, paraffin-embedded cell blocks {730,638, 696,74,503}. FISH applies well to specimens stained by ICC if 3-amino-9-ethylcarbazole is used as a chromogen {741}. If using cell blocks, the cell blocks are handled in a similar way to histopathological specimens, and the same protocols for FISH are applied {703,503}. The thickness of the paraffin sections can affect FISH results, owing to truncation artefact. Sections 5 ± 1 μm thick are recommended {966}.

The major advantages and disadvantages of different cytopathological samples for FISH analysis are shown in Table 2.04 (p. 24).

Fixation

Although formalin fixation is standard for tissues, alcohol fixatives are mostly used for non–cell block cytopathological preparations including smears or liquid-based cytopathology. However, the quality of DNA in air-dried or alcohol-fixed cytopathological samples is better than that after formaldehyde fixation {730,638,503,74,659}.

Controls

Benign cells with a regular FISH signal pattern serve as internal controls for good hybridization efficiency and a negative FISH result. Running external or on-slide control specimens is not required for FISH.

Procedures

After an appropriate area for FISH analysis is selected and marked on the stained diagnostic cytopathology specimen, the

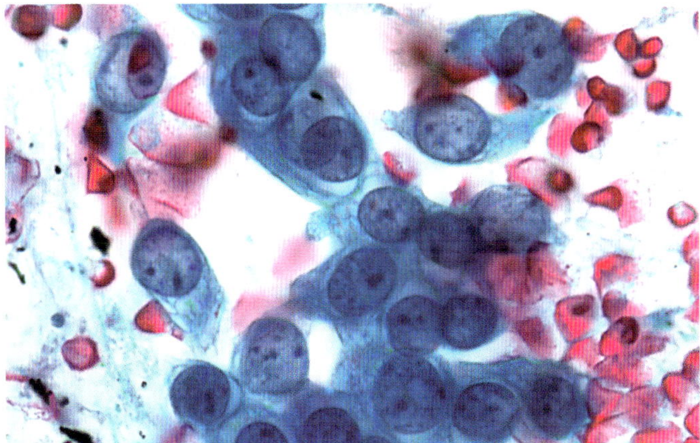

Fig. 2.05 Atypical ductal epithelium. FNAB of a pancreatic lesion in a patient with a history of pancreatitis, showing atypical ductal epithelial cells (Pap).

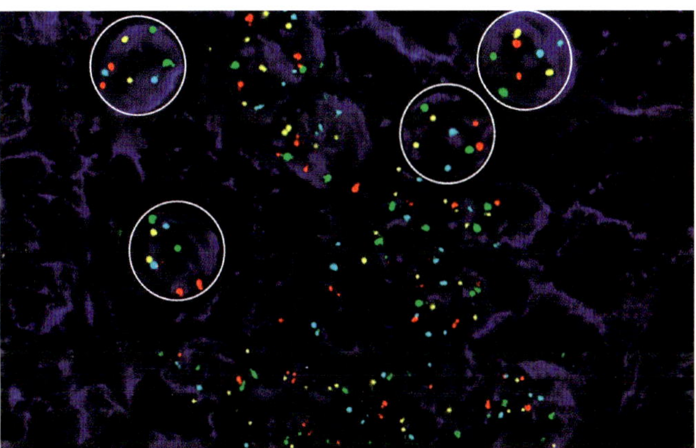

Fig. 2.06 FISH analysis. A preparation using four fluorescence-labelled DNA probes targeting the centromeric region of chromosomes 3 (SpectrumRed), 7 (SpectrumGreen), and 17 (SpectrumAqua), as well as the chromosomal locus 9p21 (SpectrumGold). Targeted FISH shows a negative result: encircled are non-overlapping cell nuclei with two signals for each probe (diploid pattern), supporting a benign diagnosis.

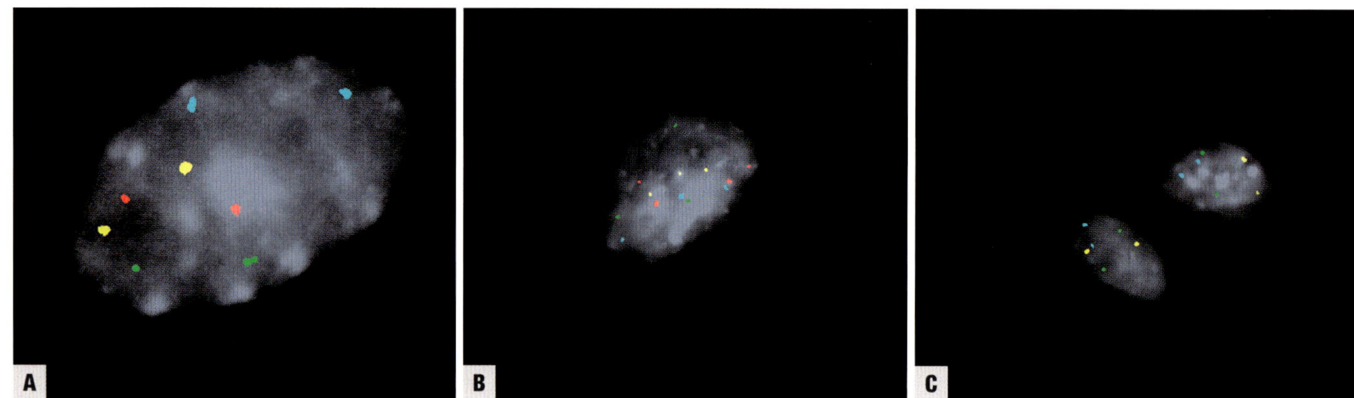

Fig. 2.07 FISH analysis, biliary brush cytology (see Fig. 2.06 for probe fluorophores and specific loci). **A** Cytology interpretation: "Atypical"; FISH result: "negative" (two copies each of probes for specific loci: 9p21, 7p12, 8q24, 1q21). **B** Cytology interpretation: "Suspicious for malignancy"; FISH result: "polysomy" (four copies of 9p21; three copies of 7p12; three copies of 8q24; three copies of 1q21). **C** Biliary brush cytology in a patient with primary sclerosing cholangitis. Cytology interpretation: "Atypical"; FISH result: "equivocal, homozygous deletion of 9p21" (two copies each of locus-specific probes 7p12, 8q24, and 1q21; no copies of 9p21).

general steps involved in FISH {410,730,688,703} include the following:

- Slide pretreatment: uncovering the coverslip, denaturing the cells using protease, applying the DNA probe
- Denaturation: heating the slide to obtain single-stranded DNA of the probe and cell
- Hybridization of the probe to the target DNA sequence
- Post-hybridization washing to remove excess probe
- Nuclear DNA counterstaining with DAPI
- FISH signal scoring and interpretation

Commercially available probes with protocols optimized for formalin-fixed, paraffin-embedded material need to be adapted for conventional cytopathology {730}. Any deviation of the protocol requires separate validation. Internal validation of FISH assays is needed and external quality assurance is advised {494,524,391}.

Scoring and interpretation of FISH signals is dependent on the FISH assay and probe design {730}. Although a few studies have developed probe sets of their own, based on known chromosomal alterations in genes associated with pancreatic carcinoma, including *TP53*, *CDKN2A* (*P16*), and *EGFR*, the most common approach is based on the multicolour UroVysion probe set (Abbott Molecular Inc.), originally developed for bladder cancer detection in urine {463}. This kit contains a probe directed at the *CDKN2A* gene located at 9p21 and chromosome enumeration probes (CEPs) directed to chromosomes 3, 7, and 17. Neoplastic cells with chromosomal alterations can be detected using the UroVysion assay {489,463}. The 9p21 FISH signal is commonly weaker than the CEP signal. Care must be taken to ensure that very weak or failed hybridization is not misinterpreted as 9p21 deletion {410,885}.

Diagnostic applications

The diagnostic challenges of routine cytopathology or small biopsy are several-fold. The pancreaticobiliary duct system is hard to access, leading to paucicellular or non-representative specimens. There can be morphological overlap between reactive conditions and malignancy {685,52}. Despite the morphological overlap, 80% of pancreaticobiliary malignancies have chromosomal abnormalities that may be detected by UroVysion FISH analysis {483}. The addition of ancillary studies to pancreaticobiliary cytopathology has the potential to improve diagnostic efficacy, with an impact on diagnostic and surveillance

Table 2.04 Advantages and disadvantages of different cytological samples for FISH analysis

Type of cytological sample	Advantages	Disadvantages
Formalin-fixed, paraffin-embedded cell block[a]	Preservation of tissue architecture No overlapping cells Cell blocks made from FNABs may be enriched in tumour cells	Probe signal loss due to nuclear truncation from sectioning Some cell blocks are poorly cellular May have autofluorescent background that obscures signals
Smears[a,b]	No nuclear truncation artefact Allows rapid onsite evaluation (ROSE) of specimen adequacy at time of procedure No alterations related to formalin fixation Smears made from FNABs may be enriched in tumour cells	Cell overlapping May have autofluorescent background that obscures signals Legal issues due to loss of diagnostic smears
Cytospins[a]	No nuclear truncation artefact Cells are concentrated in a smaller area	May have inadequate cellularity
Liquid-based cytology[a]	No nuclear truncation artefact Monolayer preparation minimizes nuclear overlap Less background Cells are concentrated in a smaller area	More expensive than other cytological preparations Special instrumentation needed for slide preparation May have inadequate cellularity

[a]Specimens after ICC are useful (see text). The area to be analysed is marked to avoid nuclear overlap and to avoid waste of the probe. [b]Pap-stained and Giemsa-stained smears, unstained smears.

screening procedures for pancreaticobiliary neoplasia {929, 928,94,563,226,251,796,689}.

Several clinical scenarios have benefited from FISH analysis in pancreaticobiliary cytopathology. Confirmation of clinically suspected malignancies, in which the cytopathology diagnosis may be equivocal because of scant cellularity or overlapping cytopathological features, was the first recognized benefit {52}.

It is also important in the setting of biliary stricture, which is difficult to recognize as benign or malignant on imaging findings alone {929,928,483}. Cytopathology and/or FISH abnormality may be the key factor in distinguishing early malignancy from a benign stricture. Finally, FISH is very useful in the setting of surveillance screening. Patients with primary sclerosing cholangitis are at increased risk for developing cholangiocarcinoma and are screened to detect early evidence of neoplasia {689,53}. The addition of FISH analysis on cytopathology brush specimens may allow early detection, with improved survival, particularly when the decision to proceed with liver transplantation is a consideration. Overall, the application of FISH on biliary brush specimens has significantly improved the diagnostic sensitivity for the detection of malignancy, which is 47–84%, while also maintaining a very high specificity (> 90%) {929,928,94,563, 226,251,796,483}.

Trisomy abnormalities or single-locus gains or losses (e.g. 9p21 loss) can be seen in both reactive and neoplastic conditions and are often viewed as equivocal findings, although 9p21 loss has been correlated with malignancy in some studies {563, 483}.

More recently, FISH has also acquired theragnostic significance, as clinical trials evaluated crizotinib safety and efficacy in patients with locally advanced cancers with *ALK*, *MET*, and *ROS1* rearrangements. The efficacy of trastuzumab and varlitinib in ERBB2-amplified biliary tract adenocarcinomas has also been investigated {43}. NTRK fusions have been detected in pancreaticobiliary malignancies, predicting a response to NTRK inhibitors {311,946}.

Molecular testing

Lozano MD
de Andrea CE
Jhala DN
Rosenbaum MW
Roy-Chowdhuri S
Singhi AD
Troncone G

Introduction

Cytopathology samples from the pancreaticobiliary tree have been utilized to perform a variety of ancillary tests including ICC and molecular testing using next-generation sequencing (NGS) {354,355,247,787}. Testing for germline mutations for hereditary cancer syndromes, tumour gene profiling including NGS for actionable somatic mutations, determinations of mismatch repair gene defects and *BRCA1* or *BRCA2* mutations are now rapidly emerging for any pancreatic ductal adenocarcinoma, as well as for bile duct cancers {921,117,435,161}. Molecular profiling for these tumours includes, but is not limited to, gene fusions (*ALK*, *NRG1*, NTRK, *ROS1*) and mutations (*EGFR*, *BRAF*, *TP53*, *SMAD4*, *BRCA1*, *BRCA2*, *ERBB2* [*HER2*], *KRAS*, *PALB2*) that could lead to personalized therapies. Furthermore, molecular analysis has made a significant impact in the diagnosis of neoplastic cysts of the pancreas. Molecular tests on pancreatic cyst fluids (*KRAS*, *GNAS*, *CTNNB1*, *VHL*, *TP53*, *PIK3CA*, *PTEN*, *AKT1*) have not only helped differentiate various neoplastic pancreatic cysts but also demonstrated association with aggressive tumour behaviour {787, 713,356,761}. In addition, for neuroendocrine tumours (NETs) of the pancreas, performance of germline testing for inherited genetic syndromes may be indicated {161,732}.

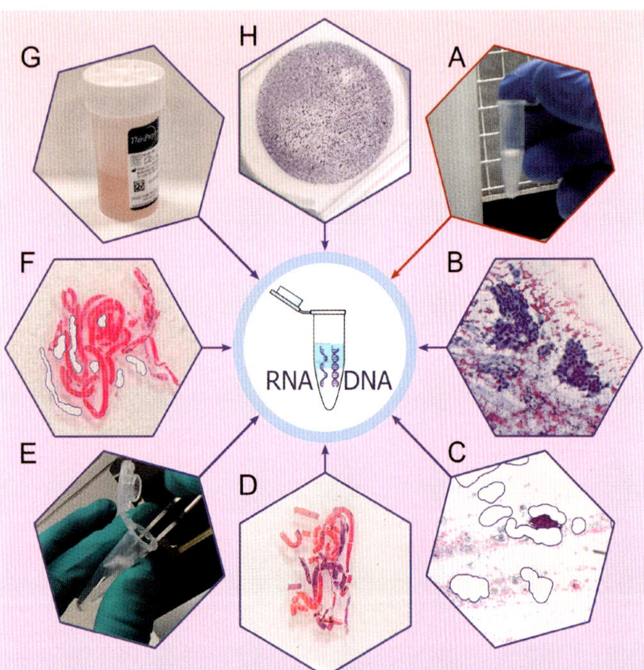

Fig. 2.08 Different types of cytological samples from solid and cystic pancreatic lesions for molecular analysis. **A** Cyst fluid. **B,C** Direct smears (with or without macrodissection/microdissection). Pap-stained and Giemsa-stained and/or unstained slides can be used. Cell scraping preferred. **D–F** Cell blocks (with or without macrodissection/microdissection). Long formalin fixation increases the risk of C>T or G>A artefacts. **G,H** Lysis buffer–derived DNA/RNA.

Technical requirements

Successful molecular testing of pancreaticobiliary samples is directly dependent on specimen adequacy and the number of tumour cells. Sequencing-based molecular testing has two input requirements, i.e. the amount of nucleic acid yield and the tumour fraction. A minimum amount of DNA/RNA is required to obtain a result and a minimum tumour to neoplastic (neoplastic nuclei) fraction is essential to detect a mutation in a background of wildtype signal {702,67,760}. When insufficient DNA/RNA occurs, no result is obtained and the result is "uninformative", but an insufficient tumour to neoplastic (neoplastic nuclei) fraction can lead to a false negative or "misinformative" result (see Table 2.05) {696,503}. Because of the low tumour fraction in many pancreatic cysts, the absence of genetic mutations is uninformative, but the detection of mutations may be diagnostic. For example, the simple detection of a *KRAS* mutation can take a biopsy from a "Non-diagnostic" or nonspecific cyst fluid interpretation to a diagnosis of a neoplastic mucinous cyst, which directly impacts patient management {364}.

Rapid onsite evaluation (ROSE) is beneficial for improving the diagnostic yield of FNAB specimens of solid masses {357} (see Box 2.02). ROSE is not advised for cysts unless there is a solid component, because cyst fluid must be conserved for ancillary studies. Standardized protocols and optimization guidelines are mandatory. Specimen collection, fixation, processing, staining, storage conditions, tumour fraction enrichment, nucleic acid quality/quantity assessment, and quality assurance/control metrics are also crucial {67,663}.

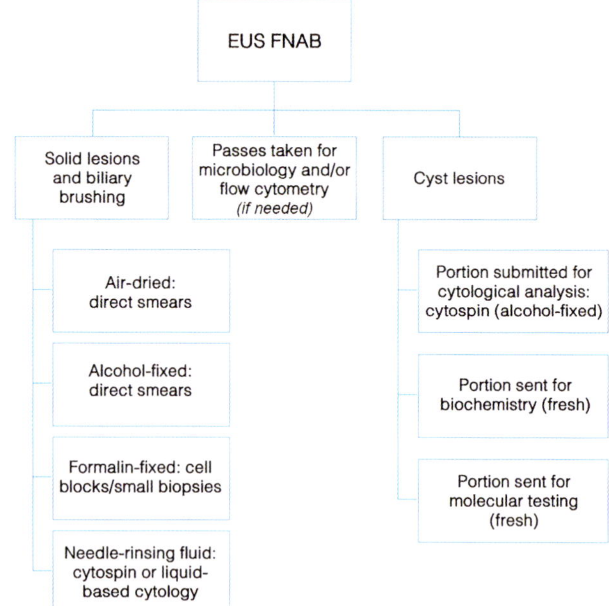

Fig. 2.09 Molecular testing. Recommended fixatives for pancreaticobiliary cytological samples.

Table 2.05 Molecular testing of cytological specimens

Basic terminology	Definition	Testing recommendation
Analytical threshold	Minimal input requirement for successful testing as determined by laboratory validation (lowest LOD)	Analytical performance of an assay is measured by its accuracy, precision, analytical specificity, and analytical sensitivity (LOD); establishment of the LOD is critical for sequencing assays used to detect the presence of low-frequency variants (SNVs, indels) and is defined as the lowest allelic frequency at which the mutant alleles can be consistently detected in ≥ 95% of the test cases LOD directly depends on the amount of amplifiable input material (DNA/RNA) that is analysed
Preanalytics	Collection, processing, and handling of specimens	
Tumour fraction (T%)	Percentage of tumour cells in a sample: the relative amount of tumour (neoplastic cell) DNA that can be reliably detected in a background of wildtype DNA T% = total number of tumour cells / total number of nucleated cells	For NGS using the Ion Torrent platform: 1. T% ≥ 20: reliable NGS readout 2. T% < 20: use one of the following: a. single-target mutation analysis of high sensitivity (PCR-based methods such as Droplet Digital PCR) b. NGS testing with enrichment of tumour cells (laser microdissection) c. NGS with molecular barcodes that label each original DNA fragment within the sample and thereby increase analytical sensitivity and specificity
Input DNA/RNA	Minimum amount of DNA/RNA to obtain valid results	Nucleic acid input for NGS testing depends on the assay and platform used, gene panel size, target enrichment method, and DNA quality DNA input requirements vary between platforms

LOD, limit of detection; NGS, next-generation sequencing.

Management of types of cytopathological specimens

Nucleic acid (DNA/RNA) can be extracted from all routine cytopathological specimen preparations, including direct smears; cytospin preparations; liquid-based cytopathology preparations; and formalin-fixed, paraffin-embedded cell block preparations {157,160,348}. Cytopathological preparations that are air-dried for Giemsa and/or alcohol-fixed for Pap provide a superior source of DNA for molecular testing when compared with formalin-fixed, paraffin-embedded preparations {286,235}. In pancreatic cyst fluids, molecular testing can be performed by extracting nucleic acid directly from fresh, unfixed cyst fluid {700,787}. Collected cyst fluid can be used for cytopathology, biochemistry testing for CEA and amylase, and molecular testing. The supernatant fluid from centrifuged pancreaticobiliary cytopathology specimens can also be used for molecular testing {216,217}.

Morphological assessment of specimen adequacy is crucial for reliable molecular results. A cytopathological slide with an area of adequate tumour is selected for macrodissection or microdissection. The coverslip is removed and the selected cells on the slide are scraped or cell-lifted into buffer medium for nucleic acid extraction. Cell block sections are processed as per standard protocols for histopathological specimens using an H&E-stained section as a guide for specimen adequacy and to extract cells from corresponding unstained sections. In cases where a single diagnostic cytopathological slide is available for molecular testing, whole slide image scanning and digital archiving of the slide for cytomorphological evidence of malignancy, before sacrificing the slide for molecular testing, can avoid medicolegal issues {67}.

Box 2.02 Advantages of rapid onsite evaluation (ROSE) for molecular testing of pancreaticobiliary cytological specimens

- Specimen adequacy
- Preliminary diagnosis
- Triage for ancillary studies
- Careful control of preanalytics
- Real-time guidance to the physician performing the FNAB procedure
- Ability to stop sampling when appropriate material has been obtained
- Clinicopathological communication
- Possibility of sampling/testing different sites

Note: ROSE is not needed in cystic lesions.

Fixation

For pancreatic cysts, fresh, unfixed, and undiluted pancreatic cyst fluid is required for molecular analysis. Direct smears from solid lesions and biliary brushing can be alcohol-fixed or air-dried. Formalin fixation is recommended for cell blocks and small biopsies that are often used to supplement bile duct brushings. Fluid can be processed as a cytospin preparation. A dedicated pass for flow cytometry can be done if a lymphoproliferative lesion is suspected.

Controls

Several single-institution studies have shown that the quality of molecular assays on pancreaticobiliary cytopathological specimens is high {166,625}. However, for NGS, multi-institutional studies are needed to exclude potential sources of inconsistent results due to differences in gene panels, target enrichment strategies, and platforms between institutions {167}. To this end, genetically engineered cell lines can be used to mimic actual clinical cytopathological samples in routine practice. However, genetically engineered cell lines have traditionally only been available as artificial formalin-fixed, paraffin-embedded histopathological sections or scrolls. The Molecular Cytopathology Meeting Group has developed molecular reference slides harbouring concurrent mutations in several genes at various allelic ratios, including low allele frequencies of 1%, to mimic actual smears {518,639}. In multicentre international studies, all participating laboratories successfully detected the mutations in the study set, despite the use of different sequencing platforms. Therefore, quantitative molecular reference slides are a

Table 2.06 The genomic alterations of the major pancreatic cysts and associated invasive adenocarcinoma

Gene(s)	IPMN	IPMN with advanced neoplasia[a]	MCN	MCN with advanced neoplasia[a]	IOPN	SCA	Cystic PanNET	SPN	Non-neoplastic cyst
KRAS	+	+	+	+	–	–	–	–	–
GNAS	+	+	–	–	–	–	–	–	–
RNF43	+	+	+	+	–	–	–	–	–
TP53	–	+	–	+	–	–	–	–	–
SMAD4	–	+	–	+	–	–	–	–	–
mTOR pathway genes[b]	–	+	–	+	–	–	–	–	–
PRKACA/PRKACB fusion gene	–	–	–	–	+	–	–	–	–
VHL	–	–	–	–	–	+	–	–	–
MEN1	–	–	–	–	–	–	+	–	–
CTNNB1	–	–	–	–	–	–	–	+	–

IOPN, intraductal oncocytic papillary neoplasm; IPMN, intraductal papillary mucinous neoplasm; MCN, mucinous cystic neoplasm; PanNET, pancreatic neuroendocrine tumour; SCA, serous cystadenoma; SPN, solid pseudopapillary neoplasm.
[a]Advanced neoplasia is defined as high-grade dysplasia and/or invasive adenocarcinoma. [b]mTOR genes include *PIK3CA*, *PTEN*, and *AKT1*.

useful tool for monitoring the performance of different multigene mutation assays, and this could lead to better standardization of molecular cytopathology procedures.

Procedures

A variety of molecular testing methodologies can be used for interrogating pancreatic and biliary cytopathology specimens. These include methods ranging from single-gene-based mutation assays such as Sanger sequencing, pyrosequencing, and real-time PCR, to multiplexed array assays, to broad, expanded molecular profiling approaches such as NGS {530,705,289, 448,365,742,787,700}. In general, targeted assays have high analytical sensitivity but limited clinical sensitivity. Testing using an expanded NGS panel approach offers the advantage of simultaneously screening multiple genes for a variety of alterations including SNVs, indels, copy-number changes, gene fusions, tumour mutation burden, and microsatellite instability, depending on the design of the assay.

Diagnostic applications

Molecular biomarkers can be used for diagnostic, prognostic, and therapeutic purposes. These assays represent an adjunct to cytomorphology evaluation and have significant value in the preoperative diagnosis of pancreatic cystic lesions {700,787}.

The detection of *KRAS* or *GNAS* mutations from pancreatic cyst fluids is highly sensitive and specific for neoplastic mucinous cysts, with *GNAS* mutations being highly specific for intraductal papillary mucinous neoplasms.

The overall diagnostic utility of molecular testing of solid lesions of the pancreas is limited, although the increasing use of broad, panel-based molecular profiling such as NGS may enable the analysis of mutations such as *TP53*, *SMAD4*, and *CDKN2A* to help in the diagnosis and prognostication of pancreatic ductal adenocarcinoma when cytopathology is indeterminate (see Table 2.06) {926,925,790,597,364,809,791,700, 787,808}.

NGS of bile duct brushings and biopsies can detect genetic alterations such as *KRAS* mutations and improve the identification of a malignant bile duct stricture with a sensitivity and specificity as high as 74% and 100%, respectively {192, 788}. Moreover, the combination of NGS and cytopathological evaluation increases the sensitivity to 85% while maintaining a high specificity. Additionally, the detection of genomic alterations can triage patients with pancreaticobiliary neoplasms to specific therapeutic regimens, such as those associated with *ERBB2* amplification or tyrosine kinase gene fusions {783,788, 616,5}.

For pancreatic neuroendocrine neoplasms (PanNENs), molecular testing can be both diagnostic and prognostic. The cytopathological distinction between WHO grade 3 (G3) pancreatic neuroendocrine tumour (PanNET) and pancreatic neuroendocrine carcinoma (PanNEC) can be problematic. G3 PanNET harbours frequent alterations in *ATRX* and *DAXX*, whereas PanNEC often has *TP53* and *RB1* mutations {360,933,842}. Molecular testing can aid in the discrimination of these two neoplasms, which is imperative when considering the differences in treatment and prognosis. Moreover, for G1 and G2 PanNETs, *ATRX* and *DAXX* alterations are prognostic biomarkers for recurrence and metastasis and are independent of histopathological grade, including Ki-67 {525,786,403,701}.

Biochemical testing of cyst fluid

Centeno BA

Introduction

Biochemical analysis is a component of pancreatic cyst fluid ancillary testing that is useful in the differential diagnosis of mucinous cysts from non-mucinous cysts. CEA and amylase are the two proteins routinely measured.

Technical requirements

A minimum of 0.3 mL is required for each test, but 0.5–1.0 mL is the optimum volume for each test. Viscous specimens are generally rejected for analysis, and dilution is not recommended because of required adjustments for the final laboratory result. Thick, viscous, white, opaque fluids correlate with a mucinous cyst, and CEA analysis does not add to this assessment {837}.

Management of types of cytopathological specimens

Biochemical analysis is indicated for the analysis of pancreatic cyst fluid and not for the analysis of needle rinsings of solid tumour FNAB. It is performed on the supernatant fluid after cytospin.

Fixation

The pancreatic cyst fluid should be kept fresh and not placed into saline, preservative, or fixative. The cyst fluid is centrifuged, and the supernatant fluid is submitted fresh and undiluted to the chemistry laboratory for testing. The cell button is processed for cytopathology.

Controls

Each laboratory must validate the assays and establish its own normal and abnormal ranges. The measured CEA and amylase values of a patient's sample can vary depending on the testing procedure used.

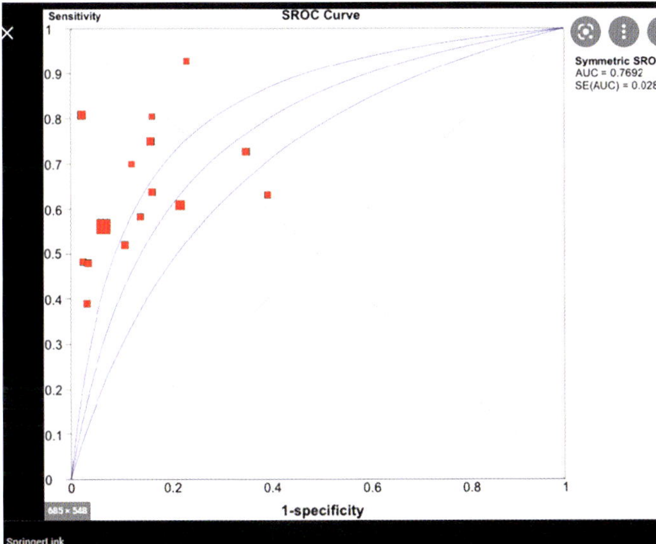

Fig. 2.10 CEA in cyst fluid. Receiver operating characteristic (ROC) curve showing utility of CEA measurement in cyst fluid in differentiating mucinous and non-mucinous pancreatic cysts, from a meta-analysis of multiple studies {396}.

Procedures

CEA

The CEA immunoassay uses the sandwich antibody method. CEA values determined on patient samples by different testing procedures cannot be directly compared with one another and could be the cause of erroneous medical interpretations. It is recommended that each laboratory establish its own cut-off level {140}.

Amylase

Amylase testing uses an enzymatic colorimetric assay to quantify α-amylase by measuring the formation of degradation products saccharogenically or kinetically with the aid of enzyme-catalysed reactions. An increase in absorbance is directly related to the colour intensity of the degradation product, which is proportional to the α-amylase activity {867}.

Diagnostic applications

CEA is measured in the pancreatic cyst fluid to establish a mucinous etiology. A multi-institutional study established a cut-off value of 192 ng/mL as the most sensitive and specific level for the diagnosis of a mucinous cyst {91}. Subsequent studies reported optimal cyst fluid CEA levels ranging from 48.6 ng/mL to 800 ng/mL {876,802,564,757,396}. As the CEA level is increased to achieve higher specificity, the sensitivity is decreased. Of note, a low level of CEA does not exclude a mucinous cyst, because pancreatic mucinous cysts may have very low CEA levels – even as low as 1.6 ng/mL {628}. A prospective study of patients with pancreatic cysts showed ranges in CEA values of 0.2–91 000 ng/mL in intraductal papillary mucinous neoplasm (IPMN) and 0–549 ng/mL in mucinous cystic neoplasm. CEA remains low in cystic pancreatic neuroendocrine tumours (PanNETs) {960}, solid pseudopapillary neoplasm, and serous cystadenoma {635}.

Cyst fluid amylase levels are very useful for differentiating a pseudocyst from other cyst types. An amylase level of < 250 U/L has a very high specificity for excluding a pseudocyst {876}. Elevated pancreatic cyst amylase fluid levels cannot be used to differentiate IPMN from mucinous cystic neoplasm {848}. In a prospective study, IPMN and mucinous cystic neoplasm showed a range of amylase levels of 0–280 000 U/L {635}.

Other recently identified markers that are promising include VEGF, the monoclonal antibody Das-1, and glucose. Measurement of VEGF in cyst fluids may detect serous cystadenomas {941,955,808}. Das-1 is a monoclonal antibody reactive to premalignant conditions of the gastrointestinal tract that can be measured in pancreatic cyst fluid to detect high-risk IPMN {162}. Measurement of glucose in pancreatic cyst fluids may be used as a supplement to CEA, because it is low in mucinous cysts and elevated in serous cystadenomas {989,100,501,687,778,555}.

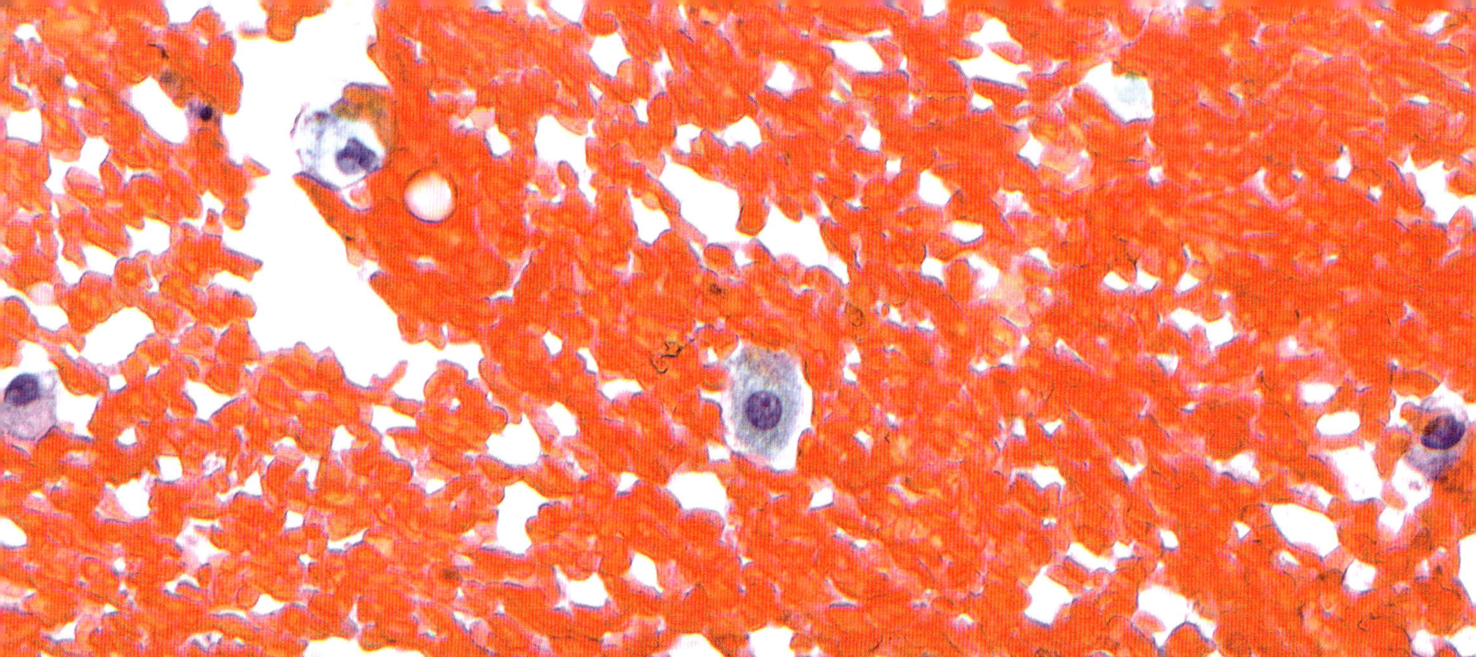

3

Diagnostic category: Insufficient/Inadequate/Non-diagnostic

Edited by: Saieg M

Introduction

Layfield LJ

The category "Insufficient/Inadequate/Non-diagnostic" is used to convey to the patient care team that the specimen obtained supplies no useful information concerning the targeted lesion and that additional sampling will be necessary. The precise terminology for this category has been controversial and not used consistently among institutions, which has resulted in three terms being offered as options {650}.

Specimens with large numbers of benign pancreatic acinar and/or ductal epithelial cells in the setting of an unexplained distinct solid or cystic lesion present on imaging can be categorized as "Insufficient/Inadequate/Non-diagnostic" rather than "Benign" because the FNAB material is clearly a sampling error and does not explain the mass. Alternatively, the interpretation can be categorized as "Benign" with an obligatory caveat or note in the report conclusion that clearly states that "the benign tissue may not be representative of the lesion depicted on imaging and further investigation and clinical correlation is required". Categorizing such cases as "Benign", however, may risk increasing the risk of malignancy for this category, and this is an area requiring further research.

An "Insufficient/Inadequate/Non-diagnostic" specimen may result from a variety of technical, preparation, and sampling issues, which obscure the cellular component. Adequacy evaluation requires correlation with the imaging findings, the gross appearance of fluid and direct smears, and when appropriate, chemical analysis of the cyst fluid. The complete absence of cells does not necessarily result in a cystic specimen being designated "Insufficient/Inadequate/Non-diagnostic". For example, the presence of background mucus or high CEA levels may be enough to diagnose a cyst fluid as mucinous, even in the absence of an epithelial component.

Definition

Layfield LJ

A specimen categorized as "Insufficient/Inadequate/Non-diagnostic" is one that for qualitative and/or quantitative reasons does not permit a diagnosis of the targeted lesion.

Discussion and background

Kurtycz D

An adequate sample is satisfactory for diagnostic purposes. However, the criteria for adequacy are a source of contention in almost all diagnostic reporting systems. Certainly, samples that are cellular, well fixed, and representative of the target lesion are adequate, and in pancreaticobiliary cytopathology correlation with imaging is virtually always available to confirm the target. Some cytopathological diagnostic systems have declared a minimum cellularity necessary for evidence of sufficient sampling and adequacy, such as in the Bethesda System for Reporting Thyroid Cytopathology (BSRTC) {138}. However, owing to the number of variables inherent in pancreaticobiliary samples, adequacy based on cell count has not been established. There is no published consensus on a minimum number of epithelial cells below which a specimen is designated as "Inadequate" or "Non-diagnostic", especially for pancreatic cysts. However, acellular specimens obtained from solid pancreatic lesions or duct strictures should certainly be placed in this category. The presence of any cellular atypia precludes categorization as "Insufficient/Inadequate/Non-diagnostic".

Paucicellular or acellular cyst fluid can provide diagnostic information from the presence of characteristic thick, colloid-like extracellular mucin or degenerated, inflammatory cyst contents characteristic of a pseudocyst {105}. On the other hand, cellular specimens composed of contaminant gastrointestinal epithelial cells from the stomach or duodenum are not adequate. In the situation where benign pancreatic tissue is found in the context of a targeted solid or cystic mass seen on imaging, some cytopathologists regard this as a "Non-diagnostic" sample, i.e. an "Inadequate" sample, because the sample does not explain the mass, whereas other cytopathologists regard this as "Benign", with the emphasis that the report requires a mandatory caveat statement that "the material may not represent the lesion seen on imaging and repeat FNAB is required". In this first WHO Reporting System for Pancreaticobiliary Cytopathology, it is recognized that both approaches are acceptable, and further use and research will establish which approach is more suitable, especially in the context of maintaining a low risk of malignancy in the "Benign" category. As with the Papanicolaou System for Reporting Pancreaticobiliary Cytology, the WHO Reporting System takes clinical and radiological findings into consideration, and a fundamental principle is that a cytopathological diagnosis is most accurate when the clinical, radiological, and cytopathological findings – the triple test of classic cytopathology – are taken into consideration {650}.

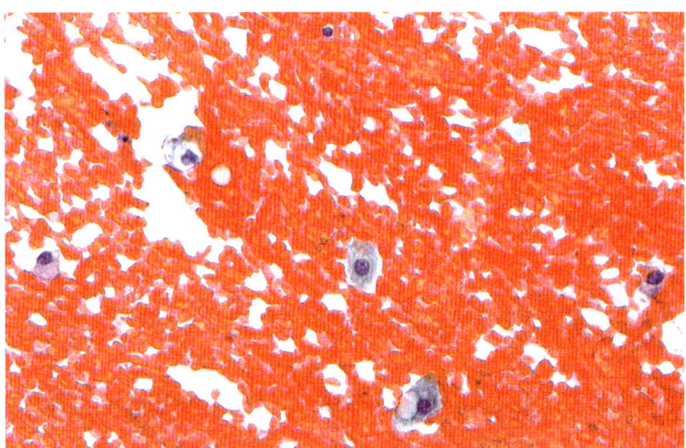

Fig. 3.02 Bloody FNAB with histiocytes, inadequate for diagnosis. This case is represented by blood only, and should be considered inadequate for diagnosis (Pap).

Reasons for an "Insufficient/Inadequate/Non-diagnostic" sample include:

- Preparation artefact including degeneration and stain precipitate
- Obscuring blood, contaminant gastrointestinal epithelium or other material

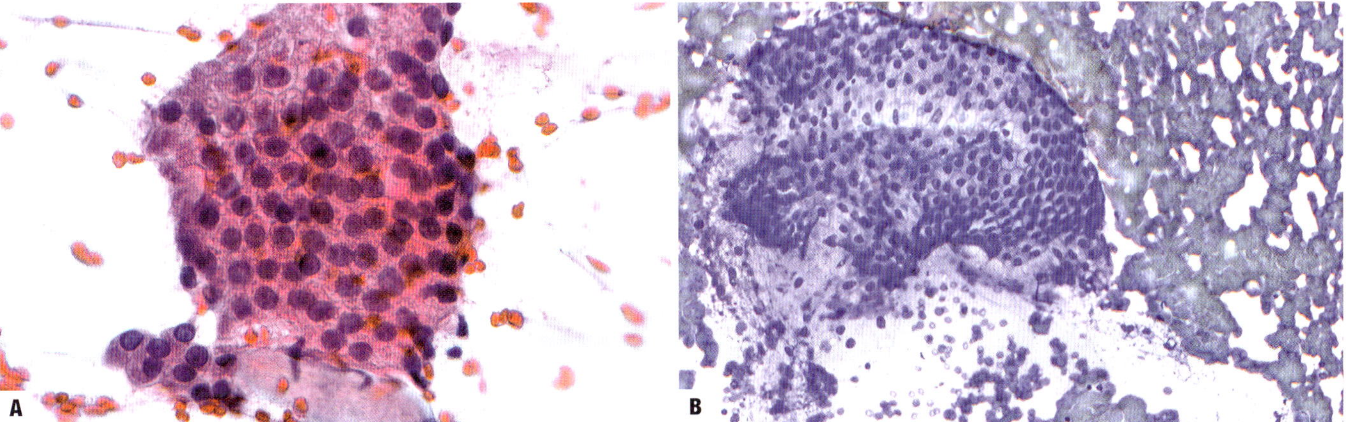

Fig. 3.01 Gastrointestinal contaminant. **A** Note the cuboidal cells with granular foamy cytoplasm and evenly spaced nuclei (Pap). **B** Gastric epithelium may be a diagnostic pitfall when a mucinous cyst is the clinical diagnosis by imaging. The benign morphology excludes adenocarcinoma from the differential diagnosis (Giemsa).

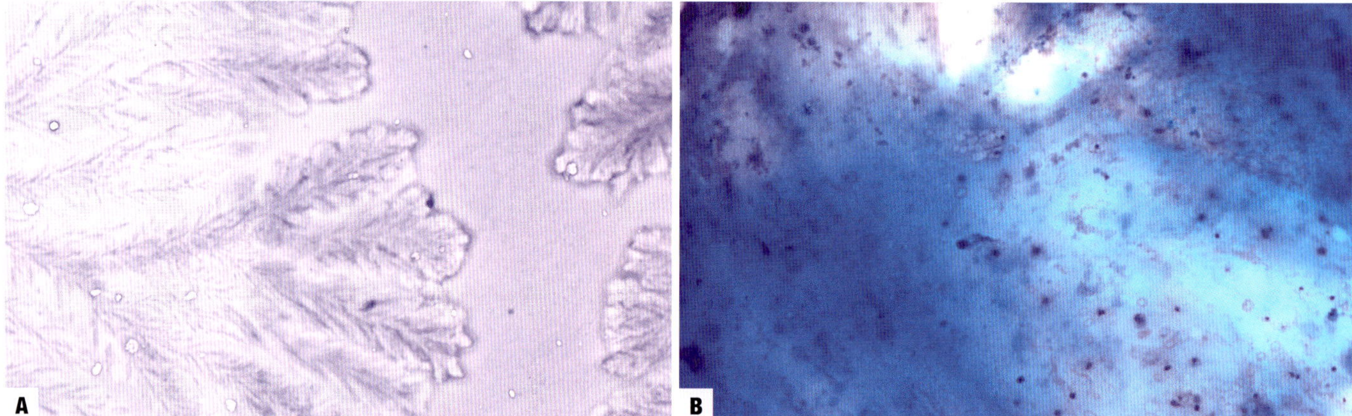

Fig. 3.03 Mucinous neoplasm. **A** Image containing only background mucus. This case cannot, therefore, be categorized as "Insufficient/Inadequate/Non-diagnostic" and should be diagnosed as a mucinous neoplasm because of the abundant mucinous background (Giemsa). **B** Another example of a sample containing only background mucus, with no epithelial cells. Because of the large quantity of mucus, however, this case should be classified as a mucinous neoplasm and should not be placed under the "Insufficient/Inadequate/Non-diagnostic" category (Giemsa).

- Normal pancreatic tissue in the context of a targeted solid or cystic mass
- Acellular FNAB of a solid mass or duct brushing
- Acellular FNAB of a cyst without evidence of a mucinous etiology such as thick, colloid-like extracellular mucin or elevated CEA (> 192 ng/mL)

Risk of malignancy and management recommendations

Kumarasinghe MP
Klapman J
Kurtycz D

Chapter 3

The risk of malignancy (ROM) for a given diagnostic cytopathological categorization provides the patient care team with reasonable management options in the context of the diagnostic category. The estimated ROMs for pancreatic FNAB are based on retrospective and prospective studies {792,307,824,711}. For the "Insufficient/Inadequate/Non-diagnostic" category, the ROM ranges from 5% to 25% {306}.

The ROM in bile duct brushing specimens in the "Insufficient/Inadequate/Non-diagnostic" category is high (28–69%) because of the sampling bias of targeting duct strictures with an inherently high risk of malignancy {875,111,192,952,658,468, 595}.

Management recommendations depend on the cause of an "Insufficient/Inadequate/Non-diagnostic" sample. The diagnostic yield depends on the operator, the technique employed, and the equipment – including the needles used and the availability of specific cytopathology expertise, including facilities with rapid onsite evaluation (ROSE) {299,551,151}. If any of the above is suboptimal, a repeat biopsy is usually needed. "Non-diagnostic" rates from published series with EUS-FNAB show an average of 12% {711}. A given procedure may therefore not produce results and may have to be repeated or give way to a different methodology in order to achieve a final definitive diagnosis.

Some processes, such as chronic or autoimmune pancreatitis, are likely to result in "Inadequate" or "Non-diagnostic" samples due to extensive fibrosis and scant material. In such situations, an empirical trial of steroids may be appropriate {560}. Brush cytopathology specimens, traditionally performed to assess bile duct strictures, are notoriously paucicellular or obscured by smearing or preparation artefact and may be deemed insufficient for accurate assessment. If there is a significant thickening of the wall, EUS-FNAB of the area may be recommended.

ROSE has proved to be effective in reducing the number of "Inadequate" samples, thereby minimizing the need for a repeat procedure. However, high cost and pathologist availability are factors hampering its broad applicability, with remote evaluation by telecytopathology proposed as an alternative {299,551,151}. There is also some recent evidence that EUS-FNAB alone is as good as EUS-FNAB plus ROSE and is associated with fewer needle passes, a shorter procedure time, and an excellent histopathological yield at a comparable cost {47,206}. Repeat procedures can be performed with an FNAB plus or minus fine core needle biopsy. In some instances, further clinical management decisions may still be made on the basis of the clinical scenario and imaging alone. Neoadjuvant therapy requires a definitive malignant diagnosis.

Sample reports: Insufficient/Inadequate/Non-diagnostic

Kumarasinghe MP
Kurtycz D
Layfield LJ

Sample report 1

Nature of specimen: FNAB 30 mm solid mass in tail of pancreas.
Specimen adequacy: Evaluation limited by non-representative specimen.
Category: Non-diagnostic.
Diagnosis: Gastrointestinal contaminants only. No lesional material is present. The biopsy does not explain the mass seen on imaging.

Sample report 2

Nature of specimen: FNAB 30 mm solid mass in tail of pancreas.
Specimen adequacy: Evaluation limited by poor cellular preservation.
Category: Inadequate.
Diagnosis: Tissue is poorly preserved, with marked air-drying artefact, and not suitable for diagnosis.

Sample report 3

Nature of specimen: FNAB 30 mm solid mass in tail of pancreas.
Specimen adequacy: Evaluation limited by non-representative specimen.
Category: Non-diagnostic.
Diagnosis: Smears contain limited pancreatic acinar material, a few scattered ductal epithelial cells, and stromal fragments. The biopsy does not explain the distinct solid mass seen on imaging.

Sample report 4

Nature of specimen: Poorly defined possible lesion in head of pancreas.
Specimen adequacy: Evaluation limited by scant cellularity.
Category: Non-diagnostic.
Diagnosis: Scattered inflammatory cells, scant pancreatic acini, and inflamed stroma with crushed cells. No specific diagnostic features are present. See comment.
Comment: Clinical and imaging suspicion of autoimmune pancreatitis is noted. Additional tissue is needed for diagnosis.

Sample report 5

Nature of specimen: FNAB 30 mm cystic lesion in head of pancreas.
Specimen adequacy: Evaluation limited by scant cellularity.
Category: Non-diagnostic.
Diagnosis: Cyst fluid contains thin proteinaceous material only. See comment.
Comment: There is no thick extracellular mucin, there are no mucinous epithelial cells, and no biochemical testing for CEA/amylase is available to support a mucinous cyst. Molecular studies are pending and may be informative.

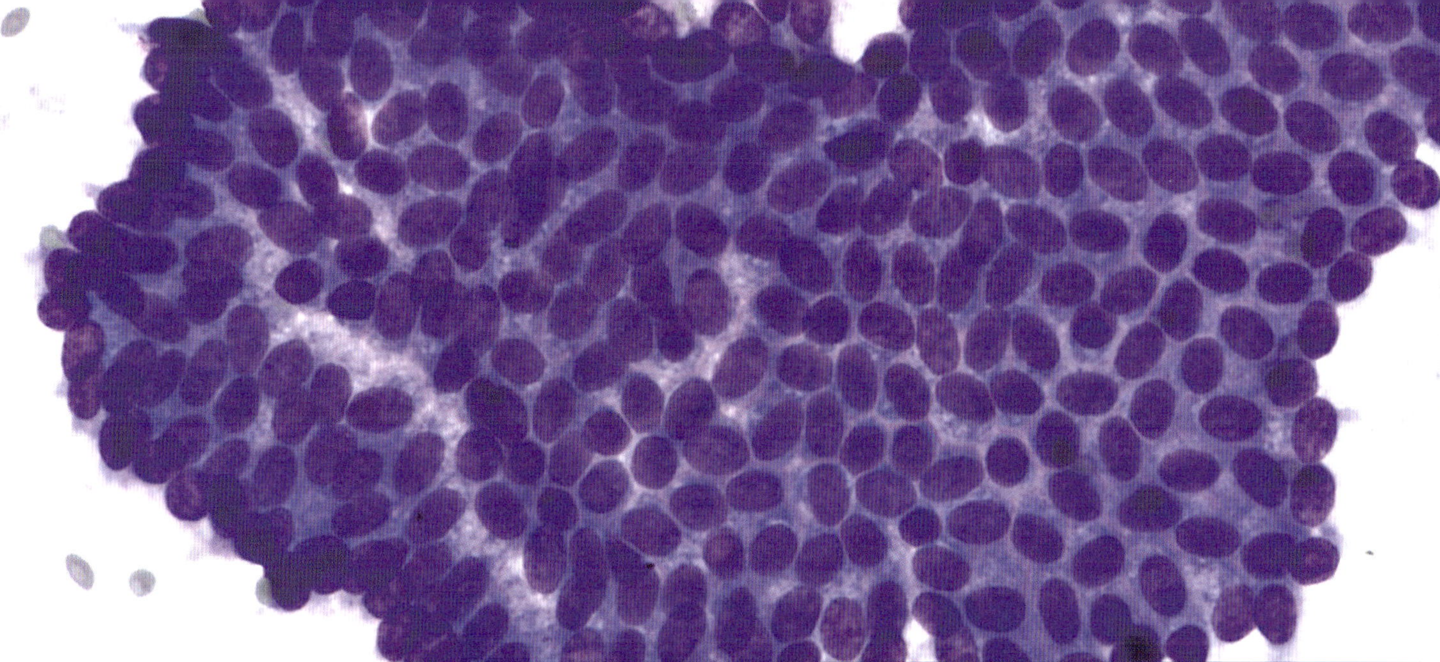

4

Diagnostic category: Benign / Negative for malignancy

Edited by: Fukushima N, Perez-Machado MA

Introduction

Saieg M
Stelow EB

The diagnostic category "Benign" or "Negative for malignancy" is used when definitive diagnoses can be made of non-neoplastic and benign neoplastic processes involving the pancreas or pancreaticobiliary tract. Such lesions include but are not limited to pseudocysts, chronic pancreatitis, cholangitis, serous cystadenomas, and benign mesenchymal neoplasms. This WHO Reporting System category includes both the "Negative for malignancy" and the "Neoplastic: benign" categories in the Papanicolaou Society of Cytopathology (PSC) System for Reporting Pancreaticobiliary Cytology, which are grouped together here to align more closely with the WHO classification of digestive system tumours {910} and with the low risk of malignancy associated with benign non-neoplastic and neoplastic lesions of the pancreas {643}.

An interpretation of "Benign" implies that the sample is adequately cellular and that no cytopathological atypia is identified in the material. Any atypia outside of what can be explained as reactive or reparative features should preclude the categorization of the biopsy within this category. The interpretation of a cytopathological sample as "Benign" without a further diagnosis of a specific condition can be used in cases where only normal pancreatic cytopathological tissue is seen and no distinct mass lesion is present on imaging. When only normal pancreatic tissue is present but a distinct mass lesion is seen on imaging, the diagnostic category can be either "Non-diagnostic" or "Benign", with a mandatory caveat note in the report conclusion stating that "the material may not represent the target lesion owing to sampling error, and clinical and imaging correlation and further investigation is warranted". Disadvantages to placing a potentially non-representative FNAB in the "Benign" category include the likelihood of a falsely elevated risk of malignancy for this category and the potential risk of improper patient management from a patient care team that does not see or read the caveat and only sees the diagnostic category of "Benign". The decision to categorize such cases as "Non-diagnostic" or "Benign", with the caveat that the sample may not represent the imaging abnormality, will be made by the cytopathologists within their institution, and this decision must be discussed with their clinicians so that there is a clear understanding of local usage.

According to published papers on the use of the PSC system, as many as 15% of all pancreaticobiliary cytopathology specimens will be categorized as "Benign" {306}. This is made possible partly by the incorporation of imaging features and biochemical cyst fluid analysis into the final diagnosis of pancreatic cysts, which reduces the number of specimens categorized as "Atypical" or "Insufficient/Inadequate/Non-diagnostic" {649,535, 633,710}.

Definition

Saieg M
Stelow EB

A specimen categorized as "Benign / Negative for malignancy" demonstrates unequivocal benign cytopathological features, which may or may not be diagnostic of a specific process or benign neoplasm.

Discussion and background

Saieg M
Stelow EB

Lesions categorized as "Benign" or "Negative for malignancy" include non-neoplastic lesions such as lymphoepithelial cyst, splenule, pseudocyst, and pancreatitis of all types, as well as benign neoplasms, most commonly serous cystadenoma. Rare neoplasms in the pancreas, such as lymphangioma {223} and schwannoma {273}, are also included in this category.

An individual cytopathologist or institution should consistently use either the term "Benign" or the term "Negative for malignancy", and this decision will be based on local practice.

A cellular sample of normal pancreatic tissue is included in this category when imaging does not show a specific solid mass or cystic lesion. An FNAB yielding only benign pancreatic tissue in the setting of a visible targeted lesion seen on imaging can be placed in the "Insufficient/Inadequate/Non-diagnostic" category, for clear communication with the patient care team that the biopsy material does not explain the target. However, including such a sample in the "Benign" category is an acceptable option as long as there is a caveat within the report and clear communication with the patient care team that correlation with imaging is required and repeat study is recommended. The report should clearly state that the cytopathological material may not represent the lesion seen on imaging. Recommendations for further diagnostic workup may also be given.

Cyst fluid analysis with biochemical testing of CEA and amylase helps categorize cystic lesions: high amylase and low CEA fluid levels are supportive of a pseudocyst, whereas a serous cystadenoma has low CEA and amylase levels {876,712}. However, lymphoepithelial cysts notoriously have elevated CEA levels {668}. This finding coupled with very degenerated keratinous debris that can mimic desiccated mucin may lead to a false positive categorization of a benign, non-neoplastic lesion as a neoplastic mucinous cyst {122}.

Benign biliary brushings are generally straightforward when they present normal-appearing ductal epithelium. However, malignancies in biliary brushing samples from inflamed and stented ducts can be extremely difficult to sample, leading to a high false negative rate {699}.

The use of ICC or molecular studies in pancreatic FNAB and biliary brushing cytopathology is discussed in more detail with each specific entity.

Risk of malignancy and management recommendations

Saieg M
Klapman J
Pitman MB
Stelow EB

The risk of malignancy (ROM) for "Benign" FNAB of the pancreas ranges from 0% to as high as 15% {792,307,824, 306}. However, the ROM for "Benign" lesions may be overestimated because it is usually calculated using histopathological confirmation, and only cases with high clinical suspicion are surgically excised after a "Benign" FNAB categorization {711}. By categorizing cellular samples of benign pancreatic tissue from an FNAB targeting a well-defined mass as "Non-diagnostic", this overestimation of the ROM can potentially be reduced. False negative interpretations represent a small percentage of cases and are related to scant cellularity or sampling error, which is common for cystic lesions {307,502, 824,712}.

ROM for samples categorized as "Benign" in bile duct brushings is particularly hard to estimate because of the small number of published studies on this topic, but it is thought to be higher than in FNAB samples from pancreatic nodules, owing to the inherently high risk of a bile duct stricture and the high morphological threshold for a "Malignant" categorization, resulting in a large number of false negative cases {352,44}. According to retrospective studies, the ROM for a "Benign" bile duct brush is as high as 55% {875,111,192,952,658,468,595}.

Patients with benign lesions can be treated medically in most instances. An accurate diagnosis of a lymphoepithelial cyst and splenule prevents unnecessary surgery for a presumed neoplasm, usually a neuroendocrine tumour (NET) owing to the round, well-circumscribed imaging features. Patients with a clinicopathological diagnosis of autoimmune pancreatitis are treated with steroids and not surgery, which is why it is very important for the cytopathologist to simply suggest the possibility of this diagnosis when inflamed, cellular stromal fragments are seen on FNAB or fine core needle biopsies, even if the features are not diagnostic {767}. Serous cystadenomas are benign and do not need to be resected, but symptomatic and/ or large and growing tumours warrant consideration of surgery, because of the potential for rupture {857}.

Normal pancreatic and biliary parenchyma and contaminants

Pitman MB
Cocker R

Definition

Pancreatic parenchyma (including acinar, endocrine, and ductal epithelium) and benign gastrointestinal tract wall contain elements that on imaging mimic a lesion, or they may contaminate the FNAB of another lesion.

Clinical features and imaging

A mass effect within the pancreas or a stricture of a bile duct caused by inflammation and fibrosis may result in sampling benign tissue. Transgastric and transduodenal biopsies may miss a small tumour, procuring benign gastrointestinal wall components from stomach or duodenum even when using a stylet. Percutaneous FNAB may sample mesothelium, and all types of biopsy may sample liver and kidney.

Histopathology

Pancreatic parenchyma is 85% exocrine acini and ducts with scant connective tissue. The endocrine component, or islets of Langerhans, are embedded throughout, predominantly in the body and tail. The ductal system comprises intercalated cells within the acinus, which progress to larger cells up to the main ducts of Wirsung and Santorini. Pancreaticobiliary ductal cells are cuboidal to low columnar, with dense, non-mucinous cytoplasm {298}.

Gastric mucosa is lined by mucous-secreting foveolar cells. Gastric pits consist of mucous, parietal cells, and chief cells. Duodenal mucosa contains numerous villi with fibrovascular cores lined by non-mucinous columnar epithelium, interspersed with goblet cells and lymphocytes. The duodenal submucosa contains Brunner glands {886}.

Mesothelial cells line the anterior surface of the pancreas. The liver is adjacent to the pancreatic head, and the kidney is adjacent to the pancreatic tail.

Key diagnostic cytopathological features

Normal pancreatic acinar cells

- High cellularity with cohesive grape-like clusters (acini) singly and in tissue fragments attached to fibrovascular stroma; single cells are few
- Round, eccentric nuclei with fine chromatin and single small nucleolus, and abundant bichromatic and granular cytoplasm

Normal pancreatic ductal cells

- Flat, cohesive sheets with even nuclear spacing
- Round to oval nuclei, inconspicuous nucleoli and fine chromatin, and non-mucinous cytoplasm

Duodenal epithelium

- Flat, monolayered honeycomb sheets
- Non-mucinous columnar glandular cells with a brush border
- Sporadic goblet cells

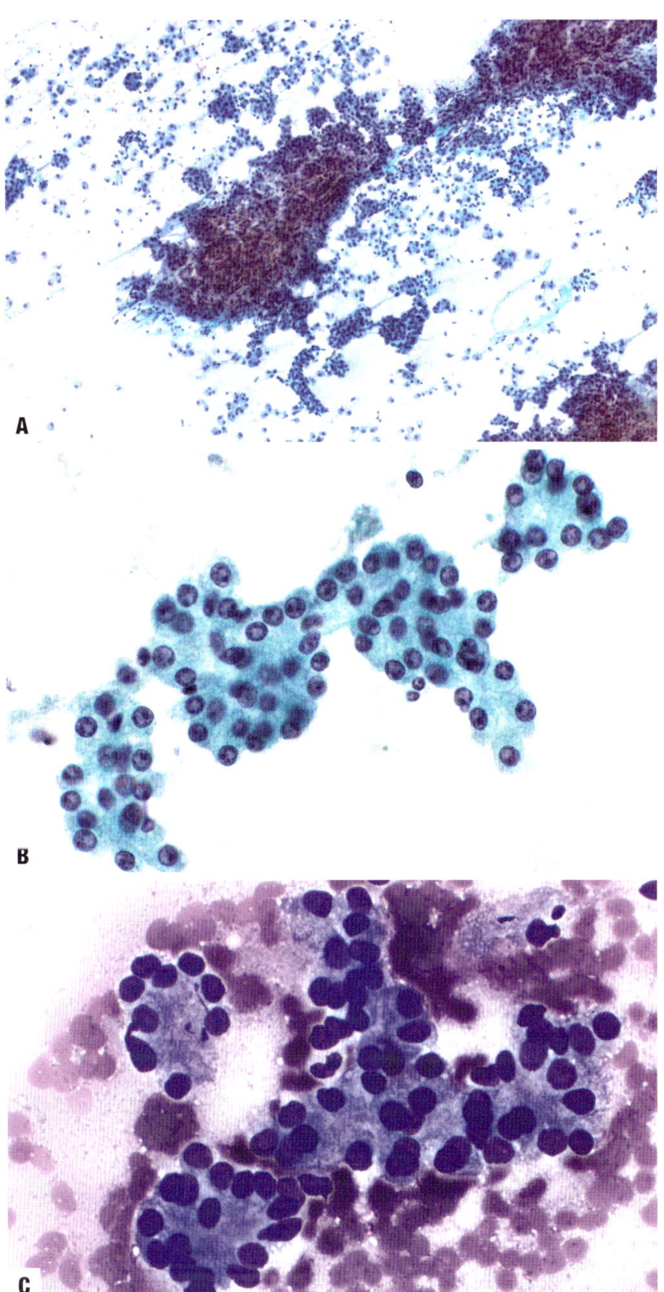

Fig. 4.01 Benign pancreatic tissue/cells. **A** Benign pancreatic tissue is dominated by acinar tissue fragments with a grapes-on-a-vine appearance at low-power magnification, with uniform acinar structures loosely tethered to connective tissue (Pap). **B** Benign pancreatic acinar cells are polygonal cells with round nuclei, small nucleoli, and granular cytoplasm, arranged in small acinar tissue fragments (Pap). **C** Benign pancreatic acinar cells are polygonal cells with round nuclei and granular eccentric cytoplasm, with negative cytoplasmic images of zymogen granules in Giemsa-stained preparations.

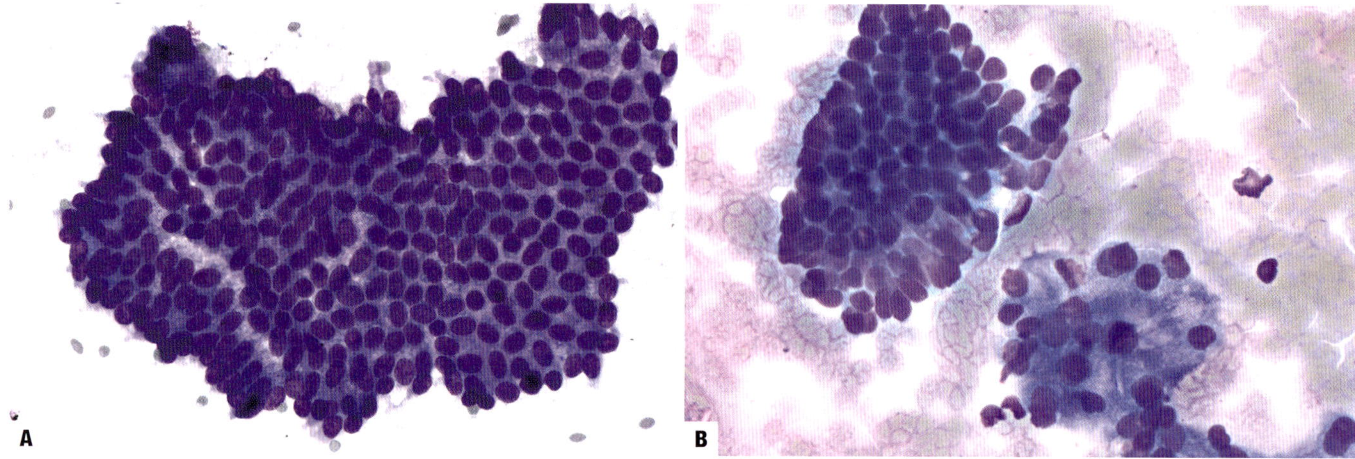

Fig. 4.02 Benign pancreatic ductal epithelium. **A** Benign pancreatic ductal epithelial cells are bland epithelial cells in cohesive tissue fragments uniformly arranged in a geometric, lattice-like, honeycombed sheet, with non-mucinous cytoplasm (Giemsa). **B** The presence of benign pancreatic ductal epithelium in the background of acinar-arranged tissue fragments favours benign parenchyma over neoplasia (Giemsa).

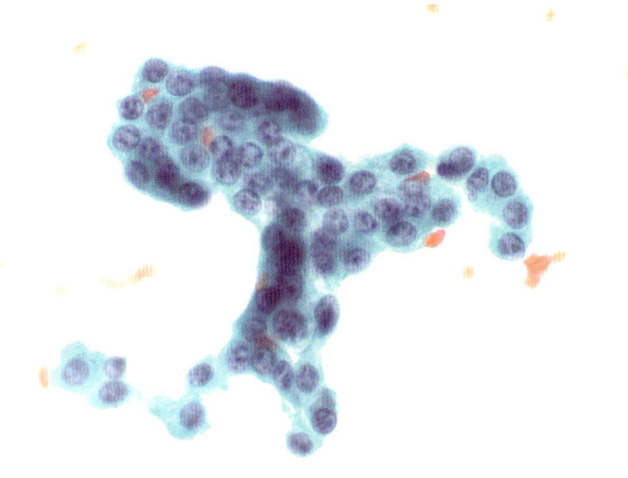

Fig. 4.03 Well-differentiated neuroendocrine tumour (NET). Well-differentiated NET cells resemble pancreatic acinar epithelium but are distinguished by their coarser stippled chromatin and less coarse granular cytoplasm (Pap).

- Lymphocytes ("sesame seeds") within epithelium

Gastric epithelium
- Small sheets, strips, single cells, and pits, with chief cells and parietal cells
- Visible cytoplasmic mucin in the upper third of the cytoplasmic compartment (mucin cup) of foveolar cells at the edge of sheets
- Naked nuclei with grooves

Mesothelium
- 2D sheets, with or without intercellular windows
- Round to oval central nuclei, conspicuous nucleoli, and moderate cytoplasm

Hepatocytes
- Polygonal with round to oval and usually central nuclei, prominent single nucleoli, and abundant cytoplasm, often with bile pigment and iron

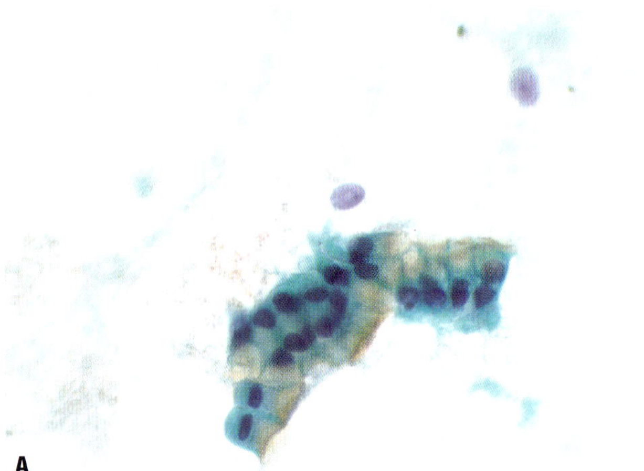

Fig. 4.04 **A** Benign gastric epithelium contaminant. Gastric epithelial contamination is recognized by the apical cups of mucin in bland columnar cells (Pap). **B** Gastric fundus contamination. Contamination by gastric mucosa, which may contain chief and parietal cells from the gastric glands (H&E).

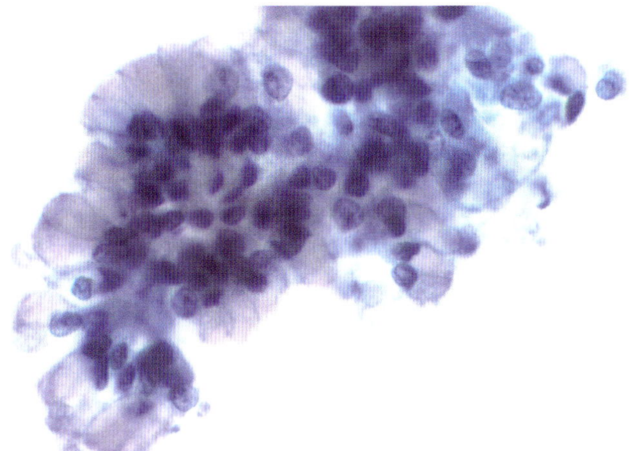

Fig. 4.05 Low-grade dysplastic epithelium of intraductal papillary mucinous neoplasm. Low-grade dysplasia in an intraductal papillary mucinous neoplasm appears similar to gastric contamination but tends to have mucin filling the cytoplasmic compartment, seen best at the edge of this tissue fragment, rather than in a well-formed, apical, smaller mucin cup as seen in gastric epithelium (Pap).

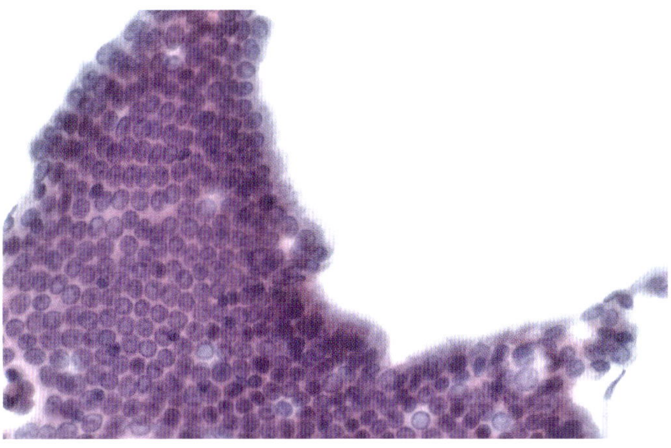

Fig. 4.06 Benign duodenal epithelium contaminant. Contaminating duodenal epithelium is often seen in large monolayered sheets composed of bland, evenly arranged, non-mucinous enterocytes studded with the cleared cytoplasm of goblet cells and small, round, dark lymphocytes (Pap).

Kidney

- Benign glandular cells representing renal tubular cells and intact glomeruli

Reference(s): {653,106}

Discussion and differential diagnosis

Smears containing cellular normal acinar tissue and contaminating tissue from the endoscopic procedure can mimic a neoplastic process. Diagnostic pitfalls include mistaking gastric foveolar epithelium for mucinous cyst-lining epithelium of a branch duct intraductal papillary mucinous neoplasm, mistaking acinar epithelium as either well-differentiated neuroendocrine tumour (NET) or acinar cell carcinoma, and mistaking reactive atypia in gastrointestinal contaminant as adenocarcinoma {770}.

Gastric foveolar–type epithelium may line a branch duct intraductal papillary mucinous neoplasm and resemble gastric epithelium. A background of thin, wispy mucin with dispersed stripped, grooved nuclei associated with columnar epithelium with superficial mucin cups supports gastric contamination {852,71}. Low-grade cyst-lining epithelium is identified by a lack of organization and uniformity and by the complete filling of its columnar cytoplasmic compartment with mucin {577}.

Benign, uniform, grape-like acini tethered to loose connective tissue produce an organoid architecture that differentiates benign acini from the discohesion and irregularity of neoplastic clusters of NET and acinar cell carcinoma {150}. Noting benign ductal epithelium in the background further supports benign tissue. The typical appearance of plasmacytoid NET cells with eccentric nuclei and coarse, stippled chromatin is absent, and the nucleoli are smaller than those noted in acinar cell carcinoma {71}.

Reactive gastric or duodenal epithelium is distinguished from adenocarcinoma by the lack of nuclear features of malignancy {590}, which are discussed in detail in the section on pancreatic adenocarcinoma.

Percutaneous FNAB may be contaminated with mesothelial cells, and kidney and liver may be inadvertently sampled with both percutaneous and EUS-guided FNAB.

Ancillary testing

ICC may be utilized if cell block material is available. See specific entities for details.

Acute pancreatitis

Naito Y
Cocker R

Definition

Acute pancreatitis is acute inflammation of the pancreas, often characterized by extensive necrosis and inflammation of the pancreatic parenchyma and the surrounding tissues.

Clinical features and imaging

Acute pancreatitis is a very common inflammatory disease of the pancreas, with a high mortality rate {927,84}. Multiple pathogenetic mechanisms have been suggested, including intra-acinar trypsinogen activation triggered by factors such as bile duct stones, alcohol, infection, trauma, and hypoxia followed by an independently driven inflammatory response {708}. This results in extensive necrosis and inflammation of the pancreatic parenchyma and the surrounding tissues.

Acute pancreatitis is characterized by the sudden onset of acute abdominal pain. Acute pancreatitis on imaging shows a homogeneous contrast effect of the pancreatic parenchyma, occasionally with the formation of cysts {629,49}. It is uncommon to FNAB acute pancreatitis unless a mass lesion is present.

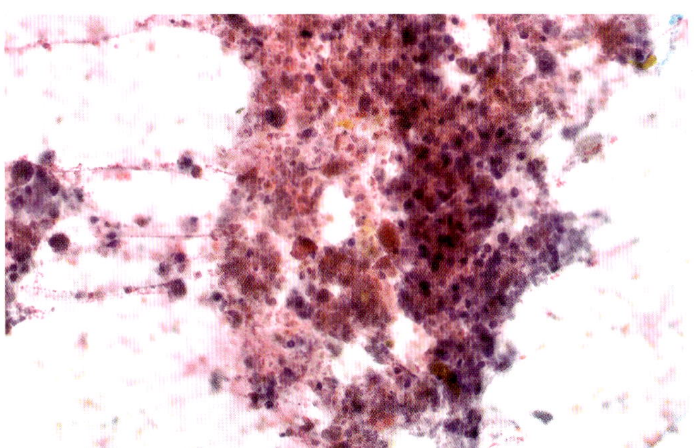

Fig. 4.07 Acute necrotizing pancreatitis. Necrotic inflammatory debris with histiocytes and haematoidin-like pigment surrounds injured acinar cells (Pap).

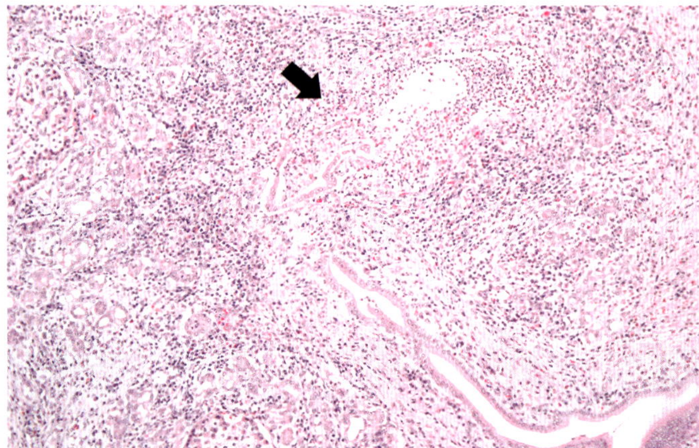

Fig. 4.09 Acute pancreatitis. Severe inflammation with focal necrosis and destruction of the pancreatic duct (arrow) (H&E).

Prerequisites for an unequivocal diagnosis of acute pancreatitis include clinical symptoms, blood amylase or lipase levels averaging more than three times the upper limit of normal, and the finding of acute pancreatitis on cross-sectional imaging using CT or MRI {84,224}.

Histopathology

Most acute pancreatitis is characterized by severe inflammation, associated with neutrophil infiltration and severe oedematous changes and haemorrhage. As the disease progresses, diffuse tissue and fat necrosis with acinar cell homogenization is observed. Calcification and abscess formation may occur early in the disease process.

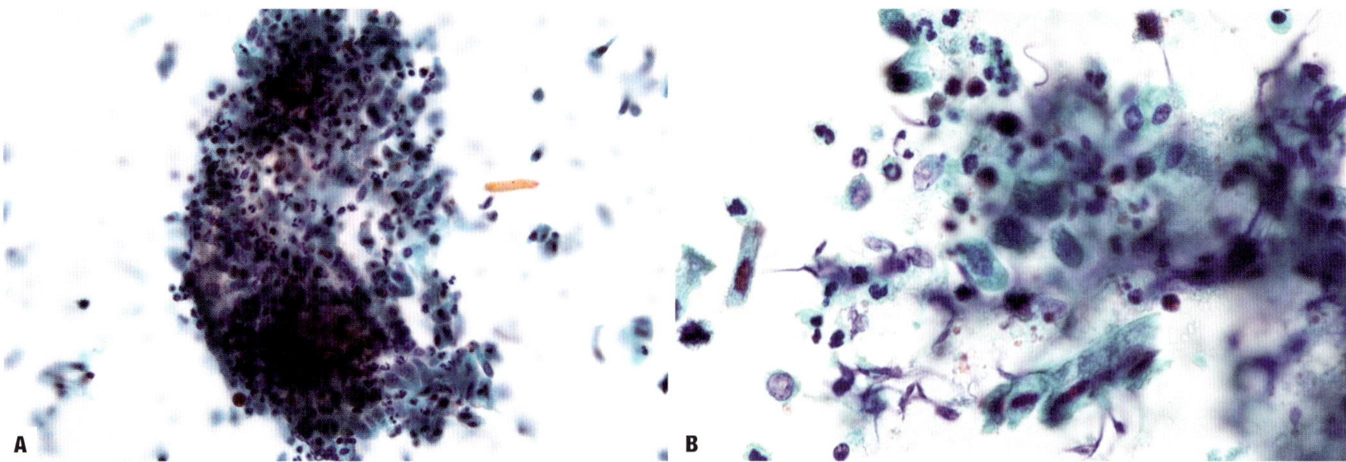

Fig. 4.08 Acute pancreatitis. **A** Tissue fragments are composed of benign epithelial cells and neutrophils with cellular debris (liquid-based cytopathology, Pap). **B** Cellular debris consists of degenerated cells, histiocytes, and neutrophils (liquid-based cytopathology, Pap).

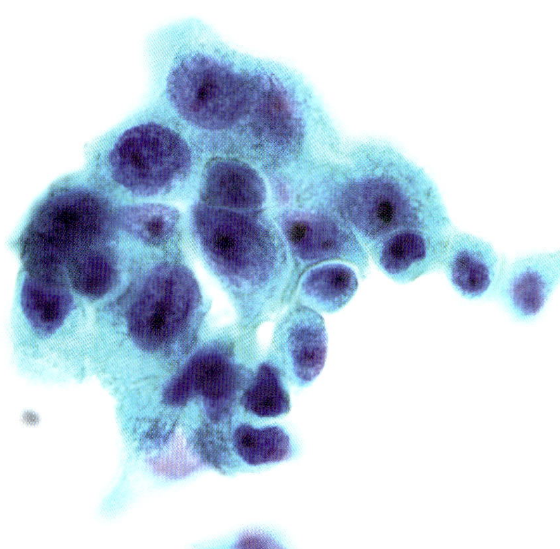

Fig. 4.10 Acute pancreatitis. Moderately atypical epithelial cells show enlarged nuclei, prominent nucleoli, and hyperchromasia. Note that the cytoplasm is not mucinous, whereas mucinous cytoplasm is typical of pancreatic ductal carcinoma (liquid-based cytopathology, Pap).

Key diagnostic cytopathological features

- Acute inflammatory cells, predominantly neutrophils
- Necrotic debris consisting of degenerated cells, fat necrosis, foamy histiocytes, and calcifications, particularly in the necrotizing type of pancreatitis
- Atypia of ductal cells, which are usually limited in number, can range from moderate to severe, showing enlarged, irregular, and hyperchromatic nuclei with conspicuous nucleoli

Reference(s): {653,106}

Discussion and differential diagnosis

Being aware of the clinical presentation and imaging findings is of paramount importance in assessing FNAB of the pancreas. Acute pancreatitis may result in inadequate material with the absence of viable cells {248,28}. Although reactive atypia can be very severe and raise the differential diagnosis of a pancreatic ductal adenocarcinoma, the presence of abundant acute inflammation and fat necrosis correlated with the findings on serology and imaging should preclude a false positive interpretation {353}.

Ancillary testing

Not relevant

Cholangitis

Zen Y
Clayton A

Definition

Cholangitis is defined as an inflammatory process focally or diffusely affecting the biliary tree. Primary sclerosing cholangitis is characterized by findings of diffuse irregular narrowing and wall thickening of the bile ducts.

Clinical features and imaging

Cholangitis can occur in any part of the biliary system, from the intrahepatic small ducts down to the intrapancreatic duct. Potential causes of cholangitis include infection, lithiasis, autoimmunity, ischaemia, drugs, and pancreatic juice reflux. Some patients, particularly those with infectious cholangitis, present with fever or abdominal pain. Incidental detection of elevated hepatobiliary enzymes may trigger the diagnosis of cholangitis, particularly in non-infectious cases such as primary sclerosing cholangitis. Finally, obstructive jaundice may be the presenting symptom in cases of localized cholangitis.

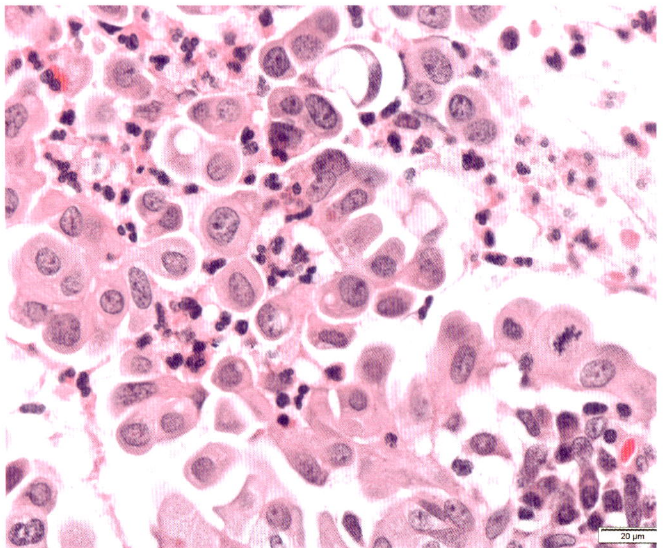

Fig. 4.11 Cholangitis. Discohesive bile duct epithelium shows nuclear enlargement but smooth nuclear membranes and homogeneous chromatin. Note the mitotic figure on the right, which is not uncommon in repair (H&E).

Biliary cytopathology is considered in patients with large duct cholangiopathy, particularly those with localized duct stricture of unknown cause or patients with primary sclerosing cholangitis with a dominant stricture, with the aim of evaluating the possibility of malignant stricture. Samples can be obtained by bile duct brushing. EUS-FNAB may also be considered in cases of mass-forming cholangitis that raises the differential diagnoses of cholangiocarcinoma, as well as IgG4-related sclerosing cholangitis and follicular cholangitis.

Imaging findings are variable and overlap with the findings found in malignancy. The bile ducts can show variable degrees of dilatation, stenosis, and wall thickening {382}. Primary sclerosing cholangitis is characterized by diffuse irregular stricturing and beading of the bile ducts {398}. Bile duct obstruction causing dilatation of the upstream ducts is commonly seen in the intrapancreatic and perihilar regions, and some cases may be associated with a pseudotumorous mass lesion {976}.

Histopathology

The bile ducts are inflamed with a mixed inflammatory infiltrate. The lining epithelium shows regenerative and hyperplastic changes such as a micropapillary architecture, nuclear pseudostratification, and enlargement. Intestinal or pseudopyloric gland metaplasia may coexist {977}. Proliferation of peribiliary glands can also be observed. Histopathological changes depend on etiologies, and characteristic features of individual conditions are summarized in Table 4.01 {975,974}.

Table 4.01 Pathological features of cholangitis

Disorder	Inflammation	Epithelial changes	Other changes
Infectious cholangitis	Predominantly neutrophilic infiltrate	Erosion; ulceration; epithelial regeneration	Infectious organisms may be identified
Ischaemic cholangitis	Neutrophilic or xanthogranulomatous inflammation around necrotic areas	Mucosal necrosis with permeation of bile contents into the stroma	None
Primary sclerosing cholangitis	Mixed chronic and acute inflammation; xanthogranulomatous foci	Ulceration; epithelial regeneration; metaplasia	Periductal fibrosis; fibro-obliteration of the bile ducts
IgG4-related sclerosing cholangitis	Lymphoplasmacytic inflammation rich in IgG4+ plasma cells; rare neutrophils	Intact bile duct epithelium	Obliterative phlebitis; storiform fibrosis
Follicular cholangitis	Lymphocytic inflammation with many lymphoid follicles	Intact bile duct epithelium	None
Eosinophilic cholangitis	Eosinophils with background of mixed inflammatory infiltrate	Intact bile duct epithelium	None
Pancreatic juice reflux (pancreaticobiliary malfunction)	Only mild, subepithelial inflammation	Papillary hyperplasia	Commonly associated with choledochal cyst

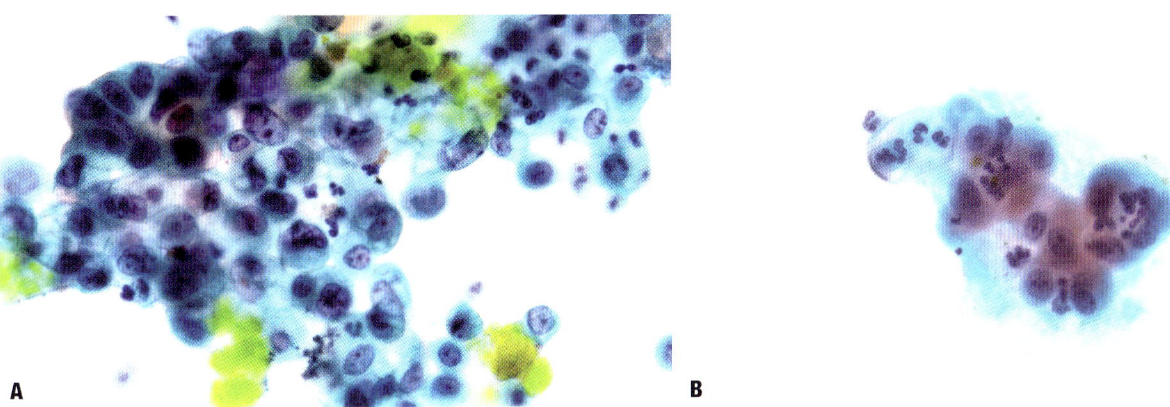

Fig. 4.12 Cholangitis. **A** Nuclear enlargement and mildly prominent nucleoli are observed. Many neutrophils are present in the epithelial tissue fragment (Pap). **B** The cell cytoplasmic borders are poorly defined, the cytoplasm is relatively dense (indicating reactive metaplastic changes), and neutrophils infiltrate the epithelium (Pap).

Key diagnostic cytopathological features

- Cohesive sheets of variable size with hyperplastic changes
- Mild anisonucleosis (2–3× variation)
- Single epithelial cells of normal size and shape
- Columnar cells with poorly defined cell–cell borders with or without dense cytoplasm indicating metaplasia
- Nuclei are enlarged with slight hyperchromasia; smooth and round nuclear membranes; and small, centrally located nucleoli
- Inflammatory background

Reference(s): {142,685,44,907,362,579}

Discussion and differential diagnosis

The main differential diagnoses are cholangiocarcinoma and biliary intraepithelial neoplasia (BilIN). Key cytopathological findings that suggest cholangiocarcinoma over cholangitis include 3D tissue fragments, nuclear pleomorphism, high N:C ratio (> 0.5), nuclear membrane irregularity, hypercellularity, atypical single cells, hyperchromasia, intracytoplasmic mucous vacuoles, prominent nucleoli, nuclear moulding, and a cell population showing two distinct cell types {44}. Although none of these are entirely specific for cholangiocarcinoma, the presence of multiple findings (usually three or more) indicates the diagnosis of malignancy {44,362,579}.

The difference between cholangitis and BilIN is more subtle. BilIN is typically diagnosed incidentally in surgically resected specimens of longstanding chronic cholangiopathy and does not cause biliary obstruction. The cytopathological diagnosis of BilIN should be made with caution and with clinical correlation.

Ancillary testing

No ancillary tests to prove the non-neoplastic nature of bile duct epithelium are currently available. There are several immunocytochemical or molecular markers suggestive of cholangiocarcinoma or premalignant lesions, and those markers are generally negative in cases of cholangitis (see relevant specific tumour discussions). Special stains or ICC may help to identify causative organisms in cases of infectious cholangitis.

Chronic pancreatitis

Yang J
Stelow EB

Definition

Chronic pancreatitis (CP) is a fibroinflammatory process characterized by the fibrotic replacement of acinar and, eventually, endocrine tissue.

Clinical features and imaging

The etiology of CP includes toxic-metabolic, idiopathic, genetic, autoimmune, and obstructive causes, as well as recurrent acute pancreatitis {153,293}. Clinically, it presents with abdominal pain, weight loss, symptoms of pancreatic exocrine insufficiency including malabsorption and steatorrhea, and diabetes. Laboratory tests may show elevated serum or urine pancreatic enzymes, and decreased serum trypsin and stool elastase {75, 636}. On cross-sectional imaging with CT or MRI, diagnostic features include pancreatic parenchymal atrophy, calcification, scarring, and duct dilatation. EUS shows hyperechoic features, shadowing, lobularity, stranding, ductal dilation, and calcification. Mass-forming CP raises the differential diagnosis of adenocarcinoma and is the primary reason for biopsy {919}. The sensitivity of imaging studies for the diagnosis of CP ranges from 75% to 81% {75,781}.

Histopathology

Cardinal features of CP on histopathology are fibrosis, loss or atrophy of acinar tissue, and duct changes. Large bands of interlobular fibrosis are present with or without obvious lymphocytic infiltration. Irregular dilated ducts and intraductal concretions are commonly seen. Other features include pseudocyst, islet aggregation, more prominent and enlarged peripheral nerves, fibrous thickening and obliteration of blood vessels, and squamous metaplasia within duct epithelium. There are no unique histopathological features that distinguish the different etiologies of CP {515,203}.

Key diagnostic cytopathological features

- Usually hypocellular and bloody
- Early stages can show abundant benign pancreatic parenchyma with acini splayed apart by fibrosis
- Fragments of fibrous tissue with or without obvious lymphocytic infiltration
- Fat necrosis, debris, and calcifications
- Islet cells, singly and in sheets of intact islets of Langerhans, may be present
- Ductal epithelium may show various degrees of reactive atypia, including loss of the normal honeycomb pattern, enlarged nuclei, prominent nucleoli, nuclear crowding, and slight anisonucleosis
- Spindle cells / myofibroblasts with plump vesicular nuclei and prominent nucleoli may be present

Reference(s): {353,137,71,131,146}

Discussion and differential diagnosis

Cytopathology is rarely used for the diagnosis of CP when clinical and imaging findings are compelling. However, CP can be associated with mass-forming fibrosis that mimics pancreatic cancer clinically and on imaging. Furthermore, CP and pancreatic cancer share risk factors, and CP itself is considered a risk factor for pancreatic cancer {412}. A workup to exclude malignancy is required in these cases, and EUS-FNAB is the initial diagnostic procedure of choice.

The major differential diagnosis of localized CP is pancreatic ductal adenocarcinoma. Reactive ductal cells can show significant cytopathological atypia in response to CP, which overlaps with well-differentiated pancreatic ductal adenocarcinoma {146}. Extensive high-grade pancreatic intraepithelial neoplasia may be present in CP and can pose a diagnostic challenge on cytopathology {71,353,131}. Cytopathological atypia seen in CP

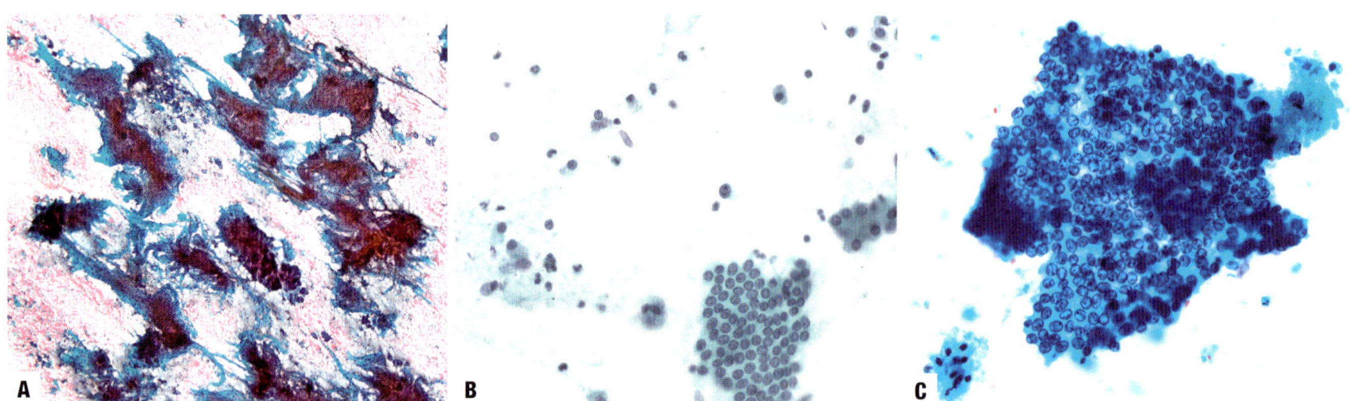

Fig. 4.13 Chronic pancreatitis. **A** Tissue fragments of fibrous tissue with lymphocytic infiltration. Acini are separated by bands of fibrosis in the tissue fragments (Pap). **B** Regularly arranged benign pancreatic ductal cells with an adjacent acinar tissue fragment in a background of inflammation support a benign process (Pap). **C** Tissue fragment of pancreatic ductal cells with enlarged nuclei, pale chromatin, prominent nucleoli, and mild loss of polarity mimics well-differentiated adenocarcinoma (Pap).

is almost always focal and limited to rare groups of ductal cells. Features diagnostic of pancreatic ductal adenocarcinoma, such as single atypical cells, significant anisonucleosis > 4:1 in the same tissue fragment, nuclear membrane irregularity, and prominent macronucleoli, are rarely seen in CP {493}.

Islets of Langerhans may remain even in the late stages of CP. The loss of acinar tissue can lead to aggregation of islets, which can result in islet cells being prominent on FNAB, posing a diagnostic pitfall for pancreatic neuroendocrine tumour (PanNET) {71,770}. The diagnosis of PanNET should be applied cautiously when only a small number of the islet cells are present in a background of CP. Correlation with imaging is helpful because PanNETs are clearly visible, round, enhancing mass lesions {137}. Spindle cells in fibrotic tissue may show plump vesicular nuclei, prominent nucleoli, and occasional mitoses, mimicking a spindle cell neoplasm.

Ancillary testing

There are currently no diagnostic biomarkers for CP. Molecular testing and cyst fluid chemistry for amylase and CEA may assist in the distinction of some neoplasms from the reactive changes and pseudocysts seen with CP {643}. ICC with IgG/IgG4 may aid in the differential diagnosis of autoimmune pancreatitis {565}.

Groove/paraduodenal pancreatitis

Reid MD
Chute DJ

Definition

Paraduodenal or groove pancreatitis is a rare form of chronic pancreatitis involving the peripancreatic soft tissues, centred on the minor ampullary papillae, with the groove representing the region between the common bile duct, pancreas, and duodenum.

Clinical features and imaging

Groove pancreatitis is most common in men in their fourth decade of life. Alcohol abuse and smoking are predisposing factors {12,571}. Patients present with abdominal pain, weight loss, jaundice, and vomiting. Inflammation of the duodenal wall or paraduodenal groove may cause stenosis and upper gastrointestinal obstruction or formation of a solid and cystic pancreatic head mass {571}. On CT, there is marked duodenal wall thickening and non-enhancing, hypodense paraduodenal soft tissue forming a mass containing small cysts {768}. On MRI, a hypointense or slightly hyperintense sheet-like mass may develop between the duodenum and pancreatic head {552}.

Because it may form an infiltrative-appearing mass that impinges on or narrows the distal common bile duct and main pancreatic duct, groove pancreatitis can mimic pancreatic ductal adenocarcinoma. However, the double-duct sign of abrupt pancreatic and bile duct cut-off, which is common in pancreatic ductal adenocarcinoma, is not seen. Instead, these ducts narrow smoothly as they traverse the mass producing the duct-penetrating sign {768,919}. Cyst-predominant groove pancreatitis can be mistaken for pseudocysts or mucinous cysts {552}.

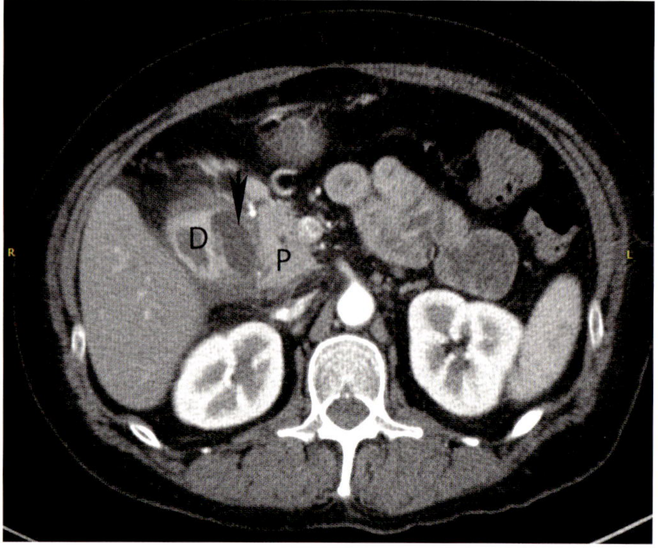

Fig. 4.14 Paraduodenal pancreatitis. CT shows a soft tissue mass with cystic change between the pancreas (P) and duodenum (D), along with near-circumferential involvement and narrowing of the duodenum by the soft tissue mass.

Histopathology

Grossly, there is a grey-white, fibrous mass with microcystic change centred on the duodenal wall or at the junction between the pancreas and the duodenum near the minor papillae {12,571}.

Histopathologically, groove pancreatitis is characterized by trabeculation of duodenal muscularis, inflammation, and myofibroblast proliferation, with thickening and fibrosis of the duodenal wall, extending into adjacent pancreas, with variably sized interspersed cysts. Cysts may be partially or completely lined by reactive ductal epithelium or granulation tissue {571}. Prominent Brunner gland hyperplasia is frequent. The inflammatory infiltrate is a mixture of acute and chronic inflammatory cells and multinucleated giant cells. Smooth muscle proliferation may be marked and can raise concern for a mesenchymal neoplasm {571,422}.

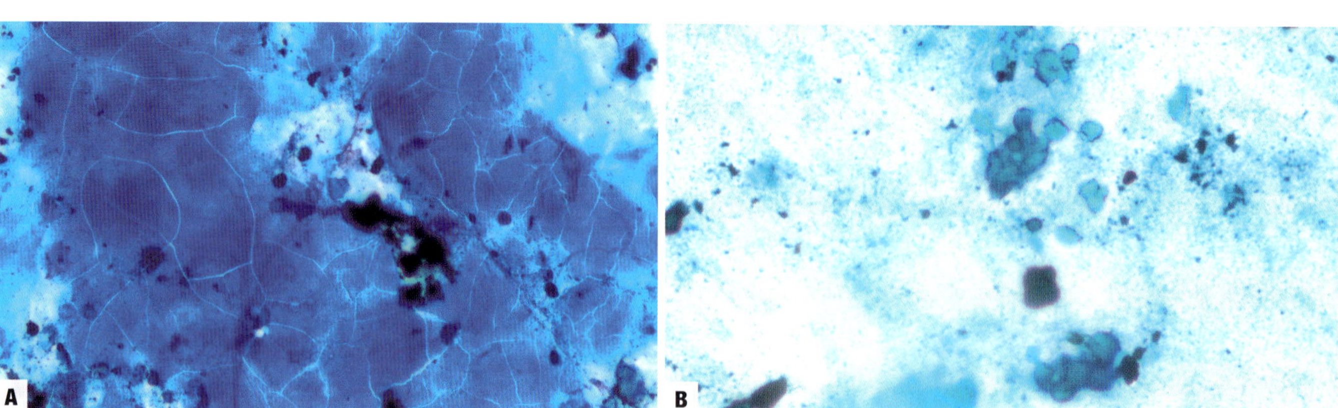

Fig. 4.15 Paraduodenal pancreatitis. **A** Dense amorphous debris with concretions produced by acinar cell enzymatic activity can show prominent cracking artefact resembling colloid (Giemsa). **B** Calcified debris in an amorphous granular background (Pap).

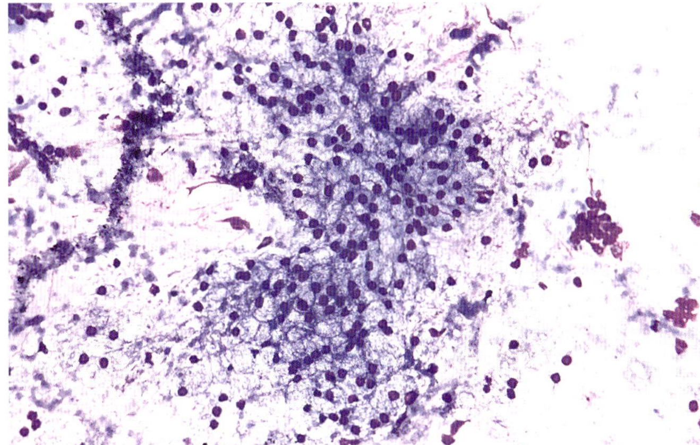

Fig. 4.16 Paraduodenal pancreatitis. Brunner glands form large sheets of bland mucinous cells with a low N:C ratio and round to oval nuclei (Giemsa).

Key diagnostic cytopathological features

- Variable cellularity
- Reactive ductal cells and granulation tissue
- Hyperplastic Brunner glands
- Mixed acute and chronic inflammatory cell infiltrate, multinucleated giant cells, and debris
- Cyst contents include amorphous proteinaceous debris, which is dense and deep-purple (Giemsa) or blue-green (Pap); can show artefactual cracking reminiscent of colloid or amyloid
- Fibrotic stroma; myofibroblasts; and bland, spindle, proliferating smooth muscle cells may be abundant and atypical

Reference(s): {87,137,480}

Discussion and differential diagnosis

The cytopathological features of groove pancreatitis have only rarely been described {87,137,480}. Depending on the region sampled, the cytopathological changes in groove pancreatitis may simulate a cystic or solid neoplasm or malignancy. Proliferating myofibroblasts and spindle cells may be abundant and mitotically active, mimicking spindle cell neoplasms {137, 480}. Multinucleated giant cells may also be abundant and have reportedly raised the differential of undifferentiated carcinoma with osteoclast-like giant cells {87}. Epithelium from hyperplastic Brunner glands may be misinterpreted as mucinous epithelium from a neoplastic mucinous cyst {137}. Unlike neoplastic mucinous cyst, the mucin in groove pancreatitis is typically watery and thin, and CEA levels are low. Inflammatory stroma, myofibroblasts, and granulation tissue in paraduodenal pancreatitis may mimic a pseudocyst, particularly when seen in conjunction with elevated cyst fluid amylase.

Ancillary testing

Ancillary testing is of limited value. Cyst fluid CA19-9 and amylase levels may be elevated, but CEA levels are normal {137,480, 102,37}.

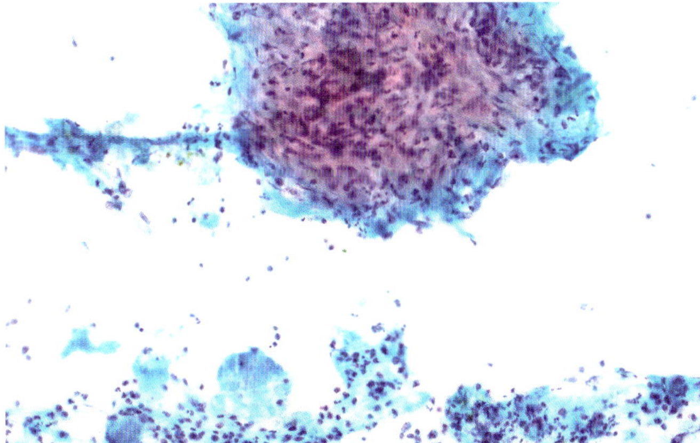

Fig. 4.17 Paraduodenal pancreatitis. A tissue fragment of spindle cells includes proliferating myofibroblasts infiltrated by neutrophils, as well as acute and chronic inflammatory cells with amorphous debris in the background (Pap).

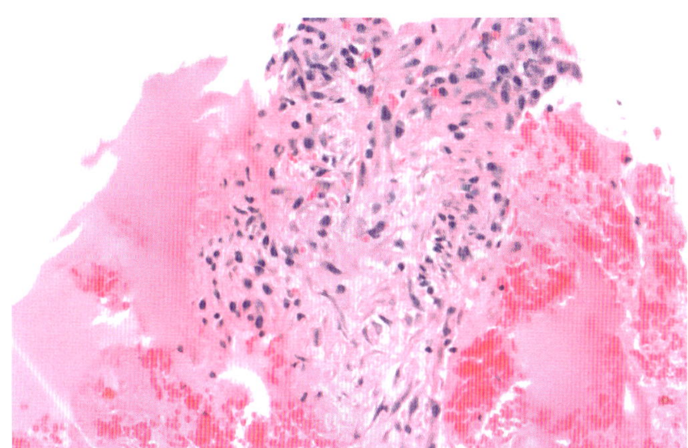

Fig. 4.18 Paraduodenal pancreatitis. Cell block with a tissue fragment consisting of mildly atypical spindle cells including proliferating myofibroblasts infiltrated by inflammatory cells, as well as bile pigment (H&E).

Autoimmune and IgG4-related pancreatitis

Notohara K
Pitman MB

Definition

Autoimmune pancreatitis (AIP) is a diffuse or focal fibroinflammatory process with two distinct types: type 1, IgG4-related pancreatitis; and type 2, associated with granulocytic epithelial lesions.

Clinical features and imaging

The clinical presentation resembles that of pancreatic ductal adenocarcinoma (PDAC). Type 1 AIP is a pancreatic manifestation of IgG4-related disease, but type 2 is not {118,864, 819,896,895}. Type 1 AIP can be diagnosed with a combination of imaging, clinical, and histopathological findings based on the international consensus diagnostic criteria (ICDC) {767} or the 2018 AIP clinical diagnostic criteria of the Japan Pancreas Society {388}. A definitive diagnosis of type 2 AIP is rendered according to the histopathological findings, because it lacks useful biomarkers and supportive clinical features except for the occasional association with inflammatory bowel disease. Type 2 AIP is diagnosed according to the ICDC.

Corticosteroid treatment is almost always effective for type 1 and type 2 AIP. If the patient shows no response, the AIP diagnosis must be reassessed. AIP may also regress spontaneously without treatment. Surgical treatment is generally not beneficial. Clinical and imaging features of types 1 and 2 are summarized in Table 4.02 {707,371,179,283,372,285,602,284, 835}.

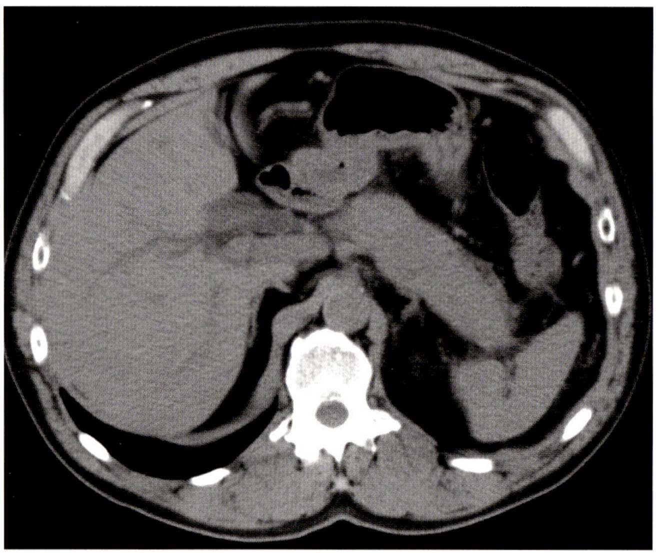

Fig. 4.19 Autoimmune pancreatitis, type 1. CT demonstrates the diffuse, sausage-like swelling of the pancreas typical of autoimmune pancreatitis.

Histopathology

Histopathological features of type 1 and type 2 AIP are presented in Table 4.02 {599,968,174,176}. Storiform fibrosis and obliterative phlebitis characterizes type 1 AIP, whereas the granulocytic epithelial lesion with neutrophilic infiltration into the acini and duct epithelium is a hallmark of type 2 AIP {118, 767}.

Key diagnostic cytopathological features

- Cellular tissue fragments of fibrous stroma with embedded inflammatory cells
- Background lymphocytes and plasma cells, as well as a variable number of normal acinar cells; plasma cells may be hard to identify
- Atypical epithelial cells containing slightly enlarged nuclei and nucleoli are present but overall show a low N:C ratio and non-mucinous cytoplasm

Reference(s): {175,310,376,377,95,444}

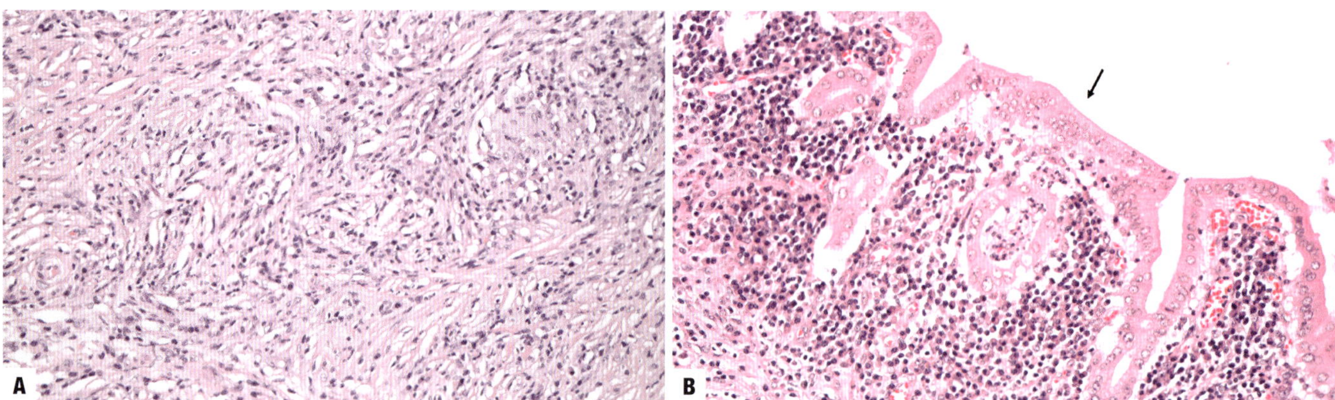

Fig. 4.20 Autoimmune pancreatitis. **A** Type 1. Storiform fibrosis infiltrated by plasma cells and lymphocytes is the classic histopathological feature of type 1 autoimmune pancreatitis (H&E). **B** Type 2. The characteristic histopathological finding of type 2 autoimmune pancreatitis is the granulocytic epithelial lesion consisting of inflamed ducts and acini filled with neutrophils (H&E).

Table 4.02 Clinicopathological features of type 1 and type 2 autoimmune pancreatitis (AIP)

Feature	Type 1 AIP	Type 2 AIP
Incidence of all AIP cases	80%	20% (even rarer in Asia)
Demographics		
Age	Common (> 50 years); uncommon (< 30 years)	All ages, including adolescents and young adults
Sex	Male predominance (70%)	No difference
Signs and symptoms		
Abdominal pain	Usually mild or absent	Common (acute pancreatitis in 30–50%)
Asymptomatic jaundice	Common	Occasional
Diabetes mellitus	Occasional worsening or presentation of new onset	Not significant
Serological examination		
Elevation of serum IgG4	Common (60–80%)	Occasional
Cross-sectional imaging		
Overall features	Diffuse or focal pancreatic swelling	Diffuse or focal pancreatic swelling
Other features	Capsule-like rim, multifocal lesions	
Cholangiopancreatogram		
Main pancreatic duct stricture	Irregular narrowing; can be multifocal	Irregular narrowing
Bile duct stricture	Common in the intrapancreatic or proximal ducts; may be multifocal in IgG4-related sclerosing cholangitis	Occasionally in the intrapancreatic portion
Lesions in other organs	IgG4-related disease, e.g. bile ducts, salivary and lacrimal glands, retroperitoneum, kidneys	Inflammatory bowel disease, which is usually ulcerative colitis
Histopathological findings		
Typical H&E findings	Diffuse lymphoplasmacytic infiltrate in storiform fibrosis occasionally with eosinophils and obliterative phlebitis	Granulocytic epithelial lesion, with neutrophils in the lumina and/or epithelium of pancreatic ducts
IgG4+ cells	> 40 IgG4+ cells/mm^2 (> 200 IgG4+ cells/mm^2 in resected specimens); IgG4:IgG+ ratio: > 0.4	< 40 IgG4+ cells/mm^2 in most cases; IgG4:IgG+ ratio: < 0.4
Steroid response and relapse		
Steroid response	Responsive in almost all cases	Responsive in almost all cases
Relapse	Common	Rare

Discussion and differential diagnosis

A definitive diagnosis of AIP is generally not possible on cytopathology alone. The suggested diagnosis can and should be based on the cellular stromal tissue fragments, which would lead to a trial treatment with steroids in the appropriate clinical setting. AIP versus PDAC is the primary differential diagnosis.

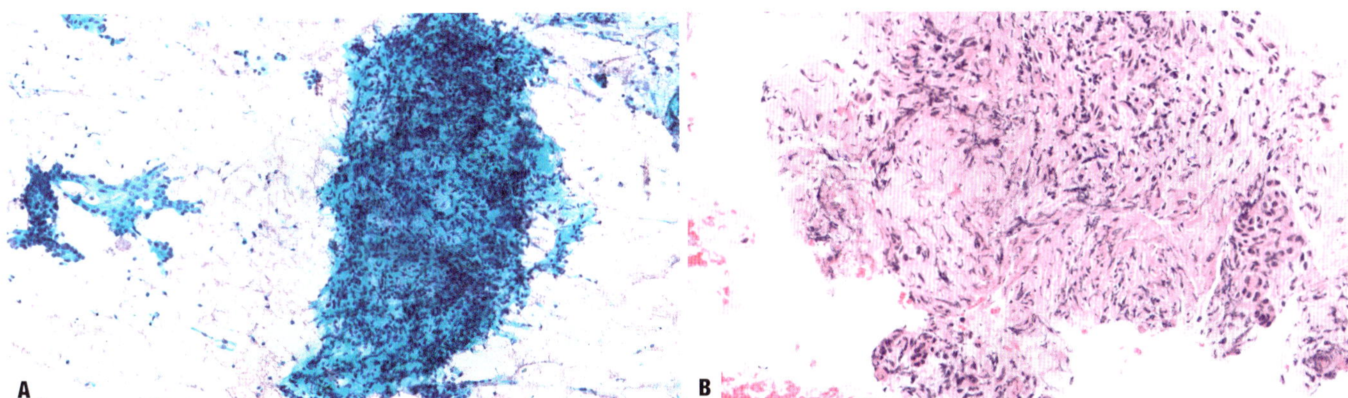

Fig. 4.21 Autoimmune pancreatitis. **A** FNAB smear shows a stromal tissue fragment that appears cellular due to an inflammatory cell infiltrate of lymphocytes and plasma cells, which is suggestive of autoimmune pancreatitis (Pap). **B** A small tissue fragment in a cell block shows a fragment of inflamed cellular stroma; the overall small size precludes assessment with IgG4 immunostains (H&E).

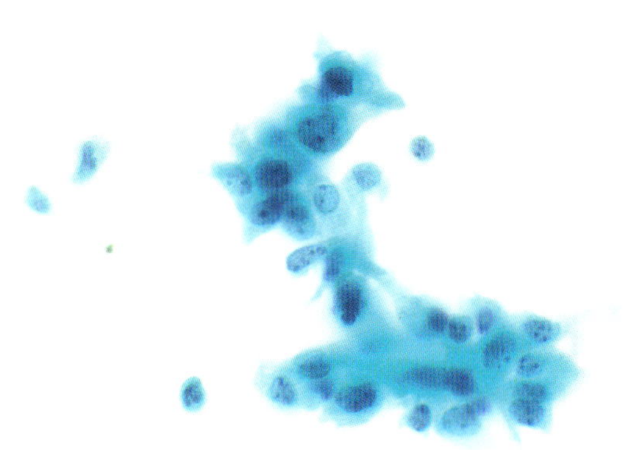

Fig. 4.22 Autoimmune pancreatitis. Atypical epithelium in autoimmune pancreatitis. These epithelial cells demonstrate enlarged nuclei and nucleoli but smooth nuclear membranes, non-mucinous cytoplasm, and a low N:C ratio (Pap).

Overdiagnosis of the atypical epithelial cells in AIP is a known pitfall {175,95,310}. These atypical cells correspond to acinar–ductal metaplasia, which occurs in the pancreatic lobules in the setting of inflammatory conditions {60,600}. Acinar–ductal metaplasia cell nuclei are smaller than those in PDAC, are round, and they lack the overt nuclear atypia (including anisonucleosis and hyperchromasia), loss of polarity, mucinous cytoplasm, and necrotic background associated with PDAC. Another pitfall is the interpretation of scattered acinar–ductal metaplasia or acinar cells as a pancreatic neuroendocrine tumour (PanNET) {771}. Cell block or core biopsy tissue will allow for ancillary studies to assess the cells.

Ancillary testing

Histopathological evaluation with immunostaining for IgG4+ plasma cells using tissue cores may aid in the diagnosis when there are > 40 IgG4+ cells/mm2 (biopsy) or when the IgG4:IgG ratio is > 0.4 {600,376,377,565,444,601}. Small tissue fragments are not suitable for this assessment. Acini stain for trypsin and BCL10, and endocrine cells stain for synaptophysin and chromogranin. Atypical ductal cells show a wildtype pattern of staining for p53 (i.e. an admixture of negative cells and weakly and strongly positive cells showing patchy and variable nuclear staining) and retain nuclear staining for SMAD4. *KRAS* mutations support neoplasia and have been reported to support the diagnosis of PDAC {395,604,626}, but the results must be evaluated cautiously because low-grade pancreatic intraepithelial neoplasia is commonly associated with type 1 AIP {373}. Diffuse nuclear staining for p53 or no staining in the null pattern and/or loss of nuclear staining for SMAD4 supports high-grade dysplasia or carcinoma.

Lymphoepithelial cyst

VandenBussche CJ
Policarpio Nicolas ML

Definition

Lymphoepithelial cyst (LEC) is a keratinous debris–filled cyst lined by benign squamous epithelium overlying benign lymphoid tissue with germinal centres.

Clinical features and imaging

Patients are often middle-aged men who are asymptomatic with an incidental finding on abdominal imaging. Some patients present with abdominal pain and other mild, nonspecific symptoms {10}. LECs can be located in any part of the pancreas and usually present as a single lesion with a median size of approximately 50 mm and with nonspecific and variable ultrasound, CT, and MRI findings, which can be cystic, solid, homogeneous, or heterogeneous {254,863,387,262}. These lesions are most often confused clinically with a neuroendocrine tumour (NET). LEC is benign and does not require resection.

Histopathology

LECs are cysts lined by benign squamous epithelium containing nucleated and more superficial anucleated squamous cells and keratinous debris. Cysts may be unilocular or multilocular. The squamous lining is surrounded by lymphoid tissue with germinal centres. Rarely, the cyst lining may include columnar rather than squamous lining {230}, sebaceous differentiation {230}, keratin granulomas {10}, goblet cells {230}, and lymphoepithelial islands {230}.

Key diagnostic cytopathological features

- Keratinous debris composed of anucleated +/− mature nucleated squamous cells present singly or in tissue fragments of stratified epithelium
- Keratinous debris may appear amorphous, fibrillar and/or granular; inspissated mucoid-appearing debris with cracking may form crystalloids and may be more easily recognized as keratin on cell block preparations

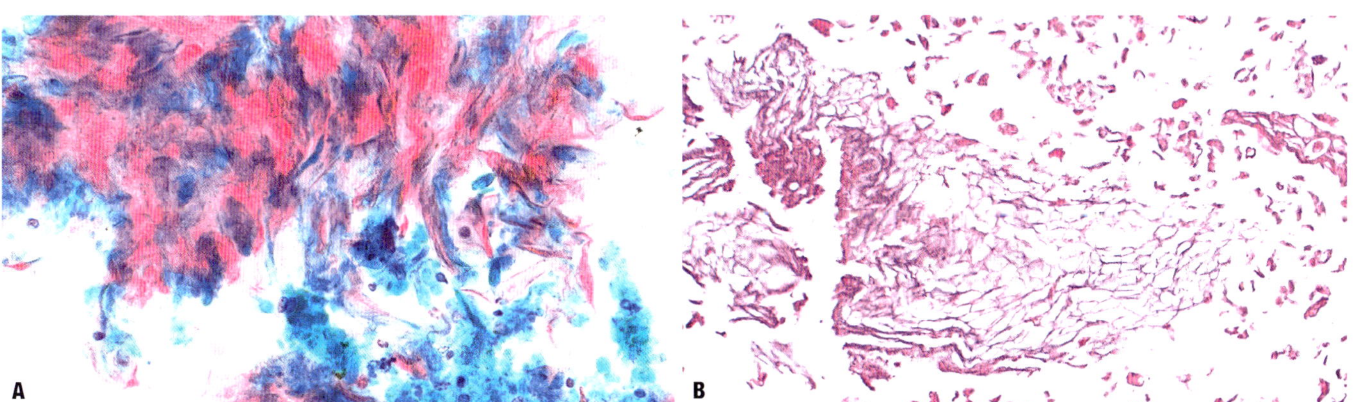

Fig. 4.23 Lymphoepithelial cyst. **A** Keratinous debris is adjacent to granular debris and intermixed with macrophages (Pap). **B** Layered keratinous debris may be more easily identified in a cell block preparation (H&E).

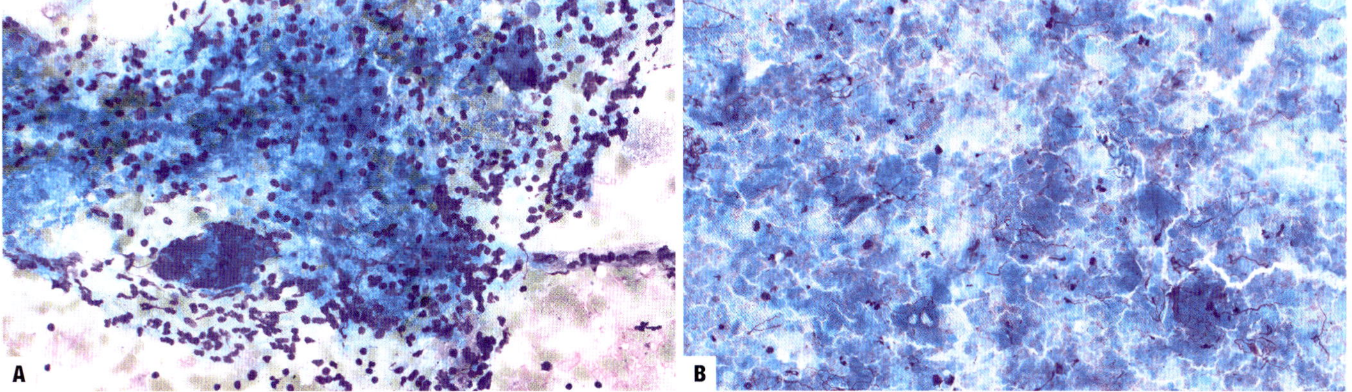

Fig. 4.24 Lymphoepithelial cyst. **A** Numerous small lymphocytes are associated with granular debris and occasional histiocytes. The lymphoid component is rarely predominant in FNAB smears (Giemsa). **B** Small lymphocytes are scattered within thick granular debris with cracking artefact resembling colloid-like mucin (Giemsa).

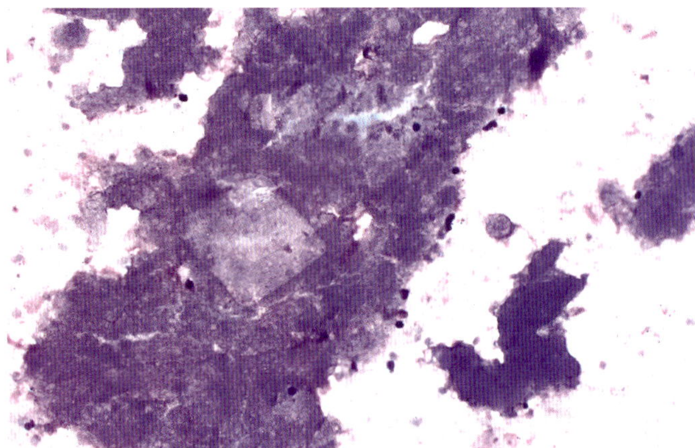

Fig. 4.25 Lymphoepithelial cyst. A rhomboid-shaped cholesterol crystal is present amid a thick layer of amorphous granular debris (Giemsa).

- Small polymorphous lymphocytes variable in number
- Cholesterol crystals, which are square to rhomboid in shape and of variable size, and which are birefringent when seen in air-dried Giemsa-stained direct smears

Reference(s): {107,586,874,668,122}

Discussion and differential diagnosis

When adequately sampled, the presence of mature squamous cells and keratinous debris indicates the presence of a benign squamous-lined pancreatic cyst, with a differential diagnosis of dermoid cyst and epidermoid cyst when seen in intrapancreatic splenic tissue, and squamoid cysts of the pancreatic duct. These entities are indistinguishable from one another on cytomorphology alone, and ancillary tests also cannot distinguish these entities.

Cyst debris may be so degenerated and amorphous that it cannot be determined to be keratinous. It may resemble crystalline material that can be seen in pseudocysts or inspissated mucin sometimes seen in neoplastic mucinous cysts such as intraductal papillary mucinous neoplasm or mucinous cystic neoplasm {122}. Careful examination of the debris usually demonstrates focal anucleated squamous morphology as seen in an epidermal inclusion cyst to suggest the diagnosis. Neoplastic mucinous cysts contain mucinous epithelial tissue fragments, whereas LEC have a squamous cyst lining. However, tissue fragments of gastrointestinal contamination may be difficult to distinguish from cyst lining and cause a diagnostic pitfall. The presence of lymphocytes, although variable, offers a clue that the debris is from a LEC. It is rare that the lymphoid component is prominent enough to cause consideration of a splenule and/or intrapancreatic lymph node. LEC do not contain CD8+ sinusoids that are seen in splenules and should not contain a predominant population of lymphocytes as seen in the sampling of lymph nodes.

Ancillary testing

ICC is not helpful for diagnosis and is typically not performed. A potential pitfall is that cells may sometimes be patchy or diffusely positive for CEA or CA19-9 {668}. CEA, CA19-9, and amylase can also be elevated in the cyst fluid {586,512,846,107,81}. An elevated CEA level, which can be in the thousands of ng/mL is a significant pitfall, because biochemical testing for cyst fluid CEA and amylase has become routine in most institutions {668} and is an ancillary test used to define a cyst as mucinous. One study showed the absence of genetic mutations associated with neoplasia {787}.

Pseudocysts

Layfield LJ
Centeno BA

Definition

Pancreatic pseudocysts are fluid-filled spaces lacking an epithelial lining and result from pancreatic tissue autolysis.

Clinical features and imaging

Pancreatic pseudocysts compose approximately 75% of all pancreatic masses and most commonly represent complications of pancreatitis or trauma {267}. Patients may present with abdominal pain or tenderness, fever, nausea, vomiting, or weight loss. Imaging discloses a well-circumscribed round or oval peripancreatic fluid collection surrounded by a well-defined thick wall on CT examination {847}. On ultrasound, pseudocysts are hypoechoic or anechoic, often with internal debris. Management can be operative or non-operative. A pseudocyst can be drained by endoscopic procedures or by external drainage, especially when infected {267}. Surgical management may involve drainage of the pseudocyst into the stomach, jejunum, or duodenum {414}. Pseudocysts can be specifically diagnosed by a combination of cytopathology and fluid biochemical analysis {267, 646}.

Histopathology

Gross examination of material obtained from pseudocysts demonstrates a dirty-appearing green/brown to brown turbid fluid. The fluid content may contain pigment-laden macrophages, acute and chronic inflammatory cells, and necrotic debris.

The pseudocyst wall is composed of granulation tissue or fibrous tissue, which is surrounded by acute or chronic pancreatitis, and necrosis may be present. No epithelial lining is present.

Key diagnostic cytopathological features

- So-called dirty proteinaceous background, often with necrosis
- Mixed inflammation dominated by lymphocytes and histiocytes
- Haemosiderin-laden macrophages
- Red blood cells, yellow-brown haematoidin-like pigment, cholesterol crystals, calcified debris, and cell debris
- No epithelial component except for gastrointestinal contaminants
- Rarely, fragments of granulation tissue may be present

Reference(s): {2,253,353}

Discussion and differential diagnosis

Pancreatic pseudocysts occur in the peripancreatic tissues, most often the lesser sac of the peritoneum. The cyst fluid contains pancreatic enzymes (particularly amylase), red blood cells, and necrotic debris, along with histiocytes and other inflammatory cells. Saponified fragments of fat may be seen.

By definition, these cysts are characterized by an absence of epithelial cells. The differential diagnosis includes the other cystic lesions of the pancreas, including serous cystadenoma, mucinous cystic neoplasm, and intraductal papillary mucinous neoplasm. Contaminating gastric or duodenal epithelium can be present, but these sheets and groups of cells will have a normal morphology from their gastrointestinal origin. Gastric contamination can pose a diagnostic pitfall with branch duct intraductal papillary mucinous neoplasm because the most common lining of this mucinous neoplasm is of the gastric type. Most branch duct intraductal papillary mucinous neoplasms do not produce much cellularity, so the abundance of gastric-type epithelium with apical mucinous cups and stripped naked nuclei in thin mucin should provide a clue to the recognition of gastric contamination, particularly when it is associated with the typical dirty cyst debris of a pseudocyst. The dirty-appearing background is composed of abundant granular necrotic debris, red blood cells, small fragments of necrotic adipose tissue, yellow or green/brown

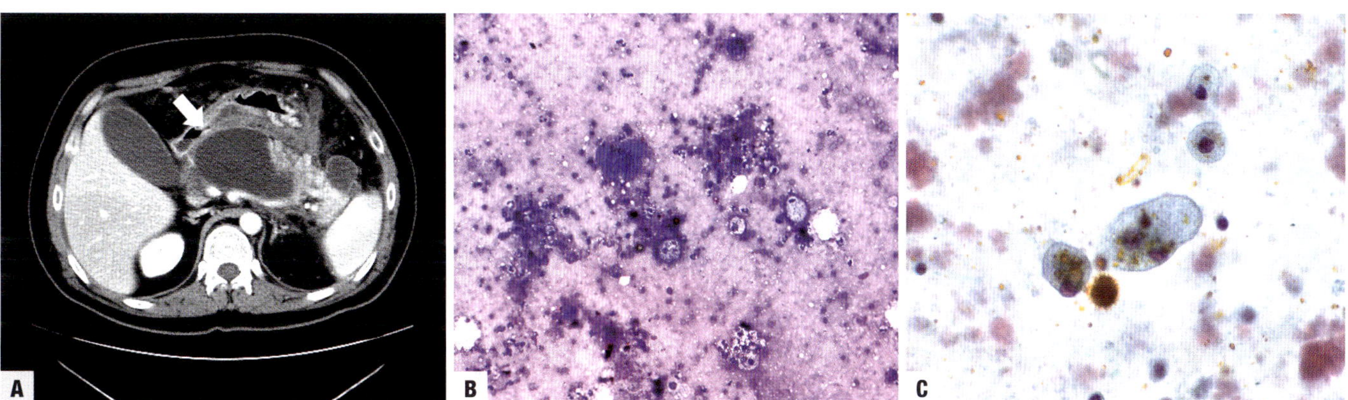

Fig. 4.26 Pseudocyst. **A** CT shows the enhanced pancreatic parenchyma of acute pancreatitis and a large, unilocular, thick-walled pseudocyst without septations or a mural nodule (arrow). **B** Pancreatic pseudocyst. FNAB smears show necrotic debris and foamy histiocytes characteristic of pseudocyst contents (Giemsa). **C** Amorphous, granular necrotic debris associated with histiocytes and yellow pigment, which may be bile or haematoidin-like material, is typical of pseudocyst (Pap).

haematoidin-like pigment, crystals, and calcifications in variable amounts {253}.

Ancillary testing

Biochemical analysis of the cyst fluid is most helpful in the differential diagnosis with other pancreatic cysts {628}. Pseudocysts always have elevated amylase levels (usually in the thousands of ng/mL) and low CEA levels (usually much lower than 100 ng/mL) {876,253,628,641,605,55,88,89}. An amylase level of < 250 U/L makes a pseudocyst very unlikely. Molecular alterations are characteristically absent in pseudocysts, except for very rare *KRAS* mutations when pancreatic intraepithelial neoplasia is inadvertently biopsied {353}.

Splenule (accessory spleen)

Perez-Machado MA
Stelow EB

Definition

Splenule or accessory spleen is normal splenic tissue that forms a small mass within the pancreatic parenchyma.

Clinical features and imaging

Nodules of heterotopic splenic tissue, known as splenules or splenunculi, derive from mesenchymal buds on the left side of the mesogastrium and are found in the left upper quadrant of the abdomen in as many as 10% of autopsies. Although most occur in the soft tissues of the splenic hilum, heterotopic spleen may be found within the pancreatic parenchyma. Intrapancreatic splenule is typically a small (< 30 mm), solid, round, well-demarcated mass, most commonly located in the pancreatic tail.

Splenules are hypervascular and therefore resemble small, solid pancreatic neoplasms, especially those with a rich vascularity such as pancreatic neuroendocrine tumours (PanNETs), sugar tumours (perivascular epithelioid cell tumours [PEComas]), or small solid pseudopapillary neoplasms. It helps the diagnosis that the signal intensity and enhancement pattern on imaging are similar to those of the patient's own spleen {390, 805,684,484}.

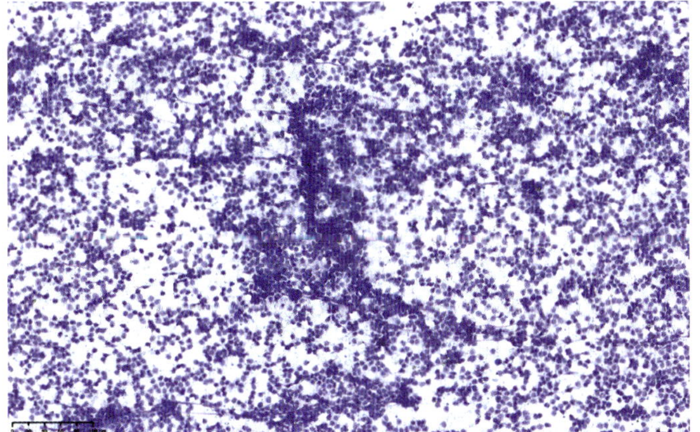

Fig. 4.27 Splenule (accessory spleen). Direct smear showing lymphocytes and thin-walled vessels lined by endothelial cells (lower centre) (Giemsa).

Histopathology

Gross examination reveals a well-demarcated dark-red mass with rich vasculature with or without cyst formation. Microscopically, splenules consist of typical splenic parenchyma, including both red and white pulp. There is a predominance of the red pulp component, suggesting that their origin was a relatively early embryonic event {332,317}. Rarely, squamous epithelial cysts arise within these nodules of splenic tissue, forming an epidermoid cyst {109,755}.

Key diagnostic cytopathological features

- Heterogeneous population of predominantly small lymphocytes and a lesser number of larger lymphoid cells
- Lymphoid cells form cohesive tissue fragments on smears and cell blocks
- Small sinusoidal vascular structures with admixed lymphocytes
- Large platelet aggregates
- No tingible-body macrophages

Discussion and differential diagnosis

Direct smears show a mixed population of inflammatory cells that includes heterogeneous lymphoid cells (with small lymphocytes predominating) admixed with plasma cells, macrophages, neutrophils, and eosinophils, embedded in a vascular meshwork and loosely dispersed throughout the smears. The main differential diagnosis includes well-differentiated PanNETs and sampling from a benign lymph node {436,309}. Recognition of the small sinusoidal vessels resembling capillaries, endothelial cells with spindle cell morphology, and large aggregates of

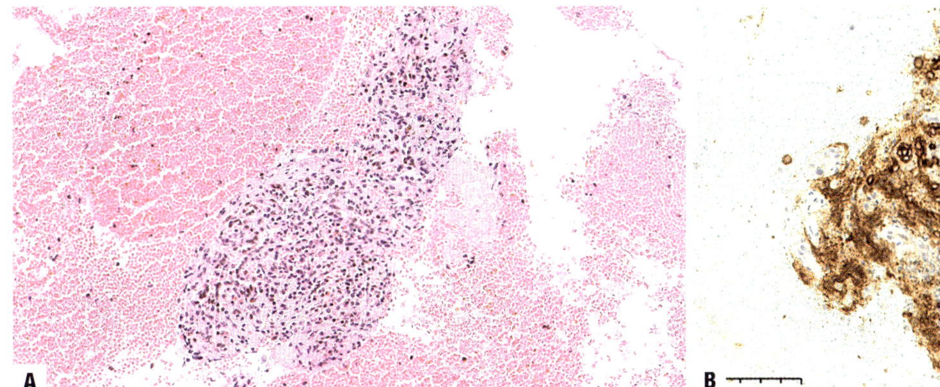

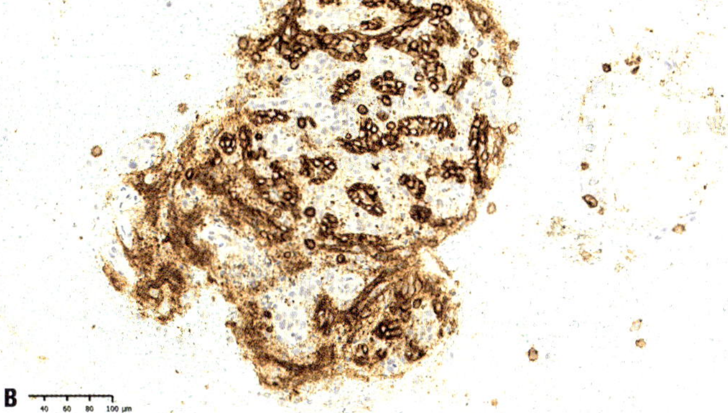

Fig. 4.28 Splenule (accessory spleen). **A** Cell block preparations are very helpful in demonstrating the red pulp architecture of thin-walled sinuses lined by endothelium and surrounded by lymphoid cells (H&E). **B** CD8 ICC highlights the splenic sinusoidal endothelial cells in a cell block tissue fragment.

platelets support the diagnosis of splenule. The tingible-body macrophages commonly seen in a reactive lymph node are absent, and the coarse stippled chromatin and plasmacytoid cytoplasm of a PanNET are not present {693,744,152,331}.

Ancillary testing

H&E slides from cell blocks allow the assessment of the architecture of the tissue that resembles the splenic parenchyma with a dense, purely lymphoid, CD45+ cellular infiltrate, consisting of a mix of CD20+ B cells and CD3+ T cells. Splenic sinusoidal endothelial cells stain for CD8, confirming the diagnosis. The neuroendocrine markers synaptophysin and chromogranin are negative {844,109,367}.

Serous cystadenoma

Reid MD
Pitman MB
VandenBussche CJ

Definition

Pancreatic serous cystadenoma (SCA) is a benign non-mucinous epithelial neoplasm composed of variably sized cysts lined by glycogen-rich cuboidal cells that produce serous fluid.

Clinical features and imaging

SCAs are the most common benign pancreatic cystic neoplasm, representing 10–16% of all surgically resected pancreatic neoplasms {791,868,433,407,787} and 1–2% of all pancreatic neoplasms. Two thirds of patients are female, and the mean patient age is 60 years {349,961,407,680}. Tumours may be sporadic or syndromic. As many as 90% of patients with von Hippel–Lindau syndrome develop SCA, which may be multifocal {272,77A,891,119,758,334}. Approximately 40% of cases are incidentally discovered on imaging studies {680}. Symptomatic patients may present with nausea, vomiting, back and/or abdominal pain, diabetes, and weight loss secondary to mass effect {147,236,961,349}. SCAs have a mean size of 60 mm, and some can be quite large (as large as 250 mm) {725,680}.

Resection is typically curative, recurrences are rare, and the prognosis is excellent {407,349,680}. Tumours may rarely extend into adjacent structures including the stomach and colon {680}, but malignant transformation into serous cystadenocarcinoma is extremely rare (0.1–0.2%).

SCAs are hyperintense on T2-weighted MRI and hypointense on T1-weighted images {985,133,369}. Classic imaging and EUS features include a well-circumscribed, lobulated, multiloculated (honeycomb) mass with a central stellate scar and calcifications {471,967,133,135,407}. Degeneration can lead to coalescence of the cysts into large cysts, creating oligocystic or (rarely) unilocular tumours, that can lead to misdiagnosis as a mucinous cyst. Unlike intraductal papillary mucinous neoplasm, SCA does not communicate with the pancreatic duct system, but it may rarely cause upstream duct dilatation {349}.

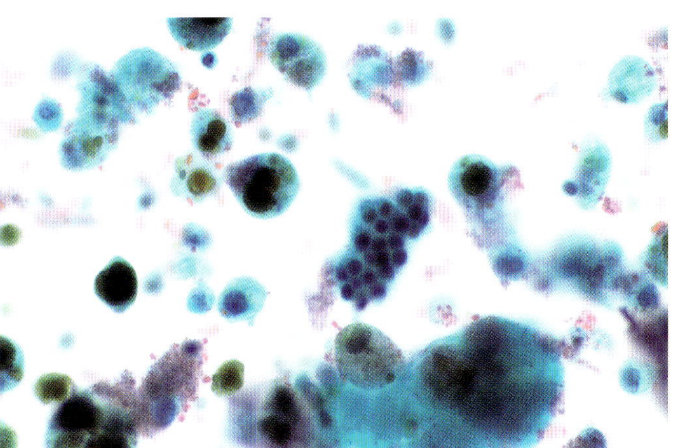

Fig. 4.30 Serous cystadenoma. A very small tissue fragment of bland, non-mucinous cuboidal epithelial cells is surrounded by numerous haemosiderin-laden macrophages (Pap).

Histopathology

On gross examination, tumours are well circumscribed with a central stellate scar and radiating hyalinized, vascular septa surrounding multiple cysts, typically microcysts. Cysts are lined by low cuboidal cells with clear cytoplasm and central round to oval nuclei with indistinct nucleoli. Tumour cells may show papillary projections or more solid growth {854}. Microcystic SCA, macrocystic or oligocystic SCA, solid serous adenoma, von Hippel–Lindau syndrome–associated serous cystic neoplasm, and mixed serous–neuroendocrine neoplasm subtypes are described {910}.

Key diagnostic cytopathological features

- Sparsely cellular and haemorrhagic, and therefore often non-diagnostic
- Bland tumour cells in loose, small tissue fragments or monolayered sheets

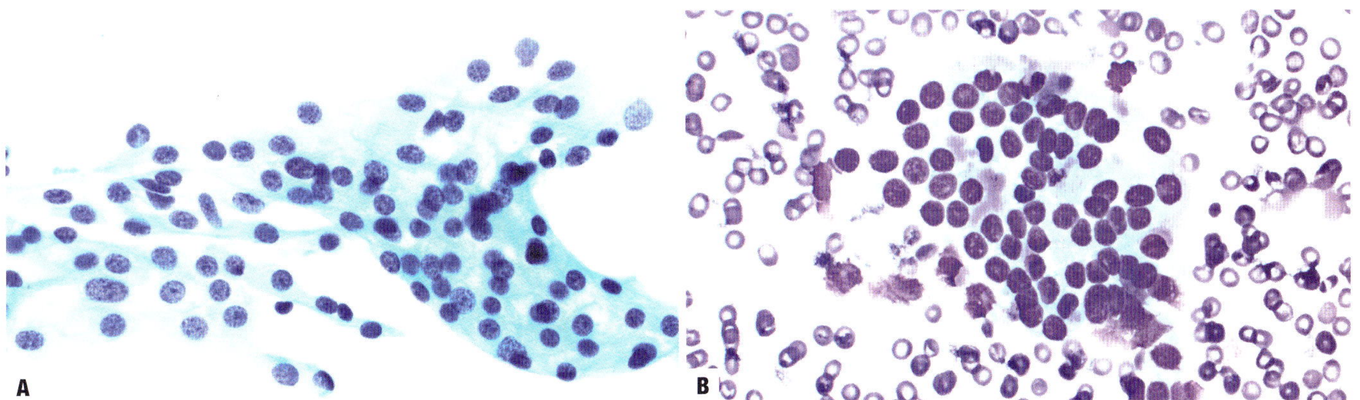

Fig. 4.29 Serous cystadenoma. **A** Tumour cells in a tissue fragment have indistinct pale to clear cytoplasm and small, round to oval nuclei with even chromatin (Pap). **B** Sheet of bland cuboidal epithelial cells with rounded nuclei and pale cytoplasm (Giemsa).

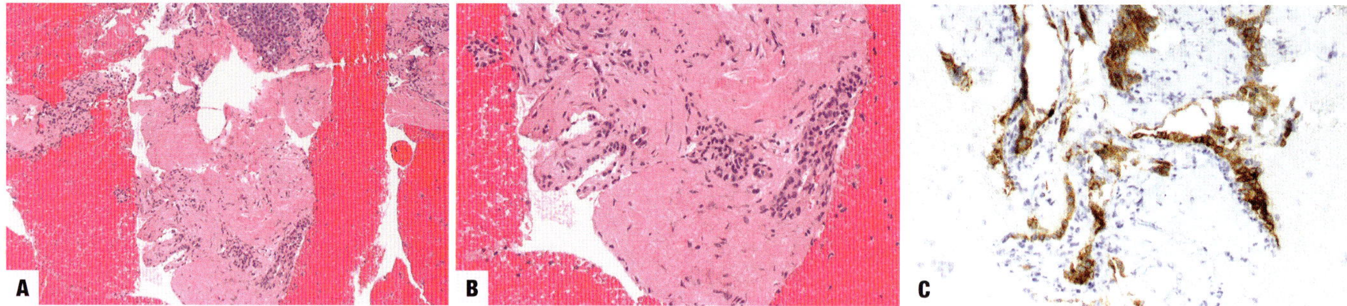

Fig. 4.31 Serous cystadenoma. **A** Cell block tissue fragments of benign pancreatic parenchyma (upper) with thick fibrotic tissue fragment (lower) and small cystic spaces lined by flat, non-mucinous cyst-lining cells (H&E). **B** Cell block tissue fragment showing hyalinized septa with small cysts lined by flat, non-mucinous cells is consistent with serous cystadenoma (H&E). **C** α-Inhibin highlights the serous cyst-lining epithelium in a cell block tissue fragment (ICC).

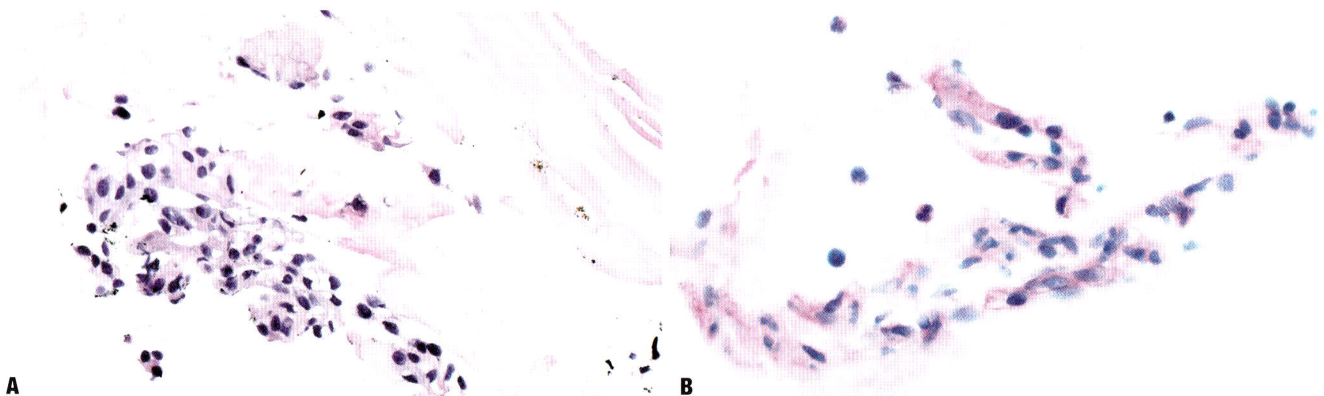

Fig. 4.32 Serous cystadenoma. **A** Cell block showing a tissue fragment of serous epithelium with round to oval nuclei with dark, even chromatin (H&E). **B** Cell block showing a tissue fragment of tumour cells with glycogenated cytoplasm which is positive for PAS. A PAS stain with diastase removes the staining (not shown).

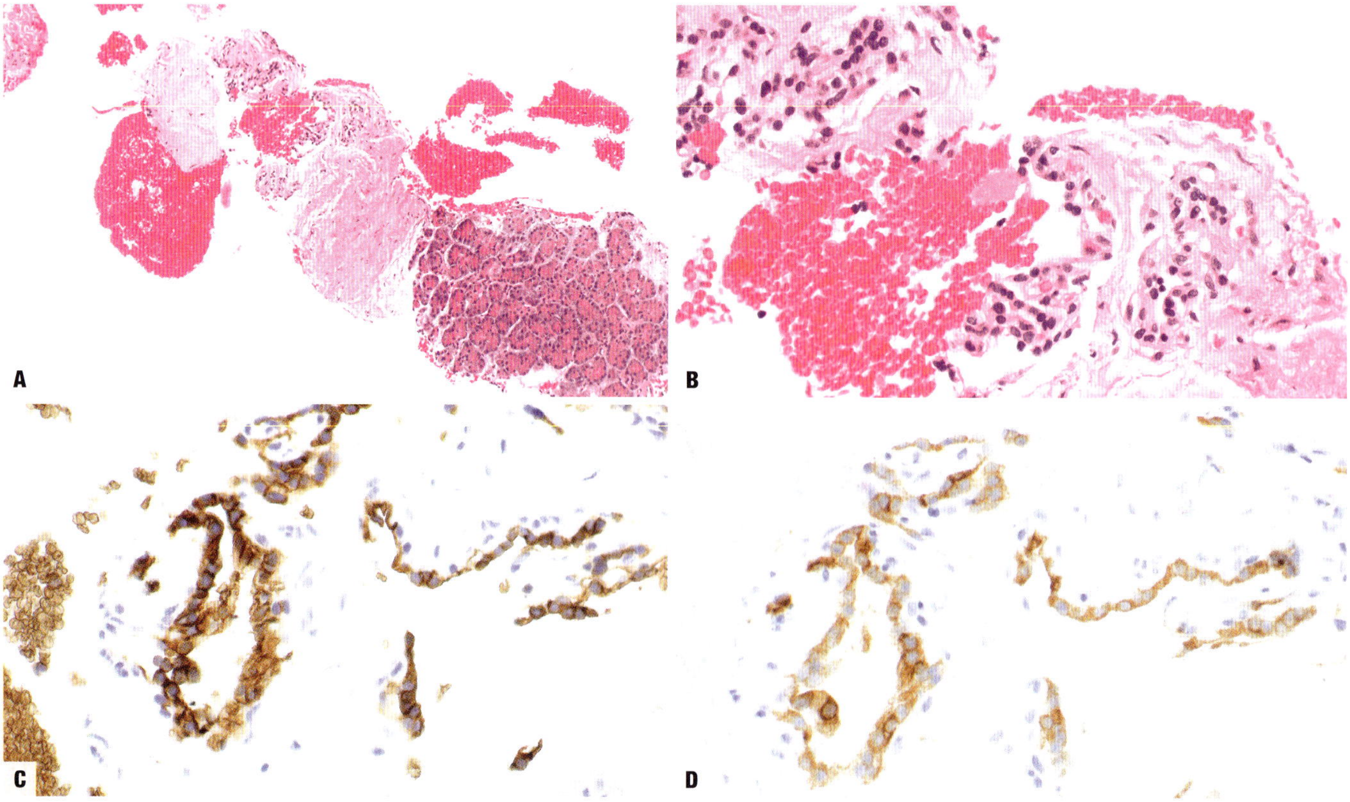

Fig. 4.33 Serous cystadenoma. **A** Bland, non-mucinous cuboidal epithelial cells line thick fibrous septa adjacent to normal pancreatic tissue. **B** The cyst-lining cells have clear cytoplasm containing glycogen, not mucin. Note the cuboidal shape and bland round nuclei (H&E). **C,D** Cyst-lining cells show cytoplasmic staining for GLUT1 (**C**) and α-inhibin (**D**).

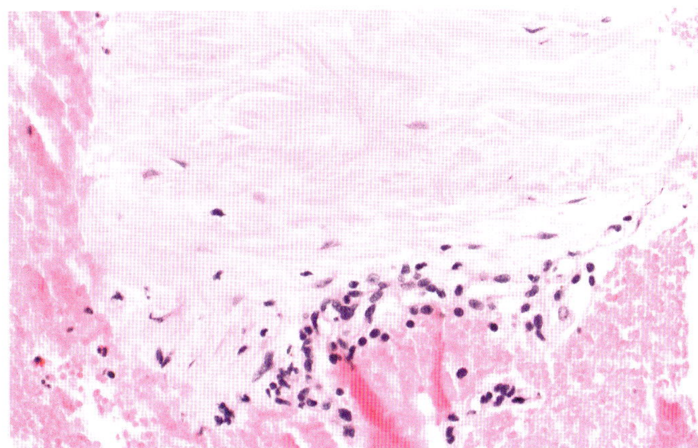

Fig. 4.34 Serous cystadenoma. This fork-tipped fine core biopsy shows predominantly hyalinized stroma with only a minute strip of serous epithelium at one end (H&E).

- Clean or granular background without extracellular mucin
- Cuboidal cells typically have indistinct cell borders and granular or clear cytoplasm, and/or stripped nuclei can be present
- Haemosiderin-laden macrophages
- Nuclei are small and round, with coarse chromatin and indistinct nucleoli
- No mitotic activity or nuclear atypia
- Hyalinized stromal fragments may be the predominant finding, with only minute strips of serous epithelium hugging their edges
- No necrosis or mucin in the background

Reference(s): {329,491,144,716,69}

Discussion and differential diagnosis

FNAB may not produce cyst fluid due to microcysts. Direct smears often result in scant, non-diagnostic tissue composed of denuded fibrous septa and no intact epithelial cells, owing to mechanical crush artefact on the delicate and fragile cyst-lining cells. Oligocystic SCA may produce clear or serosanguineous fluid with only histiocytes and haemosiderin-laden macrophages, also leading to a "Non-diagnostic" interpretation {69,144}. Cyst-lining cells are bland, cuboidal, non-mucinous epithelial cells and are often absent or scant. The use of larger-bore needles and microforceps devices improves the diagnostic yield by sampling more of the cyst-lining cells and providing tissue for ancillary testing {982,56}.

The presence of contaminating gastrointestinal epithelium and/or mucin can lead to misdiagnosis as a mucin-producing neoplastic cyst, either intraductal papillary mucinous neoplasm or mucinous cystic neoplasm {329}. Unilocular or oligocystic SCAs with increased haemorrhage, granular material, and haemosiderin-laden macrophages may be misdiagnosed as pseudocysts {491}.

Ancillary testing

α-Inhibin is a sensitive marker for SCA, with positive staining in as many as 88% of cases {716}. Tumour cells are also positive for pancytokeratin and GLUT1, and the subepithelial capillary meshwork is highlighted by CD31 {680}. Cytoplasmic glycogen results in positivity for PAS, and PASD is negative after digestion with diastase {329}.

Cyst fluid analysis shows low or undetectable levels of CEA and CA19-9, and low levels of amylase {329}. CEA levels < 5 ng/mL and amylase levels < 250 U/mL are helpful in excluding a mucinous cyst and pseudocyst, respectively {491}. VEGF protein levels are also elevated in the cyst fluid {955}.

SCAs have *VHL* gene alterations, which are not found in other pancreatic cysts {891,809,561}. *VHL* (3p25) mutations or loss of heterozygosity are detectable in SCA cyst fluid {809, 491,787}. Other alterations include aneuploidy of chromosome 3p {809}.

Schwannoma

Fonseca R
Ozretić L

Definition

Pancreatic schwannoma is a rare benign neoplasm arising from Schwann cells of the peripheral nerve sheath.

Clinical features and imaging

Pancreatic schwannomas are usually asymptomatic tumours, most commonly located in the head of the pancreas {202}. Symptomatic patients most commonly present with abdominal pain; other symptoms include back pain, weight loss, nausea, vomiting, melena, anaemia, or jaundice {566}.

On ultrasound, schwannomas appear as well-defined, hypoechoic lesions with poor contrast uptake and are hypoenhanced compared with the surrounding pancreatic parenchyma {506}. Cystic change is noted in a high percentage of cases {828}. On unenhanced CT, pancreatic schwannomas usually present as low-density or cystic masses {828,899}. Contrast-enhanced CT findings correlate well with histopathological features, with well-enhanced areas corresponding to hypercellular and more vascular (Antoni A) areas, whereas unenhanced areas correspond to hypocellular (Antoni B) areas {828,506}. On MRI, these tumours appear hypointense on T1-weighted images, inhomogeneously hyperintense on T2-weighted images, and hyperintense on diffusion-weighted images {764}.

Histopathology

On gross examination, pancreatic schwannomas are well-circumscribed, usually encapsulated, homogeneous tumours with a yellow-tan cut surface. Degenerative changes are often seen, usually in the form of haemorrhage, hyalinization, calcification, or cystic degeneration. Microscopically, schwannomas often show a biphasic architecture, with alternating hypercellular areas of spindle cells (known as Antoni A areas) and hypocellular areas with myxoid stroma (i.e. Antoni B areas). There is minimal atypia, a low mitotic count, and an absence of cellular necrosis.

Key diagnostic cytopathological features

- Variably sized cohesive spindle cell tissue fragments
- Biphasic pattern, with regions showing more nuclei and regions showing fewer nuclei in a myxoid stroma
- Variable cellular density
- Nuclear palisading can be absent
- Bland spindle cells with abundant syncytial-appearing wavy cytoplasm
- Elongated, wavy nuclei with tapered ends
- Mitotic figures are absent
- Clean background with no evidence of necrosis or atypical single cells

Reference(s): {485,882,825,190}

Discussion and differential diagnosis

Pancreatic schwannomas with a cystic component account for almost 60% of cases {905}. Hence, clinically, the differential diagnosis is with other cystic lesions of the pancreas. The spindle cell morphology is unique to schwannoma relative to other primary cysts in the pancreas. Smooth muscle tumours and gastrointestinal stromal tumour are the primary spindle cell lesions to consider in the differential diagnosis of other spindle cell neoplasms {485,825, 190}. Perinuclear vacuoles are a feature of gastrointestinal stromal tumour but may not be appreciated on cytopathology. The blunt-ended, elongated nuclei of leiomyoma are distinctly different to the tapered, wavy nuclei of schwannoma, but ancillary studies confirming the nature of the spindle cell lesion are warranted for accuracy, given the overlapping morphology of these lesions {913,379,882}.

Ancillary testing

Schwannomas show diffuse and strong positivity for S100, and they are also positive for SOX10. They are negative for markers of smooth muscle differentiation such as desmin and SMA, as well as markers supportive of a gastrointestinal stromal tumour, including DOG1 and KIT (CD117) {190}.

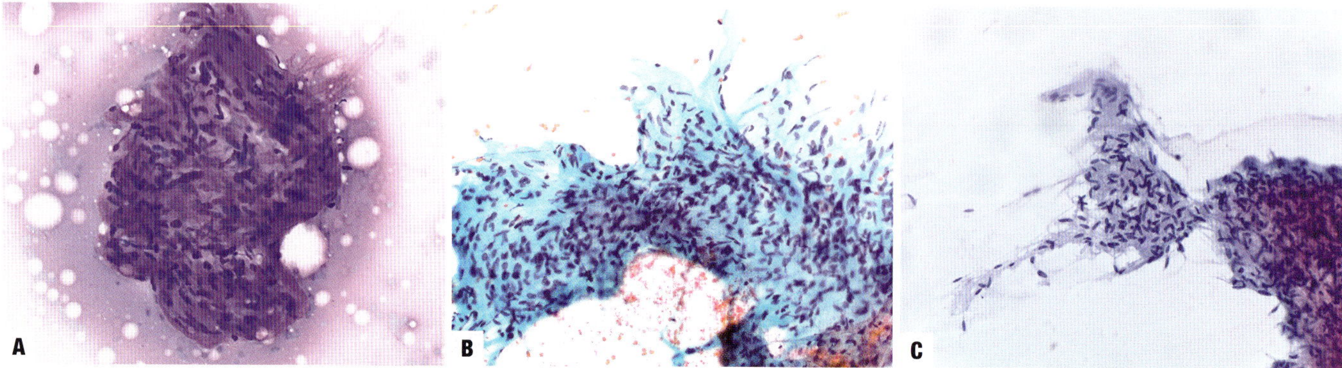

Fig. 4.35 Schwannoma. **A** Spindle cell proliferation composed of cells with wavy nuclei unevenly distributed in myxoid stroma (Giemsa). **B** Spindle cell proliferation composed of unevenly distributed cells with wavy nuclei without atypia and without mitotic activity (Pap). **C** Variably sized cohesive tissue fragments of bland spindle cells showing elongated, wavy nuclei with tapered ends and thin, drawn-out cytoplasm when seen singly, and less well defined in the tissue fragments (Pap).

Lymphangioma

Fonseca R
Ozretić L

Definition

Lymphangioma is a rare benign congenital malformation of the lymphatic system.

Clinical features and imaging

Lymphangiomas can occur within the pancreatic parenchyma or peripancreatic soft tissue or be connected to the pancreas by a pedicle. Pancreatic lymphangiomas are rare, accounting for < 1% of all lymphangiomas, and they represent only 0.2% of all pancreatic lesions {621}. In most cases, pancreatic lymphangiomas are asymptomatic. Symptoms can occasionally occur in response to the size, location, and mass effect of the lesion and include gastrointestinal discomfort, vomiting, and abdominal pain {148}.

Pancreatic lymphangiomas are far more common in women than in men, and they have a wide age range (2–61 years, mean: 29 years) {108}. Most lymphangiomas are large (30–200 mm, mean: 127 mm) {621,887}, solitary, unilocular to multicystic lesions occurring in the distal pancreas, making their distinction from other pancreatic cystic lesions challenging with imaging studies alone.

Ultrasound shows multiple hypoechoic or anechoic cysts with thin intervening septa, and very rarely calcifications. Contrast-enhanced CT shows a well-circumscribed, thin-walled, low-density, homogeneous cystic mass, unilocular or multilocular, with multiple fine septa that may enhance {511}. On MRI, the lesion appears hypodense on T1 sequences and hyperintense on T2, with mild septal enhancement {380}. The presence of infection or haemorrhage may alter the appearance of the cysts {520}. MRI is most useful for excluding communication between the cystic lesion and pancreatic duct {884}.

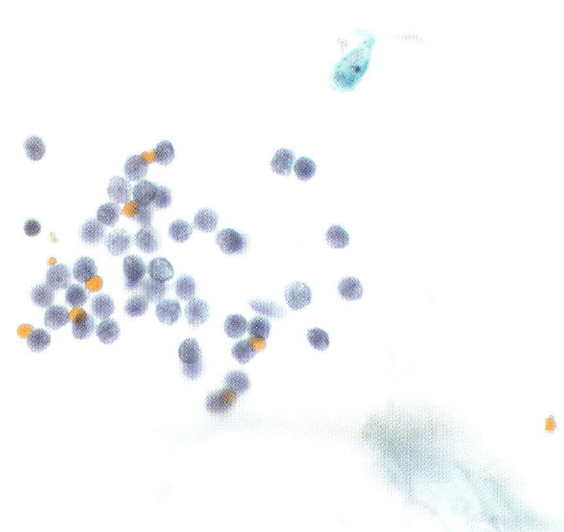

Fig. 4.36 Lymphangioma. A cytospin preparation shows small mature lymphocytes (Pap).

The prognosis of pancreatic lymphangiomas is excellent with complete resection, but recurrence may occur in cases that are incompletely resected {2}. There are no reported cases of malignant transformation of pancreatic/peripancreatic lymphangiomas.

Histopathology

On gross examination, pancreatic lymphangiomas are macrocystic masses, usually multilocular, containing watery to milky fluid. The inner lining of the cysts is smooth.

Lymphangiomas are characterized by thin-walled, enlarged lymphatic vessels of different sizes, lined by a flattened or low cuboidal endothelium. The cyst walls frequently contain lymphoid aggregates and variable amounts of collagenous connective tissue (particularly in larger cysts), as well as smooth muscle cells, adipose tissue, and histiocytes.

Key diagnostic cytopathological features

- Chylous/yellow/turbid/serosanguineous non-mucinous cyst fluid
- Small mature lymphocytes with no atypia
- Background of amorphous proteinaceous material with scattered histiocytes.

Reference(s): {223,2,108}

Discussion and differential diagnosis

FNAB of lymphangiomas is often characterized by nonspecific features including scattered mature lymphocytes with proteinaceous debris and no epithelial cells. The differential diagnosis includes other cystic pancreatic lesions including pseudocyst, lymphoepithelial cysts, dermoid cyst, epidermoid cyst, and serous cystadenoma in cases with scant material. Chemical analysis of the fluid helps in the differential diagnosis. The presence of contaminating gastrointestinal epithelium or a misinterpretation of the background amorphous proteinaceous material as mucin can lead to a misdiagnosis of a mucin-producing neoplastic cyst, i.e. intraductal papillary mucinous neoplasm or mucinous cystic neoplasm {223}.

Ancillary testing

The high triglyceride content of the cyst fluid can confirm a diagnosis of lymphangioma but is not always present {2}. Special stains for mucin, such as mucicarmine, are negative. Chemical analysis of the cyst fluid shows low levels of CEA (< 5 ng/mL). The amylase level may show mild elevation (in the low thousands) which could suggest, by itself, the diagnosis of a pseudocyst {108}. Flow cytometry of the cyst fluid shows a predominance of T lymphocytes with a mature phenotype (CD2+, CD3+, CD5+, and CD7+) and a balanced CD4:CD8 ratio. The endothelial cyst-lining cells are typically positive for D2-40 and CD31, occasionally positive for CD34, and negative for cytokeratin and PAS.

Other rare benign neoplasms

Stelow EB
Fabre M

Very uncommonly, benign mesenchymal tumours other than those discussed specifically in this volume may arise in the pancreas, including but not limited to haemangiomas, granular cell tumours, neurofibromas, paragangliomas, leiomyomas, solitary fibrous tumours, and lipomas {557,834,859,726,384,667,695}. Additionally, sclerosing epithelioid mesenchymal neoplasm of the pancreas is a recently described neoplasm that may be unique to the pancreas {62}. Granular cell tumours, leiomyomas, and sclerosing epithelioid mesenchymal neoplasms of the pancreas are solid, well-circumscribed tumours that most frequently are found incidentally. Neurofibromas most often present in patients with neurofibromatosis. Haemangiomas may appear more cystic and can resemble lymphangiomas or serous cystadenomas radiographically and grossly.

Histopathology

The histopathology of these tumours varies greatly. Solitary fibrous tumours show a haphazard arrangement of bland ovoid to spindled cells arranged around a branching and dilated vasculature within a variably collagenous stroma. Sclerosing epithelioid mesenchymal tumours of the pancreas are composed of nests, sheets, and linear arrays of epithelioid to spindled cells with scant cytoplasm and round to oval nuclei.

Key diagnostic cytopathological features

Like the histopathology, the cytopathology will vary depending on the tumour type. Typically, cytopathological features of malignancy, including pleomorphism, necrosis, and mitotic activity, are not present.

Discussion and differential diagnosis

The differential diagnoses for these lesions vary. Sclerosing epithelioid mesenchymal neoplasms of the pancreas must be distinguished from other epithelioid mesenchymal neoplasms including gastrointestinal stromal tumours, solitary fibrous tumours, sclerosing epithelioid fibrosarcomas, and melanomas. ICC and molecular studies may be used. Leiomyomas and neurofibromas should be distinguished from other bland spindle cell tumours. Lipomas should be distinguished from both fatty infiltration of the pancreas and well-differentiated liposarcomas.

Ancillary testing

Ancillary testing may be required to definitively categorize a tumour as "Benign". For example, it may be necessary to perform MDM2 testing to show that a tumour composed of mature adipose tissue is definitively a lipoma.

Benign mesenchymal tumours will show only limited or no expression of cytokeratins. This is in contrast to most primary epithelial neoplasms, except for some undifferentiated carcinomas and solid pseudopapillary neoplasms. Undifferentiated carcinomas are high-grade malignancies and typically have severe cytopathological atypia and are associated with necrosis and abundant mitotic activity. Solid pseudopapillary neoplasms show strong, diffuse β-catenin nuclear expression, in contrast to benign mesenchymal neoplasms. Solitary fibrous tumours show nuclear STAT6 expression. Sclerosing epithelioid mesenchymal neoplasms of the pancreas express CD99 and do not express CD34, STAT6, DOG1, KIT (CD117), or MUC4.

Sample reports: Benign / Negative for malignancy

Reid MD
Fonseca R
Perez-Machado MA

Sample report 1

Nature of specimen: FNAB 30 mm mass in head of pancreas.
Specimen adequacy: Considerable normal pancreas components.
Category: Benign.
Diagnosis: These highly cellular smears show pancreatic acini, stromal fragments with mild chronic inflammation, and duodenal epithelial contaminants. See comment.
Comment: There is a large amount of pancreatic parenchyma. But there is a concerning solid irregular pancreatic head mass seen on imaging and the FNAB material may not represent the target lesion. Correlation with imaging is required and repeat FNAB may be warranted in this case.

Editorial note:
Some cytopathology services or institutions may regard this case as "Non-diagnostic" because there may be sampling error. A cytopathology service or institution should decide how it will report cases where considerable benign pancreatic FNAB or benign bile duct brushing material is present on the slides but does not appear to represent the lesion seen on imaging; i.e. the service should decide to report these cases either as "Non-diagnostic" or as "Benign" with a mandatory caveat in the report conclusion that "the material may not represent the lesion seen on imaging, and repeat FNAB/brushing is recommended".

Sample report 2

Nature of specimen: FNAB possible cystic mass in body of pancreas.
Specimen adequacy: Satisfactory for evaluation.
Category: Benign.
Diagnosis: Acute inflammatory infiltrate, reactive ductal cells, debris, necrotic acini, calcific deposits, and amorphous proteinaceous material are present, consistent with acute pancreatitis. Clinical correlation required.

Sample report 3

Nature of specimen: FNAB poorly defined lesion in head of pancreas. History of high alcoholic consumption and pancreatitis.
Specimen adequacy: Satisfactory for evaluation.
Category: Benign.
Diagnosis: Mixed acute and chronic inflammatory infiltrate, amorphous proteinaceous material, and benign pancreatic acini consistent with chronic pancreatitis. See comment.
Comment: The patient's history of chronic alcoholic pancreatitis and imaging showing a poorly defined pancreatic head lesion are noted. Clinical and imaging correlation is recommended to ensure that the biopsy is representative of the lesion.

Sample report 4

Nature of specimen: FNAB possible mass lesion head of pancreas with bile duct obstruction.
Specimen adequacy: Satisfactory for evaluation.
Category: Benign.
Diagnosis: Mixed acute and chronic inflammatory infiltrate, amorphous proteinaceous material, stromal fragments, and benign pancreatic acini consistent with chronic pancreatitis. See comment.
Comment: The presence of mixed microcysts and solid pancreatic head/groove enhancement on imaging is noted. These cytopathological changes are consistent with groove/paraduodenal pancreatitis. Clinical and imaging correlation is recommended.

Sample report 5

Nature of specimen: Diffuse enlargement of pancreas. FNAB of head of pancreas.
Specimen adequacy: Satisfactory for evaluation.
Category: Benign.
Diagnosis: Pancreatic acini and dense fibrotic stroma with increased plasma cells and lymphocytes, findings suggestive of autoimmune pancreatitis. See comment.
Comment: A chronic plasma cell–predominant inflammatory infiltrate is noted along with fragments of fibrosis. The plasma cells are positive for IgG with increased IgG4+ plasma cells. Although concerning for autoimmune pancreatitis, a definitive diagnosis cannot be rendered on limited cytopathological samples. Clinical correlation recommended.

Sample report 6

Nature of specimen: FNAB of rounded lesion in pancreatic body.
Category: Benign.
Diagnosis: Lymphoepithelial cyst. See comment.
Comment: Nucleated and anucleated squamous cells, laminated keratin, keratinous debris, and scattered small lymphocytes are present, diagnostic of a lymphoepithelial cyst. Cyst fluid CEA is markedly elevated (5102 ng/mL), a common finding in this lesion.

Sample report 7

Nature of specimen: 60 mm cyst in the pancreatic tail of a patient with alcohol abuse.
Specimen adequacy: Satisfactory for evaluation.
Category: Benign.
Diagnosis: Pseudocyst. See comment.
Comment: Granular debris, yellow-brown pigment, lymphocytes, and haemosiderin-laden macrophages are seen. Biochemical analysis reveals markedly elevated cyst fluid amylase (6300 U/L) and low CEA (13 ng/mL), findings that support the diagnosis.

Sample report 8

Nature of specimen: 15 mm round mass in the pancreatic tail, clinically consistent with a neuroendocrine tumour (NET).
Specimen adequacy: Satisfactory for evaluation.
Category: Benign.
Diagnosis: Splenule. See comment.
Comment: Polymorphous lymphoid population with scattered plasma cells and branching capillaries, which on the cell block are CD8+ endothelial cells, consistent with a splenule.

Sample report 9

Nature of specimen: FNAB and fine CNB of multicystic, lobulated mass in the head of pancreas.

Part A – FNAB, pancreatic head mass:
Specimen adequacy: Evaluation limited by scant cellularity.
Category: Benign.
Diagnosis: Cyst contents with haemosiderin-laden macrophages and low CEA and amylase, findings suggestive of serous cystadenoma. See comment.

Part B – Fine CNB, pancreatic head mass:
Diagnosis: Serous cystadenoma. See comment.

Comment: The smears are paucicellular and show blood and haemosiderin-laden macrophages. CEA is 1 ng/mL and amylase is 25 U/L. The cell block shows fibrous tissue focally lined by bland cuboidal, non-mucinous epithelial cells that are positive for pancytokeratin, α-inhibin, and GLUT1. The cytomorphology and immunoprofile support the diagnosis of serous cystadenoma.

Sample report 10

Nature of specimen: FNAB of rounded tumour in posterior mid-pancreas.
Specimen adequacy: Specimen limited by scant cellularity.
Category: Benign.
Diagnosis: Low-grade spindle cell neoplasm consistent with schwannoma.
Microscopic findings: Smears and cell block show few fragments of bland-appearing, elongated spindle cells with wavy nuclei and filamentous cytoplasm, associated with cellular myxoid stroma.
Ancillary testing: Spindle cells are positive for S100 and SOX10, and negative for KIT (CD117), DOG1, desmin, CD34, and STAT6. The cytomorphology and immunoprofile support the diagnosis of schwannoma.

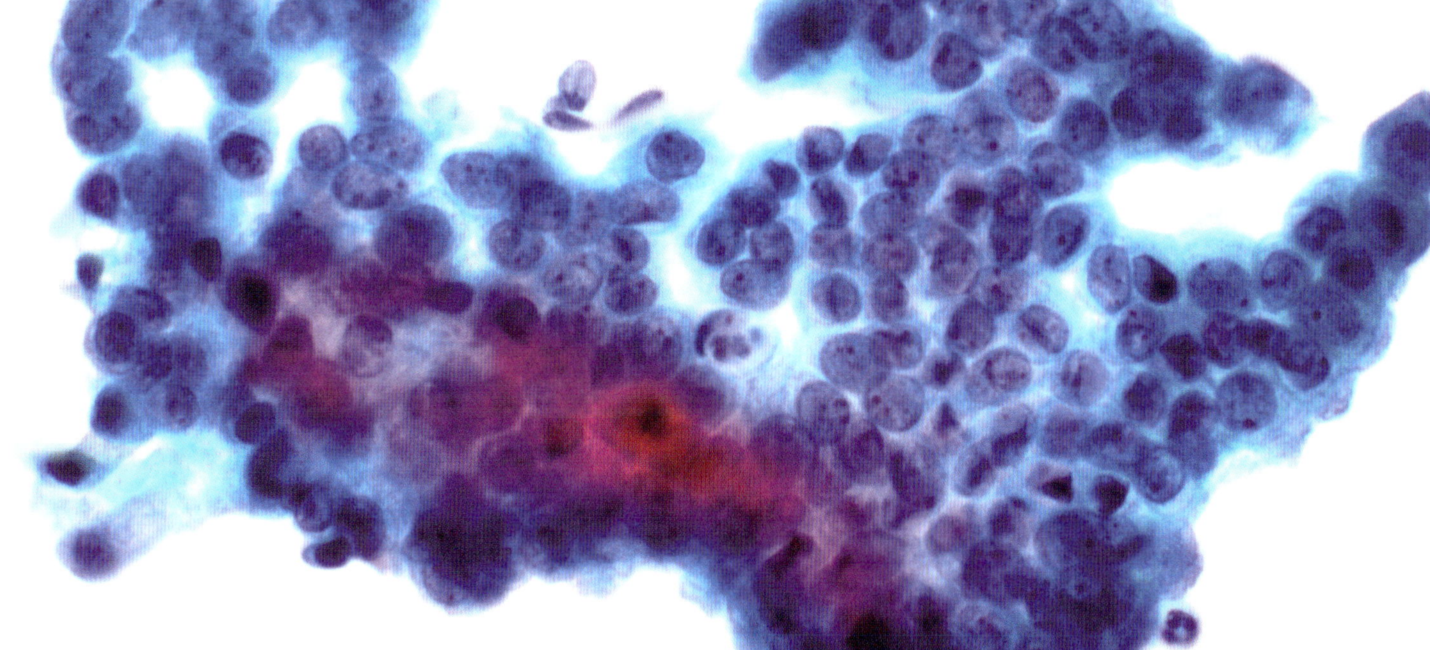

5

Diagnostic category: Atypical

Edited by: Siddiqui MT

Introduction

Yang J
Heymann JJ
Roy-Chowdhuri S

"Atypical" is an indeterminate category characterized by cells with a spectrum of architectural and/or cellular atypia that cannot be confidently ascribed to benign entities or to malignancy. Historically, the cytopathological criteria and nomenclature defining the "Atypical" category have varied widely among cytopathologists, some using only the one term, "Atypical", and others using two categories, termed "Atypical" and "Suspicious for malignancy", to represent the benign and malignant ends of the spectrum of indeterminate cases. The reported frequency of the "Atypical" category in EUS-FNAB of the pancreas ranges from 0% to 14%, with an average of 5.5% {1,711}. The frequency in bile duct brushings is higher, ranging from 11% to 39.8%, which may be partially due to the challenge in recognizing reactive atypia inherent to primary sclerosing cholangitis, stents, or biliary stones {111,268,890,30}. Common reasons reported for "Atypical" categorization include low cellularity and poor preservation and the high threshold for a "Malignant" categorization in the interpretation of bile duct brushing specimens.

Guidelines for reporting pancreaticobiliary cytopathology developed by the Papanicolaou Society of Cytopathology (PSC) have previously provided objective cytopathological criteria and incorporated imaging features and biochemical and molecular analysis of cyst fluid into the final diagnosis {643}. This multimodal approach redistributed many "Atypical" cases into either "Benign" or "Neoplastic" categories. Most FNABs previously categorized as "Atypical" utilizing this system were reclassified as "Neoplastic: other" because they were cystic lesions with mucinous epithelium and no clear high-grade epithelial atypia. FNAB with no supportive evidence of neoplasia remained in the "Atypical" category.

Based on the different risks of malignancy, the current WHO Reporting System for Pancreaticobiliary Cytopathology divides the neoplastic category into two distinct categories: "Pancreaticobiliary neoplasm, low-risk/grade (PaN-low)" and "Pancreaticobiliary neoplasm, high-risk/grade (PaN-high)". Specimens containing cells diagnostic of low-grade dysplasia that were otherwise placed in the "Atypical" category using the PSC system are now included in the "PaN-low" category.

In the PSC system, indeterminate FNABs not diagnostic of a well-differentiated neuroendocrine tumour (NET) or solid pseudopapillary neoplasm, which were tumours that were in the "Neoplastic: other" category rather than the "Malignant" category, were categorized as "Atypical" rather than "Suspicious for malignancy". A significant change in categorization with the WHO Reporting System is that these tumours are now categorized as "Malignant", in line with the fifth-edition WHO classification of digestive system tumours {910}. Therefore, if an FNAB is not diagnostic of one of these tumours, but one of these tumours is suspected, then the interpretation should be "Suspicious for malignancy" and not "Atypical". The "Atypical" category is appropriate when the differential diagnosis of finding a few endocrine cells includes islet cell hyperplasia in the clinical setting of chronic pancreatitis {110,649}.

Definition

Yang J
Heymann JJ
Roy-Chowdhuri S

A specimen categorized as "Atypical" demonstrates features predominantly seen in benign lesions and minimal features that may raise the possibility of a malignant lesion, but with features insufficient in either number or quality to diagnose a process or lesion as "Benign", "Pancreaticobiliary neoplasm, low-risk/grade (PaN-low)", "Pancreaticobiliary neoplasm, high-risk/grade (PaN-high)", or "Malignant".

Discussion and background

Gan Q
Heymann JJ
Roy-Chowdhuri S

The WHO Reporting System for Pancreaticobiliary Cytopathology revises the six-tiered Papanicolaou Society of Cytopathology (PSC) System for Reporting Pancreaticobiliary Cytology but retains the two indeterminate categories, "Atypical" and "Suspicious for malignancy" {649}. One of the benefits of implementation of the PSC system is the decreased number of "Atypical" determinations, especially for cystic lesions, which is accomplished by the integration of imaging findings and ancillary tests into the final diagnosis {649}. The "Atypical" category is applied to a variety of cases where cellular or architectural abnormalities are beyond the cytopathological features observed in reactive processes in the pancreas or biliary tract, and are insufficient to render a more definitive diagnosis, including "Pancreaticobiliary neoplasm, low-risk/grade (PaN-low)", "Pancreaticobiliary neoplasm, high-risk/grade (PaN-high)", or "Malignant", owing to scant cellularity, degenerative changes, inflammatory conditions, and previous stenting.

The histopathological outcome of this category ranges from benign to premalignant and malignant entities {134,307,338, 610,712,824,924}. Reasons for using the "Atypical" category are multiple. The inherent characteristics of the pancreaticobiliary lesion, low tumour cellularity, and anatomically challenging tumour sites may all preclude a more definitive classification. Technical factors, such as the endosonographer's skill in procuring adequately cellular and representative samples, specimen preparation artefact, and the availability of rapid onsite evaluation (ROSE) {195,434} will all also influence the quality of the specimen. Moreover, because of different levels of experience and expertise, training, and institutional case volume, there is significant interobserver and intraobserver variability in the use of the "Atypical" category {466}.

Because of the change in categorization and the fact that the "Atypical" category is heterogeneous in nature, an easy way to delineate the "Atypical" category is to divide it into three different scenarios: EUS-FNAB of a pancreaticobiliary mass lesion,

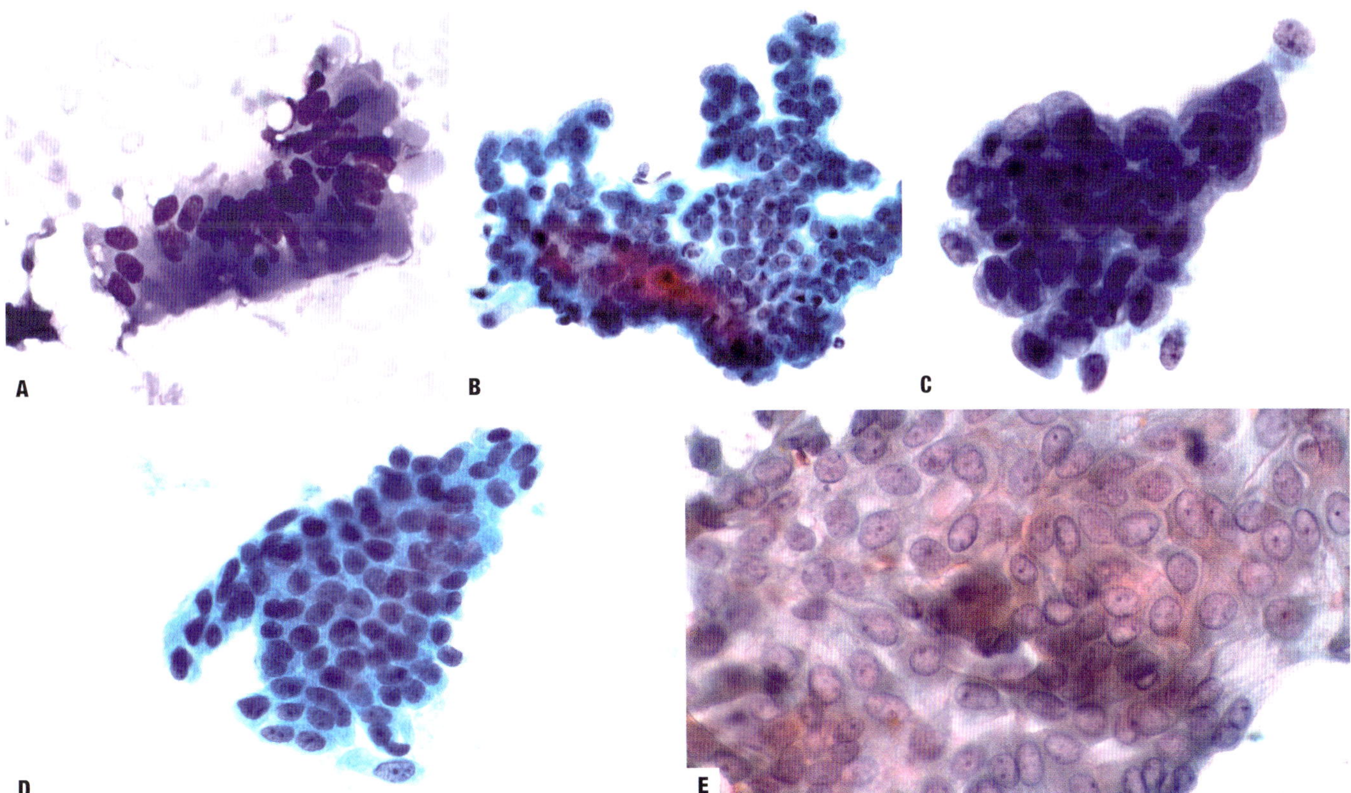

Fig. 5.01 Diagnostic category: "Atypical". **A** Ductal cells from a pancreatic FNAB show elongated and pseudostratified nuclei but maintain a low N:C ratio (Giemsa). **B** Atypical ductal epithelium in bile duct brushing. Fragment of epithelium showing loss of architectural polarity, minor anisonucleosis, small nucleoli, and parachromatin clearing (Pap). **C** Atypical ductal epithelium. Bile duct brushing in liquid-based preparation. Small tissue fragment of epithelial cells demonstrating focal mucinous metaplasia and nuclear membrane irregularity (Pap). **D** This sheet of bile duct epithelium shows nuclear enlargement with anisonucleosis of 2× and mild crowding. Nuclear membranes are smooth, chromatin is even, and nucleoli are small (Pap). **E** Ductal cells from a pancreatic FNAB show nuclear enlargement and pallor with mild anisonucleosis and only focal nuclear membrane irregularities. No uneven nuclear arrangement (drunken-honeycomb architecture) or mucinous cytoplasm is seen (Pap).

EUS-FNAB of a pancreatic cystic lesion, and bile duct brushing (BDB). It is important to understand that "Atypical" should be used judiciously and as little as possible, because an "Atypical" report may lead to unnecessary additional investigation. In EUS-FNAB of a pancreaticobiliary mass lesion, the "Atypical" category may be related to reactive atypia in pancreatitis, low-grade pancreatic intraepithelial neoplasia, well-differentiated adenocarcinoma, or scant or poorly prepared samples of other malignant entities. In EUS-FNAB of a pancreatic cyst, low-grade intraductal papillary mucinous neoplasm or mucinous cystic neoplasm could be categorized in the "Pancreaticobiliary neoplasm, low-risk/grade (PaN-low)" category with the integrated approach in a majority of cases. The "Atypical" category should be reserved for cytopathology specimens that are not diagnostic of a low-grade neoplasm.

To align classification with the fifth-edition WHO classification of digestive system tumours {910}, low-grade biliary intraepithelial neoplasia and intraductal papillary neoplasm of the bile duct, which were included in the "Atypical" category in the PSC system, are now included as "Pancreaticobiliary neoplasm" categories if they are diagnostic. Because these lesions are either a microscopic lesion not associated with imaging findings (biliary intraepithelial neoplasia) or have not been clearly defined on cytopathology (intraductal papillary mucinous neoplasm of the bile duct), it is likely that sampling of these lesions will continue to be categorized as "Atypical" {71,353}.

For BDB, the "Atypical" category is applied to cases for which the atypia observed is beyond that seen in reactive/inflammatory changes while being quantitatively and qualitatively insufficient for categorization as "Suspicious for malignancy". Although low-grade biliary intraepithelial neoplasia and intraductal papillary mucinous neoplasm of the bile duct are entities included in the "Pancreaticobiliary neoplasm, low-risk/grade (PaN-low)" category in this WHO Reporting System, the atypia present on cytopathology without histopathological correlation will be categorized as "Atypical" because the atypia is mild.

In order to improve the reproducibility of cytopathological evaluation of the "Atypical" category, the PSC system proposed the following cytopathological criteria for ductal epithelium, because the majority of malignancy in the pancreaticobiliary system originates from ductal epithelial cells. The findings listed below are common causes of an "Atypical" interpretation and are applicable to both EUS-FNAB of pancreaticobiliary lesions and BDB specimens {60}:

1. Loss of architectural polarity
2. Minor degree of nuclear crowding
3. Mild alteration of the honeycomb pattern
4. No 3D tissue fragments
5. No true nuclear moulding
6. Pseudostratification within the lower two thirds of cell strips
7. Near-normal N:C ratio
8. Slight nuclear membrane irregularity without marked clefting
9. Parachromatin clearing without other cytopathological features of adenocarcinoma
10. Small nucleoli without true macronucleoli
11. Minor anisonucleosis, 2:1
12. Clean background without necrosis, which might not be important in BDB because necrosis is not helpful in identifying malignancy in BDB {28}

Risk of malignancy and management recommendations

Gan Q
Heymann JJ
Klapman J
Roy-Chowdhuri S

The primary goal of the WHO Reporting System for Pancreaticobiliary Cytopathology is to standardize the categorization of various diseases of pancreaticobiliary system and to guide clinical management according to the risk of malignancy (ROM) {711}. Since the implementation of the Papanicolaou Society of Cytopathology (PSC) reporting system, studies have shown a large range in use of the "Atypical" category among institutions, from as little as 0% to as much as 13.9% {28,71,124,338,461, 610,502,134,268,307,752,824,883,918,924}. The use of "Atypical" in bile duct brushing (BDB) cytopathology is very high, owing to the high threshold required for the diagnosis of malignancy with this specimen type. The known overlap between the morphology of reactive and reparative changes in bile duct epithelium from stents, stones, and inflammation, and the morphology of well-differentiated adenocarcinoma leads to a high use of indeterminate interpretations {699}. The ROM associated with the diagnostic categories of the PSC system has been refined by series of studies since its implementation {338,268,752,924}.

The ROM of the "Atypical" category is different for BDB and EUS-FNAB of pancreatic lesions. There is a remarkable range in the ROM for BDB and pancreas FNAB depending on the type of study, date of the study (e.g. pre-PSC system), and experience of the institution reporting the study. From studies carried out after the establishment of the PSC system, where the category "Neoplastic: other" provided a home for non-malignant neoplasia that otherwise would have been categorized as "Atypical" or "Suspicious for malignancy", the ROM of the "Atypical" category for pancreas FNAB is 30–40% and for BDB is 25–61% {792,307,824,875,111,192,952,306}

Management of an "Atypical" categorization should include multidisciplinary discussion, consensus review, expert consultation, ancillary tests, and repeat sampling with rapid onsite evaluation (ROSE). In recent years, evolving technologies such as multifocal FISH {54,113,447,585} and molecular tests with genetic sequencing have been reported to improve the classification of pancreatic cysts {700,787} and the sensitivity of detection of malignancy in BDB {281,788,856,192}. Molecular testing using either otherwise discarded cytocentrifuged BDB specimens {281} or paired specimen collection has significantly increased the sensitivity of detecting malignancy to 93%, while maintaining a specificity of 100% and also identifying markers potentially predictive of response to targeted therapy {788}. Therefore, molecular tests increase the information available for clinical decision-making. Precisely defining the correct categorization and specific diagnosis of pancreaticobiliary cytopathology is challenging, so consensus review or second opinion from experienced pancreaticobiliary cytopathologists may be cost-effective and is recommended {883}. If ancillary testing is not available and multidisciplinary discussion is inconclusive, further workup may include repeat sampling with ROSE. Depending on the three different scenarios discussed above, management may differ slightly.

Sample reports: Atypical

Roy-Chowdhuri S
Gan Q
Heymann JJ
Yang J

Sample report 1

Nature of specimen: Bile duct brushings.
Specimen adequacy: Satisfactory for evaluation.
Category: Atypical.
Diagnosis: Rare ductal epithelial cells with loss of architectural polarity, mild anisonucleosis, and prominent nucleoli are present.

Sample report 2

Nature of specimen: FNAB of mass in body of pancreas.
Category: Atypical.
Diagnosis: Scant endocrine cells. See microscopy report below.
Microscopic description: There is a scant population of loosely cohesive, monomorphic cells with occasional stippled chromatin and varied amounts of cytoplasm consistent with neuroendocrine cells. The scant endocrine-type cells are too few to suspect a neuroendocrine tumour (NET) and may be the result of islet cell aggregation. Correlation with imaging is recommended.

Sample report 3

Nature of specimen: Bile duct brushings.
Specimen adequacy: Satisfactory for evaluation.
Category: Atypical.
Diagnosis: Atypical biliary epithelium. See comment.
Comment: The epithelium shows a loss of cell polarity, nuclear enlargement, and crowding, and prominent nucleoli are present. The features favour reactive changes, given the associated history of stent placement.

Sample report 4

Nature of specimen: Bile duct brushings in a patient with primary sclerosing cholangitis.
Specimen adequacy: Satisfactory but limited by scant cellularity.
Category: Atypical.
Diagnosis: Atypical biliary ductal epithelial cells. See comment.
Comment: The cells show nuclear crowding, nuclear enlargement, hyperchromasia. Background inflammation is present. Definitive features of dysplasia and malignancy are not present. Molecular testing is pending and will be reported separately.

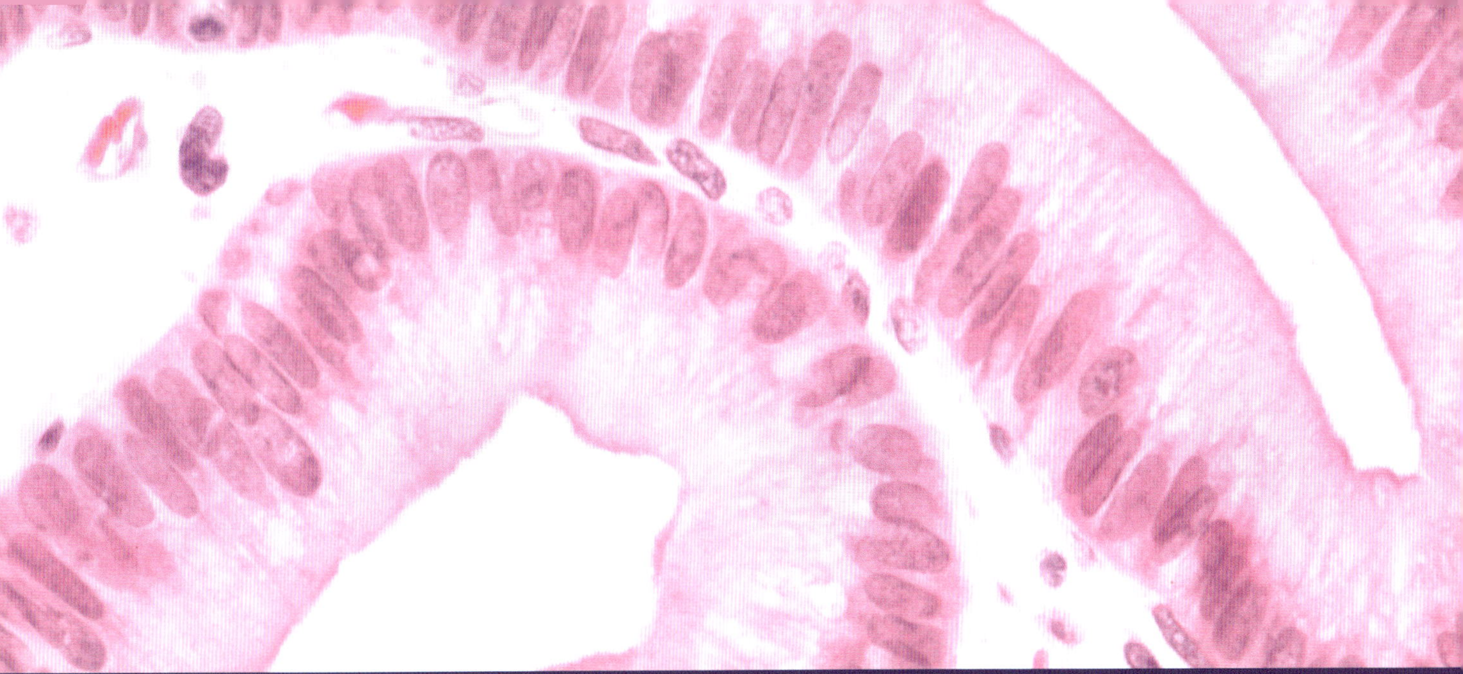

6

Diagnostic category: Pancreaticobiliary neoplasm, low-risk/grade

Edited by: Fukushima N, Weynand B

Introduction

Centeno BA
Pitman MB

The category "Pancreaticobiliary neoplasm, low-risk/grade (PaN-low)" is extracted from the "Neoplastic: other" category of the Papanicolaou Society of Cytopathology (PSC) System for Reporting Pancreaticobiliary Cytology {643}, which included intraductal papillary mucinous neoplasm and mucinous cystic neoplasm and the low-grade malignancies pancreatic neuroendocrine tumour (PanNET) and solitary pseudopapillary neoplasm {643}. This new category is limited to intraductal and cystic neoplasms with low-grade epithelial atypia {543,644}, and it classifies the epithelium as neoplastic rather than indeterminate. It is preferred to "Atypical", which would require repeat biopsy, or "Suspicious for malignancy", which implies the probable presence of an invasive carcinoma.

A two-tiered categorization system for epithelial atypia has been proposed for FNAB of pancreatic cysts, to stratify the risk for high-grade dysplasia or carcinoma within a given lesion {645}. Low-grade epithelial atypia encompasses low-grade and intermediate-grade dysplasia and has a low risk of disease progression. The two-tiered categorization of epithelial atypia in pancreaticobiliary cytopathology samples matches the two-tiered histopathological classification of intraepithelial and cystic neoplasia in the fifth-edition WHO classification of digestive system tumours {910,60}. A two-tiered system is more easily reproducible, although intermediate-grade dysplasia may sometimes be categorized as either low-grade or high-grade epithelial atypia {645}.

Definition

Centeno BA
Pitman MB

A specimen categorized as "Pancreaticobiliary neoplasm, low-risk/grade (PaN-low)" has features of an intraductal and/or cystic neoplasm with low-grade epithelial atypia.

Discussion and background

Centeno BA
Klapman J
Pitman MB

The primary differential diagnosis for low-grade intraductal papillary mucinous neoplasm (IPMN) is gastrointestinal contamination. Mucin that is thick, copious, tenacious, and colloid-like is diagnostic of neoplastic mucin even without mucinous epithelium {253}. Thin, wispy mucin is indeterminate for origin, and in liquid-based preparations it is attenuated, making distinction from fibrin difficult. Low-grade neoplastic epithelial cells have evenly spaced nuclei with cytoplasmic mucin that may be apical and nearly identical to gastric foveolar epithelium. Features supporting a neoplasm include nuclear crowding, mild nuclear enlargement, mild to moderate cytopathological disorganization, and papillary fragments. Low-grade IPMN is not readily distinguished from low-grade mucinous cystic neoplasm {645}.

Intermediate-grade epithelium shows moderate atypia with pseudostratification, nuclear crowding, focal loss of polarity, a higher N:C ratio, and diminished cytoplasmic mucin. This epithelium straddles the morphology of both low- and high-grade atypia {645}.

In the Papanicolaou Society of Cytopathology (PSC) System for Reporting Pancreaticobiliary Cytology, bile duct brushings with low-grade atypia were categorized as "Atypical", because clear cytopathological criteria for a definitive diagnosis of biliary intraepithelial neoplasia with low-grade dysplasia were not well defined. In this WHO Reporting System these features are defined, and these lesions are placed in the "Pancreaticobiliary neoplasm, low-risk/grade (PaN-low)" category. Similarly, a definitive diagnosis of low-grade pancreatic intraepithelial neoplasia on FNAB is not well defined, but features described in this WHO Reporting System can be used to place such lesions in the "PaN-low" category, which is used to encompass low- and intermediate-grade dysplasia. More likely than not, most of these low-grade, non-cystic, intraductal lesions will still be placed in the "Atypical" category.

Ancillary tests are often critical for the diagnosis of a low-grade mucinous cyst because of the paucicellularity and thin mucin of most branch duct IPMNs. Cyst fluid CEA levels > 192 ng/mL are approximately 80% accurate for a mucin-producing neoplasm {91} and have been shown to be the best test for classifying a cyst as mucinous {140}. Molecular assays performed on cyst fluid or supernatant material can identify mutations correlating with mucinous neoplasia, such as *KRAS*, *GNAS*, and *RNF43* mutations, which are seen in as many as 75%, 60%, and 70% of IPMNs, respectively {925,926}.

Risk of malignancy and management recommendations

Centeno BA
Klapman J
Pitman MB

The risk of malignancy (ROM) for the "Neoplastic: other" category in the Papanicolaou Society of Cytopathology (PSC) system ranged from 14.2% to 100% {124,792,461,924,824,711}.

This wide range of ROM was due to the broad group of lesions in this category, from low-grade to high-grade premalignant lesions to low-grade malignancies. With pancreatic cysts, the cytopathological ROM is directly related to the epithelial atypia in the cyst fluid. A study that focused on the ROM in cysts with high-grade epithelial atypia (HGEA) identified a ROM of 80% in this category {308}. In a follow-up study from the same group, cases in the "Neoplastic: other" category with low-grade epithelial atypia (LGEA) had an absolute ROM of 4.3%, compared with 90% for those with HGEA {307}. The absolute ROM was 19.0% for LGEA and 95.2% for patients with HGEA in a further study, published in 2020 {824}.

A recent study using a prior study cohort {307} to evaluate the ROM using the WHO Reporting System categories {306} shows a ROM for "PaN-low" at 5–20%. There are no current data on ROM with bile duct brushing samples.

Management options for "PaN-low" include clinical correlation with repeat sampling, preferably with ancillary studies such as FISH {603,979,411,445} or next-generation sequencing {788, 281,192,699}.

There are five published guidelines for the management of pancreatic cysts. They include the revised international consensus Fukuoka guidelines for the management of intraductal papillary mucinous neoplasms {839}, the European evidence-based guidelines on the management of pancreatic cystic neoplasms {204}, the American Gastroenterological Association (AGA) guidelines on the management of asymptomatic neoplastic pancreatic cysts {878}, the American College of Gastroenterology (ACG) clinical guidelines on the diagnosis and management of pancreatic cysts {201}, and the American College of Radiology (ACR) white paper on the management of incidental pancreatic cysts {537}.

All these guidelines use a combination of clinical and imaging findings as absolute or relative indications for surgery, surveillance protocols, and indications for EUS-FNAB for patients with intraductal papillary mucinous neoplasm. Four guidelines include the cytopathological findings in the decision algorithm, and the presence of a "Positive" or "Suspicious" cytopathology sample with high-grade dysplasia will lead to surgical intervention. The white paper published by the ACR is the only one that does not include cytopathology as an integral part of the algorithm {537}.

Management has shifted from resecting all intraductal papillary mucinous cysts and mucinous cystic neoplasms (MCNs), due to their premalignant nature, to the conservative management and surveillance of intraductal papillary mucinous neoplasm and MCN with low-risk/grade features. This is because most of the lesions are on the very early spectrum of progression to carcinoma, and most patients are elderly with comorbid conditions, making the patient a high-risk surgical candidate {836}.

Cytopathology is the best test to accurately distinguish low-grade from high-grade cysts on the basis of the epithelial atypia in the cyst fluid {140}. Stratifying epithelial atypia into high-grade or low-grade leads to better patient management, because pancreatic cyst fluid FNABs are rarely interpreted as suspicious or diagnostic for malignancy owing to their scant cellularity. In the absence of cytopathological HGEA and the presence of LGEA, the patient has the option of surveillance depending on the clinical and imaging features {839,648,652}.

MCNs have been considered an absolute indication for surgery in older management guidelines and in some recent ones {839,878,748}, because of the ease of the usual distal pancreatectomy versus a lifetime of surveillance for progression to carcinoma. More recently, however, there is a move to refer patients for surveillance on the basis of their clinical and imaging findings {204,201,537}. Patients with MCN and LGEA on cytopathology can be referred for surveillance in the absence of other high-risk factors {201,748}.

Pancreatic intraepithelial neoplasia, low-grade

Tanaka M
Fukushima N
Stelow EB

Definition

Low-grade pancreatic intraepithelial neoplasia (LG-PanIN) is a microscopic, non-invasive, flat or micropapillary epithelial neoplasm with low- to intermediate-grade dysplasia.

Clinical features and imaging

Pancreatic intraepithelial neoplasia (PanIN) lesions are common in the older population {528}. LG-PanIN lesions are present in ≥ 80% of patients with pancreatic ductal neoplasia, in about 60% of patients with pancreatitis, and in about 30% of non-tumorous and non-pancreatitis glands {673,32}. Furthermore, PanIN is common in patients with familial pancreatic cancer and hereditary pancreatitis. It can be sometimes multifocal, and it occurs in younger patients {762,672}. LG-PanIN lesions are asymptomatic and not detected by imaging studies. However, because PanIN, even low-grade, is associated with pancreatic fibrosis {178}, multifocal PanIN lesions may be detected by EUS through parenchymal change adjacent to PanIN, such as multifocal parenchymal atrophy {762}.

Histopathology

Macroscopically, LG-PanIN lesions are not visible, but some cases are associated with lobulocentric atrophy because of regional ductal strictures.

Microscopically, LG-PanIN lesions are flat or papillary, with basally located nuclei (mild dysplasia) or pseudostratified nuclei (intermediate dysplasia) with mild to moderate cytopathological atypia. Marked architectural alterations are absent and mitoses are not frequent. Most LG-PanIN lesions consist of gastric foveolar or pyloric gland–type epithelium.

In contrast to high-grade PanIN lesions, LG-PanIN lesions never progress to pancreatic ductal adenocarcinoma (PDAC) {910}.

Key diagnostic cytopathological features

- Low cellularity of the atypical ductal cells
- Background of normal pancreatic acini or with some features of pancreatitis
- No nuclear atypia (mild dysplasia) to mildly enlarged to elongated, minimally irregular nuclei (intermediate dysplasia)
- Increased N:C ratio (intermediate-grade dysplasia)
- No background necrosis

Discussion and differential diagnosis

The size of PanIN lesions is usually ≤ 5 mm; therefore, these lesions are not targeted with FNAB but found incidentally on FNAB of other lesions. The background of pancreatitis may provide support for the diagnosis of LG-PanIN because this lesion is often found in patients with chronic pancreatitis {325}.

The differential diagnosis includes the following:

1. Simple mucinous cyst, low-grade intraductal papillary mucinous neoplasm (IPMN), and low-grade mucinous cystic neoplasm (MCN): The cells of simple mucinous cyst, IPMN, and MCN have the same morphology as LG-PanIN and are indistinguishable. Correlation with imaging findings is mandatory because the targeted lesion for the diagnosis of PanIN is not a cyst.
2. Normal gastric epithelium: Gastric-type epithelium raises the possibility of gastric contamination. The presence of gastric parietal cells may help to make this distinction.
3. High-grade intraductal lesions (high-grade PanIN [HG-PanIN], IPMN, and MCN) and well-differentiated PDAC: Cells with high-grade dysplasia are small (< 12 µm duodenal enterocyte) with a high N:C ratio, loss of the mucinous

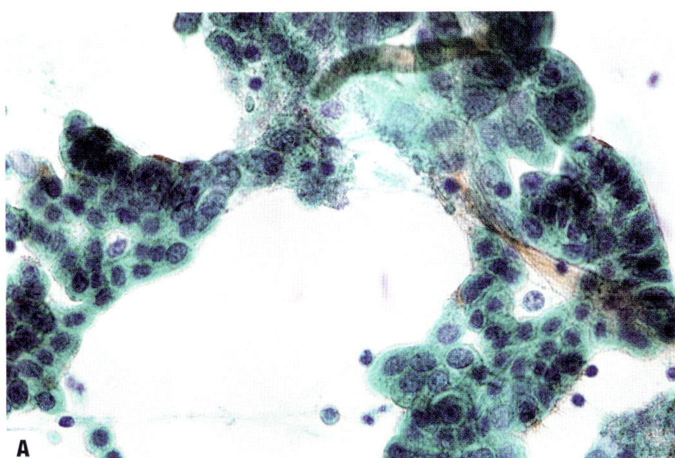

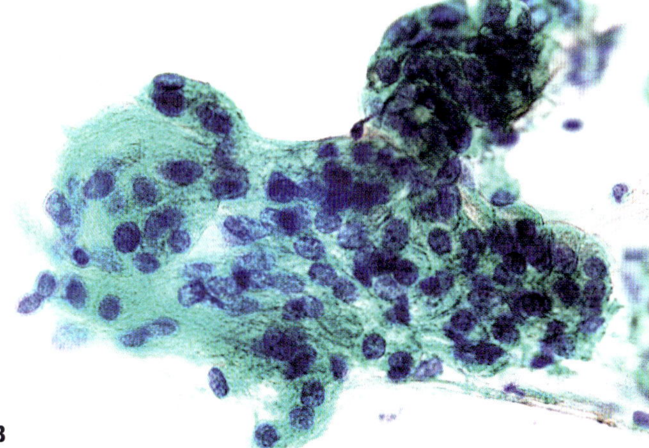

Fig. 6.01 Low-grade pancreatic intraductal neoplasm. **A** Pancreatic duct brushing cytopathology shows tissue fragments of mildly atypical epithelium with increased cellularity, nuclear pseudostratification, and nuclear irregularities (liquid-based cytopathology, Pap). **B** Pancreatic duct brushing cytopathology shows a cohesive tissue fragment of ductal epithelial cells with mild disorganization, nuclear crowding, and mild nuclear atypia in a clean background (Pap).

cytoplasmic compartment, nuclear irregularity, and abnormal chromatin distribution {644}.

Moderate to high cellularity, crowded sheets of disordered ductal cells (drunken honeycomb), and isolated cells are seen in PDAC. The foamy gland subtype of PDAC can be deceptively bland but the key feature here is the rounded cells with finely vacuolated, lacy cytoplasm, in contrast to the columnar mucinous cytoplasm in low-grade PanIN. Correlation with imaging is also important because FNAB of PanIN is not likely when the targeted lesion is visible as a mass.

These differential diagnoses should be carefully considered, especially in patients with a strong clinical suspicion of malignancy and in high-risk individuals. Repeated sample collections should be performed in cases of clinicopathological discordance.

Ancillary testing

Mutations in *TP53* and *SMAD4* are late events in pancreatic carcinogenesis and rare in LG-PanIN lesions {320}, but ICC for p53 and SMAD4 is helpful in the differential diagnosis between PDAC and LG-PanIN. The Ki-67 labelling index is also helpful in the differential diagnosis between high-grade lesions (including PDAC) and LG-PanIN.

Activating mutations of *KRAS* are common (> 90%) in LG-PanIN lesions {374} and other precancerous lesions of the pancreas and PDAC. The frequency of variant allele *KRAS* mutations is low in LG-PanIN and gradually increases in HG-PanIN {374}. Oncogenic mutations of *KRAS* may be useful for the detection of neoplastic epithelium, but they do not stratify grade. Activating mutations of *GNAS* and inactivating mutations of *RNF43* are common in IPMN and MCN, respectively, but rare in PanIN lesions {374}. Next-generation sequencing testing for these mutations may be helpful for the differential diagnosis.

Biliary intraepithelial neoplasia, low-grade

Tanaka M
Layfield LJ
Zen Y

Definition

Biliary intraepithelial neoplasia, low-grade (BilIN-low) is a microscopic, non-invasive neoplasm with a flat, micropapillary, or pseudopapillary architecture with low-grade dysplasia.

Clinical features and imaging

BilIN-low is often found in patients with chronic biliary disease such as hepatolithiasis, primary sclerosing cholangitis, IgG4-related sclerosing cholangitis, congenital biliary dilation, or anomalous union of pancreaticobiliary ducts. It can also be seen in patients with non-biliary disease such as chronic hepatitis B or C or alcoholic cirrhosis {18,409,727,383}. The incidence of biliary intraepithelial neoplasia (BilIN) in the general population is unknown. BilIN-low lesions are asymptomatic and cannot be detected by current imaging modalities.

Histopathology

The biliary tract mucosa with BilIN is macroscopically unremarkable or displays only subtle changes such as mild granularity or a thickened, velvety texture {18}.

Microscopically, BilIN-low is a flat or micropapillary lesion with a mildly increased N:C ratio, focally distorted polarities, mild irregularities of the nuclear membrane, nuclear elongation, and variations in nuclear size and shape. Nuclear pseudostratification is sometimes observed, but reaching to the luminal surface is not common. Mitoses are rare. In addition to the biliary phenotype, gastric (foveolar, pseudopyloric gland) and intestinal (goblet cells) phenotypes can also be recognized. Multifocal lesions can be observed.

Key diagnostic cytopathological features

BilIN-low does not have a defined cytopathological description and is found incidentally, rather than targeted. By analogy to low-grade pancreatic intraepithelial neoplasia, mild atypia and focally distorted nuclear polarity might be observed. Most cases will be interpreted as "Atypical", owing to the low-grade atypia defined by mucinous cytoplasm and mild nuclear atypia.

Discussion and differential diagnosis

These premalignant lesions potentially progress to cholangiocarcinoma in a multistep manner. BilIN is divided into low and high grades on the basis of the highest degree of cytoarchitectural atypia.

The main cytopathological differential diagnosis of BilIN-low includes reactive atypia. Intraductal papillary neoplasm of the bile duct and mucinous cystic neoplasm can display similar cytopathological features, but, unlike BilIN-low, they present with characteristic imaging abnormalities.

Discrimination between reactive atypia and BilIN-low is virtually impossible, particularly in patients with chronic cholangiopathy. Reactive bile duct epithelium demonstrates nuclear enlargement and mild variation in nuclear size, but the nuclei are round to oval in shape, with a smooth nuclear membrane, fine chromatin, and visible nucleoli. Intraepithelial neutrophils are common in tissue fragments of reactive biliary epithelium.

The cytopathological diagnosis of BilIN-low is not likely to be made, given the lack of defined criteria and imaging correlates.

Ancillary testing

Diffuse expression of p53 or the loss of SMAD4 expression suggests cholangiocarcinoma over BilIN-low, given that mutations in *TP53* and *SMAD4* are late events in biliary carcinogenesis and absent in BilIN-low. The diffuse expression of maspin

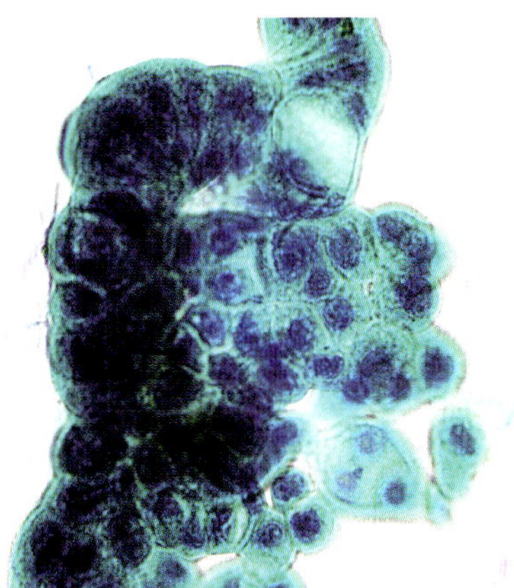

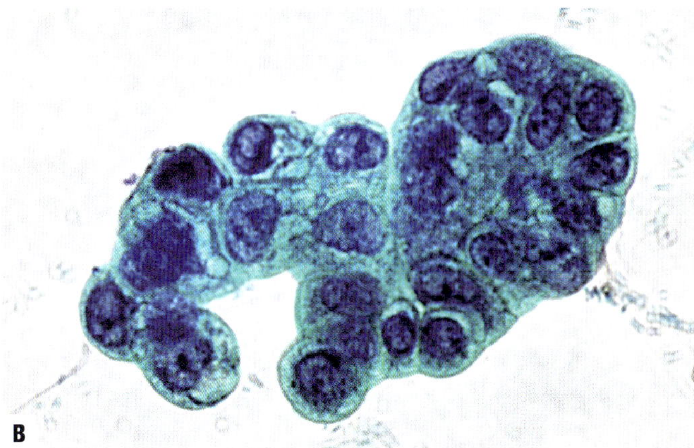

Fig. 6.02 Low-grade biliary intraepithelial neoplasia. **A** Bile duct exfoliative cytopathology shows a micropapillary epithelial tissue fragment with mildly increased N:C ratio and mucin production (liquid-based cytopathology, Pap). **B** Bile duct exfoliative cytopathology from a 37-year-old man with IgG4-related sclerosing cholangitis. An atypical epithelial tissue fragment with mildly increased N:C ratio and mildly irregular nuclear membranes (liquid-based cytopathology, Pap).

or nuclear expression of S100 can be observed in BilIN-low but not in reactive biliary epithelium {378,19}.

Aneuploidy detected by FISH probes targeting chromosomes 3, 7, 9p21, and 17 or the pancreaticobiliary-specific FISH probe directed against chromosomes 1q21, 7p12, 8q24, and 9p21 suggests high-grade BilIN (BilIN-high) or malignancy rather than BilIN-low {54}.

KRAS sequencing does not assist in the differential diagnosis between BilIN-low and BilIN-high or malignancy {326}.

These ancillary tests help to define a low-risk and high-risk ductal lesion but are not specific for a diagnosis of BilIN.

Pancreatic intraductal papillary mucinous neoplasm, low-grade

Cai G
Pitman MB
Sigel C

Definition

Low-grade pancreatic intraductal papillary mucinous neoplasm (IPMN) is a mucin-producing epithelial neoplasm of the main and/or branch ducts of the pancreas with low-grade dysplasia.

Clinical features and imaging

Low-grade IPMNs constitute approximately 40% and 80% of main duct and branch duct IPMNs, respectively {156}. CT and endoscopic imaging show multiloculated cysts that may be seen connecting to the main pancreatic duct {80}. Compared with high-grade IPMN, low-grade IPMN occurs in younger patients (with an average age 5 years younger), is asymptomatic, and is less likely to present with high-risk stigmata as described by the Fukuoka guidelines {839,798}. Progression to invasive carcinoma is slow, requiring many years {717,473}. Because most cases of branch duct IPMN are low-grade and found in elderly patients with comorbid conditions, conservative, observational management is preferred over surgical resection, making cytopathological distinction between low- and high-grade IPMN essential for patient care.

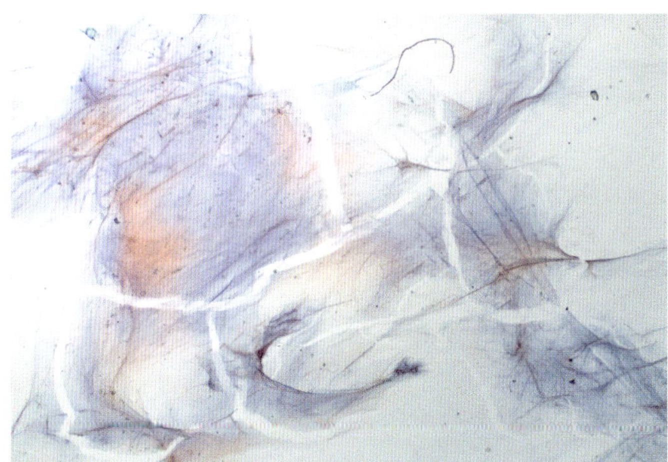

Fig. 6.03 Mucinous cyst NOS, low-grade. Even if acellular, the presence of thick, colloid-like mucin supports the diagnosis of a neoplastic mucinous cyst. Clinical and imaging information can help to add specificity to the diagnosis. Although no epithelium is present to grade the cyst, such an FNAB should be categorized as low-grade, with a caveat stating that correlation with imaging is required (Pap).

Histopathology

Low-grade IPMNs are characterized as an intraductal proliferation of columnar mucinous epithelium with mild to moderate cytoarchitectural atypia, lining cystically dilated ducts with or without intraductal papillae. Low-grade neoplasms typically consist of gastric and/or intestinal-type epithelium {60,910}.

Key diagnostic cytopathological features

- Generally low cellularity
- Mucin, thick or thin, and often acellular or with histiocytes and scant epithelium
- Columnar epithelial cells about the size of a duodenal enterocyte in small tissue fragments, which may be papillary or occur as single cells
- Polarized nuclei, which are evenly spaced to mildly crowded with mild atypia, or pseudostratified and crowded with moderate atypia
- Intranuclear inclusions may be seen
- Moderate to abundant cytoplasmic mucin
- Round to ovoid nuclei with mild to moderate nuclear enlargement and atypia but generally smooth nuclear membranes
- Even chromatin

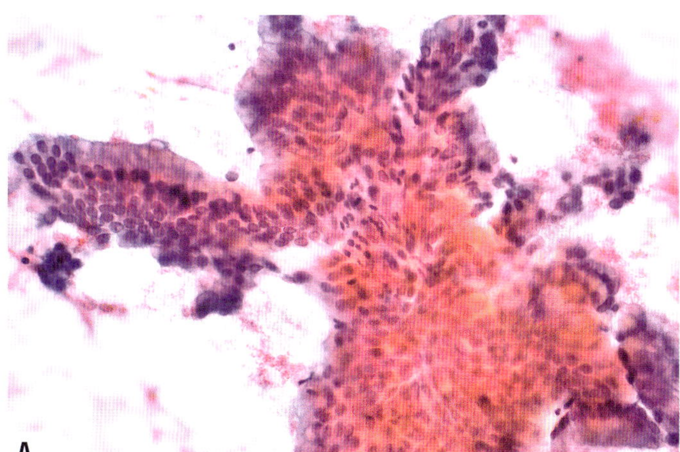

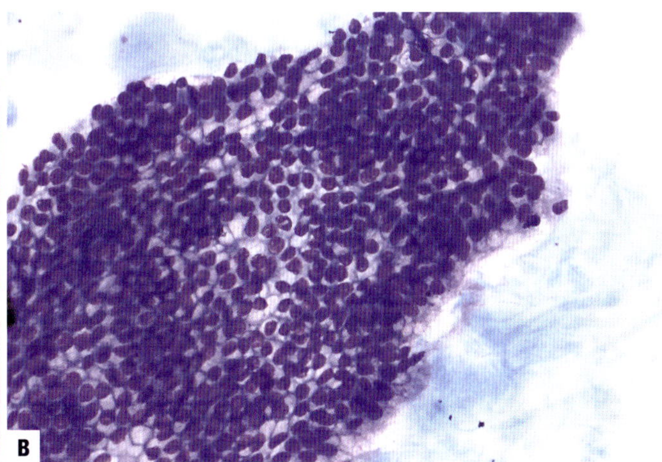

Fig. 6.04 Low-grade intraductal papillary mucinous neoplasm. **A** An irregular tissue fragment of slightly disorganized gastric-type epithelial cells with crowded nuclei, nuclear membrane irregularities, evenly distributed chromatin, and small nucleoli (Pap). **B** Tissue fragment of gastric-type epithelial cells with mildly crowded nuclei and apical mucin caps seen best at the tissue fragment edge (Giemsa).

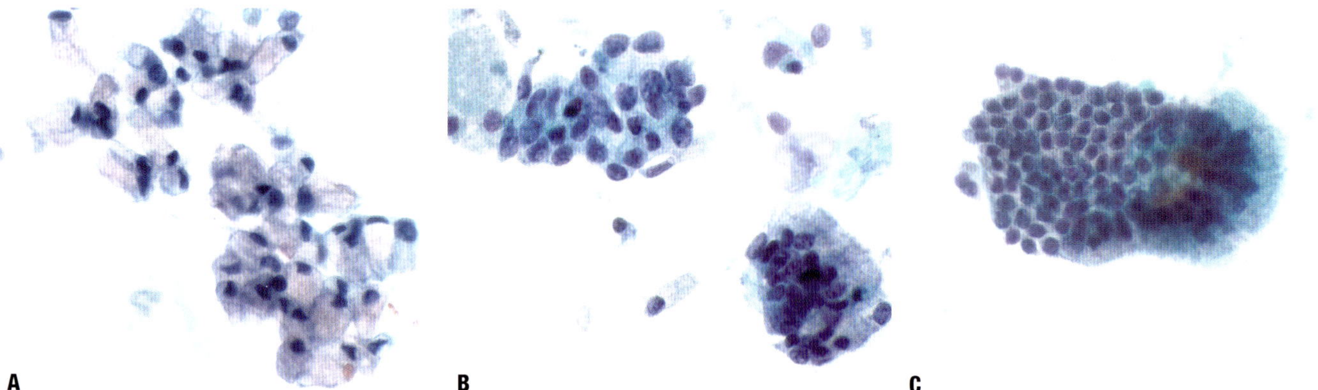

Fig. 6.05 Low-grade intraductal papillary mucinous neoplasm. **A** Discohesive tissue fragments of irregularly arranged columnar cells with low N:C ratios; abundant faintly pink mucinous cytoplasm that fills the cytoplasm; and relatively small, pleomorphic, occasionally indented hyperchromatic nuclei with few nucleoli (Pap). **B** Columnar glandular epithelium in small tissue fragments, which show a columnar arrangement, with crowded, moderately atypical, overlapping nuclei but abundant mucinous cytoplasm, is consistent with intermediate (low-grade) dysplasia (liquid-based cytopathology, Pap). **C** Mucinous glandular epithelium, regularly arranged in a honeycomb-like sheet, with uniform nuclei and abundant cytoplasmic mucin that fills the cytoplasmic space, seen particularly at the right edge of the sheet, supports a low-grade mucinous cyst (liquid-based cytopathology, Pap).

- Absent or inconspicuous nucleoli
- Absent or scant background necrosis

Reference(s): {543,477}

Discussion and differential diagnosis

The primary differential diagnosis for low-grade IPMN is gastrointestinal contamination. Mucin that is thick, copious, and colloid-like is diagnostic of a mucinous neoplasm even without mucinous epithelium {253}. Thin, wispy mucin or mucin attenuated in liquid-based preparations may be difficult to distinguish from fibrin or gastrointestinal mucin contaminant. The epithelial cells of low-grade IPMN are of a similar size to duodenal enterocytes and may contain apical cytoplasmic mucin, which is nearly identical to gastric foveolar epithelium {645}. The presence of intranuclear inclusions is reported to be a specific feature in support of IPMN on gastrointestinal contamination {477}. The presence of an apical mucin cup in the upper third of the columnar cytoplasm or stripped naked nuclei in thin extracellular mucin favours gastric contamination. When a cyst is classified as mucinous on the basis of extracellular mucin or elevated CEA (> 192 ng/mL) and mucinous epithelium is absent, the cyst should be categorized as low-grade with a caveat in a comment/note stating that point and stating that correlation with imaging is required.

Features supporting a neoplasm include irregularly spaced nuclei, mild nuclear enlargement, and papillary fragments. Low-grade IPMN with moderate atypia may be more readily distinguishable from gastrointestinal contaminants due to pseudostratification, nuclear crowding, focal loss of polarity, a higher N:C ratio, and diminished cytoplasmic mucin. Distinction of intermediate-grade atypia from high-grade atypia is often difficult but is important, because this distinction determines patient management {645}. When in doubt, categorize as low-grade and raise the question of the possibility of a higher-grade lesion in a comment or note.

Low-grade IPMNs are not readily distinguished from low-grade mucinous cystic neoplasms. Subepithelial ovarian-type stroma is very rarely sampled with FNAB and aspiration of cyst fluid alone. Microforceps biopsy before cyst aspiration may be able to sample the subepithelial-type stroma {982}.

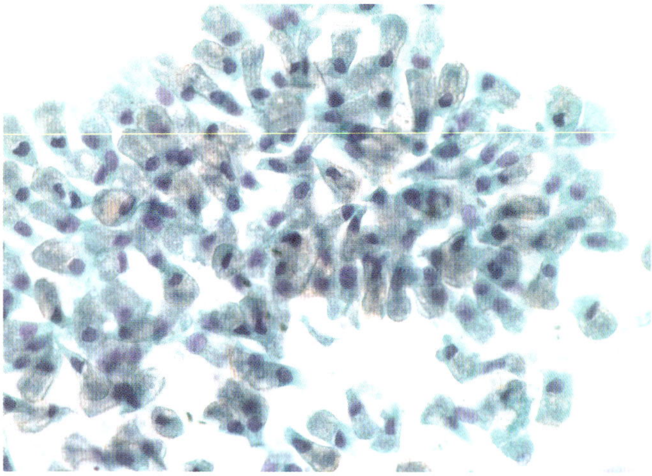

Fig. 6.06 Gastric contaminant. Gastric contaminant shows uniform gastric foveolar epithelial cells that may be discohesive or in loosely cohesive tissue fragments. Note the irregularity of cytoplasmic mucin, often confined to the upper third of the cytoplasmic column (Pap).

Ancillary testing

Ancillary tests are often critical for the diagnosis of a low-grade IPMN, because of the paucicellularity and thin mucin of most branch duct IPMNs. A cyst fluid CEA level of > 192 ng/mL is approximately 80% accurate for a mucin-producing neoplasm {91} and has been shown to be the best test for classifying a cyst as mucinous {140}. The use of mucin stains, including mucicarmine and Alcian blue pH 2.5, can also be used to confirm the presence of extracellular mucin, but these stains must be interpreted with caution, because both mucicarmine and Alcian blue stains have been demonstrated to label mucin trapped in pseudocysts {253}. ICC is not helpful in the distinction of cyst-lining epithelial cells from gastrointestinal contamination {910}.

Single-gene and targeted molecular-based assays performed on cyst fluid or supernatant material can identify mutations correlating with mucinous neoplasia, such as *KRAS*, *GNAS*, and *RNF43* mutations, which are seen in as many as 75%, 60%, and 70% of IPMNs, respectively {925,926}.

Intraductal papillary neoplasm of the bile duct, low-grade

Cai G
Sigel C

Definition

Low-grade intraductal papillary neoplasm (IPN) of the bile duct is a grossly visible premalignant epithelial neoplasm with intraductal papillary or villous growth, mucin production, and low-grade dysplasia.

Clinical features and imaging

Low-grade IPNs of the bile duct account for about 10% of all IPNs. They are more likely to involve intrahepatic ducts and are associated with mucin supersecretion {441,583,584}. Imaging studies show the filling defect in the biliary duct often associated with dilatation of the proximal duct due to obstruction from a polypoid tumour and/or mucin secretion {624,39}.

Histopathology

Low-grade IPNs show prominent papillary architecture, with fine fibrovascular cores lined by biliary epithelium {582,624}. Tubular or glandular formation may be focally present. Low-grade IPNs often demonstrate intestinal and/or gastric-type differentiation with mild to intermediate cytoarchitectural atypia, which consists of nuclear enlargement and nuclear stratification while maintaining a relatively low N:C ratio, absence of nuclear pleomorphism, and preservation of polarity {583,765,910}.

Key diagnostic cytopathological features

- Epithelial cells arranged in flat sheets, tubules, and papillary tissue fragments
- Variable amount of background mucin with possible acute or mixed inflammation
- Cuboidal or columnar cells that may contain intracytoplasmic mucin and exhibit intestinal or gastric epithelial differentiation
- Oval nuclei with mild nuclear membrane irregularities, fine chromatin, and inconspicuous nucleoli
- Necrosis usually absent

Discussion and differential diagnosis

Because of the rarity of this neoplasm, the cytomorphological criteria for IPN are not well established and, in part, are extrapolated from its counterpart in the pancreas {97,858,643}.

IPN with moderate atypia can show nuclear enlargement and nuclear stratification and should be differentiated from high-grade IPN. Other differential diagnoses include reactive bile duct epithelial hyperplasia, biliary intraepithelial neoplasia, metastases, and colonization (cancerization of the duct) by adjacent tumours.

Ancillary testing

Neoplastic cells show a variety of mucin core protein expression profiles, which are dependent on epithelial differentiation. Gastric-type epithelial cells frequently express MUC5A and MUC6, whereas intestinal epithelial cells show positive staining for MUC2 {582}. The clinical utility of ancillary testing is yet to be validated {33,583}.

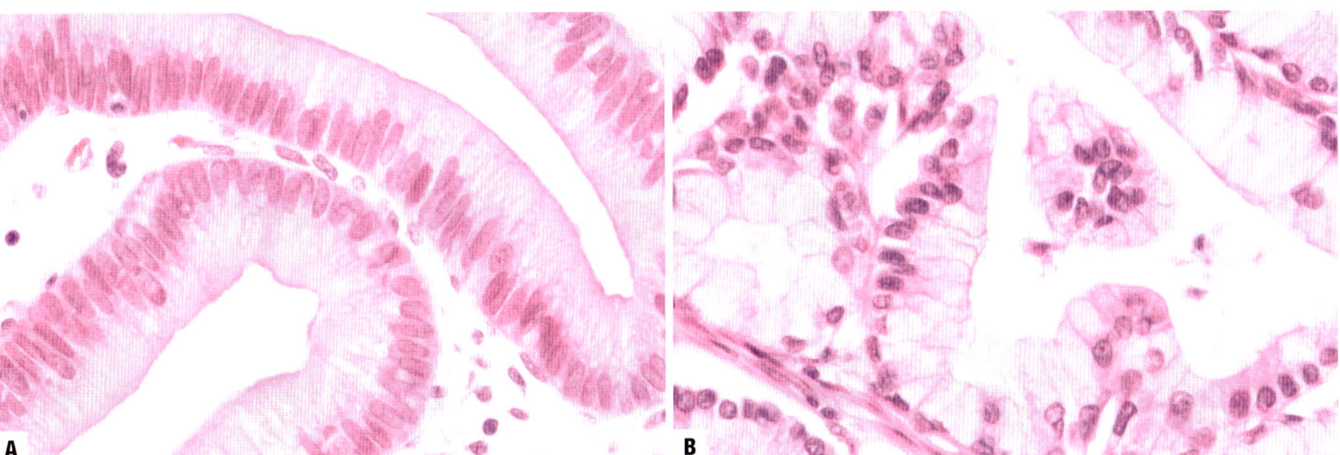

Fig. 6.07 Intraductal papillary neoplasm of the bile duct. **A** Low-grade epithelium of intestinal type with basally located, slightly elongated nuclei and mild nuclear atypia without copious cytoplasmic mucin (formalin-fixed, paraffin-embedded tissue; H&E). **B** Low-grade epithelium of gastric type shows basally located round nuclei with mild nuclear atypia and abundant cytoplasmic mucin (formalin-fixed, paraffin-embedded tissue; H&E).

Mucinous cystic neoplasm, low-grade

Cai G
Stelow EB

Definition

Low-grade mucinous cystic neoplasm (MCN) is a cyst-forming and mucin-producing epithelial neoplasm with distinctive ovarian-like subepithelial stroma and low-grade dysplasia.

Clinical features and imaging

Low-grade MCN almost exclusively occurs in middle-aged women and predominantly involves the body or tail of the pancreas or the intrahepatic biliary system. Imaging studies show a multiloculated, thick-walled cystic lesion without connection to the pancreatic duct or biliary duct {433,940}. The features suggestive of invasive carcinoma, such as irregular thickening of the cyst wall and intracystic mural nodules, are absent {351}.

Histopathology

MCNs arising in the pancreas and hepatobiliary duct system share the same histopathological features. The tumours are multilocular cysts lined by epithelium and underlying ovarian-type stroma. The lining cells are predominantly columnar mucin-producing cells, although non-mucinous cuboidal cells can be seen in as many as 50% of MCNs arising in the hepatobiliary system {984}. Attenuation of the epithelium from pressure can also diminish the cytoplasmic mucin and reduce the cyst-lining epithelium to flat to cuboidal non-mucinous cells. Erosion of the lining is also not uncommon. Low-grade MCNs show mild to moderate cytoarchitectural atypia without complex papillary projections or severe cytopathological atypia {324}. The presence of ovarian-like stroma is required for the diagnosis, which is characterized by densely packed spindle-shaped cells with round or elongated nuclei and scant cytoplasm.

Key diagnostic cytopathological features

- Usually low cellularity
- Variable amount of thin or thick mucin with histiocytes
- Bland or mildly atypical epithelial cells in small sheets and tissue fragments or singly
- Columnar or cuboidal cells that may or may not contain cytoplasmic mucin
- Round or oval nuclei with smooth or mildly irregular nuclear membranes, evenly distributed chromatin, and inconspicuous nucleoli
- Background coagulative-type necrosis is absent, but erosion can cause the cyst fluid to be inflammatory with degenerated cells

Reference(s): {748}

Discussion and differential diagnosis

A variable amount of background mucin and sparse mucin-containing columnar cells are the classic cytopathological findings, which along with the imaging finding of a multiloculated, thick-walled cyst in the body or tail of the pancreas in a middle-aged woman support the diagnosis of MCN {649,244, 748}. In cases with no or scant mucin identified, a high CEA level (≥ 192 ng/mL) in cyst fluid supports the diagnosis of a mucinous cyst {91}. MCNs share similar cytopathological features with intraductal papillary mucinous neoplasms (IPMNs), especially side-branch IPMN, and distinction between the two is difficult if not impossible in the absence of ovarian-like stroma; thus, it is acceptable to render a cytopathological diagnosis of "neoplastic mucinous cyst", to include MCN and IPMN, in the differential diagnosis {14}. The use of microforceps biopsy that obtains a bite of the cyst wall can help make a specific diagnosis of MCN by obtaining a tissue sample demonstrating the ovarian-type stroma {982}.

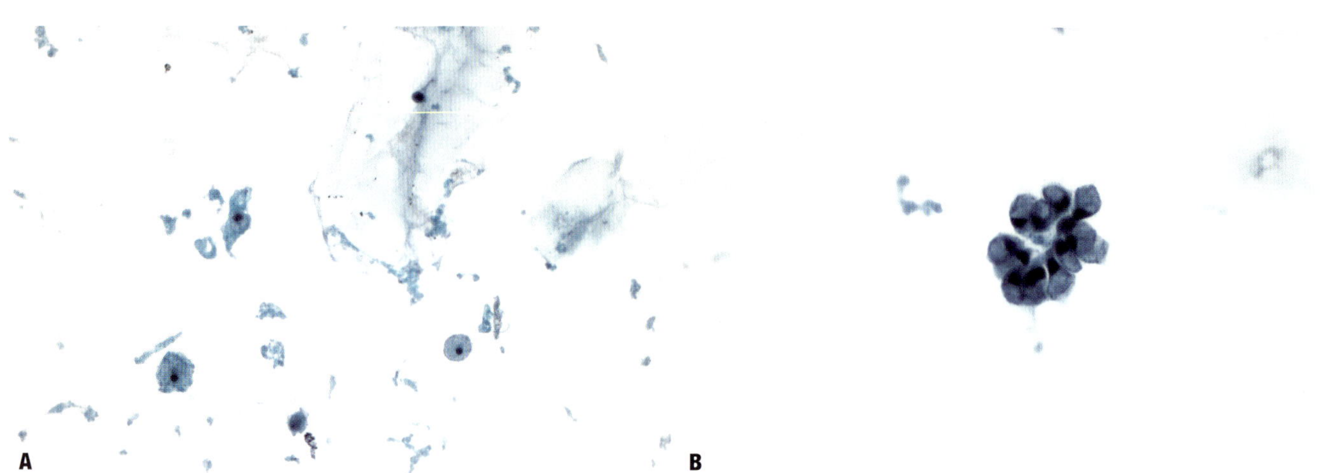

Fig. 6.08 Mucinous cystic neoplasm, low-grade. **A** Extracellular mucin, somewhat attenuated due to liquid-based cytopathology processing, with scattered histiocytes (liquid-based cytopathology, Pap). **B** A small discohesive tissue fragment of uniform mucinous epithelial cells with apical mucin (liquid-based cytopathology, Pap).

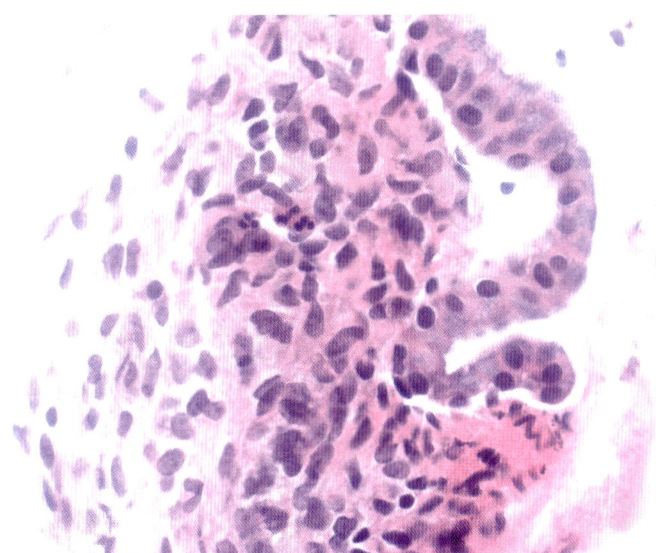

Fig. 6.09 Mucinous cystic neoplasm, low-grade. A microforceps biopsy highlights the subepithelial ovarian-type stroma (left), allowing for a specific diagnosis of mucinous cystic neoplasm. Note the attenuation of the cytoplasmic mucin (right) (H&E).

It is critically important to differentiate low-grade MCN from high-grade MCN. The FNAB material should be carefully examined to assess the degree of cytoarchitectural atypia, although it is well known that high-grade atypia can be underrepresented in the FNAB of MCN {308,644,244}. MCN may undergo substantial degenerative changes and mucin-producing cells may be absent, making it difficult to distinguish from a pseudocyst {344,2}. Other entities in the differential diagnosis include serous cystadenoma, lymphoepithelial cyst, and secondary dilatation of the duct due to proximal obstruction {815}.

Ancillary testing

Cyst fluid chemical analysis is helpful in the differential diagnosis between MCN and a non-mucinous cyst, including pseudocysts. A high CEA level (≥ 192 ng/mL) supports a mucinous cyst, whereas a low amylase level (< 250 U/L) helps to exclude a pseudocyst {91,605}. Elevated pancreatic cyst fluid levels of amylase cannot be used to differentiate IPMN from MCN {848}. In a prospective study, IPMN and MCN showed a range of amylase levels from 0 to 280 000 U/L {635}.

Molecular testing may have a potential role in the diagnosis of low-grade MCN. MCNs harbour *KRAS* mutations; however, *KRAS* mutations are identified in only a small subset of low-grade MCNs {654,923}. Other gene alterations such as *TP53* and *SMAD4* mutations are absent in low-grade cysts. Identification of *GNAS* mutation supports the diagnosis of IPMN {926,789}.

Other lesions (including spindle cell tumours)

Stelow EB
Fabre M

The diagnostic category "Pancreaticobiliary neoplasm, low-risk/grade (PaN-low)" can be used for FNAB of uncommon bland spindle cell neoplasms and other uncommon tumours for which a definitive and specific diagnosis cannot be made but for which a benign diagnosis is expected. Such cases may include but are not limited to FNAB of schwannomas, neurofibromas, lipomas, leiomyomas, paragangliomas, fibromatosis, haemangiomas, and lymphangiomas. FNAB of such lesions may show very scant, bland spindle cells with or without fat. Without ancillary testing, however, a definitive and specific diagnosis of one of these lesions may be impossible. For example, S100 expression would need to be shown to diagnose a schwannoma, and further ICC, such as MUC4, may be needed to exclude bland spindle cell malignancies such as low-grade fibromyxoid sarcoma. MDM2 testing may be necessary to show a lack of amplification before definitively categorizing a bland fatty lesion of the pancreas as "Benign".

Sample reports: Pancreaticobiliary neoplasm, low-risk/grade

Cai G
Sigel C
Tanaka M

Sample report 1

Nature of specimen: FNAB of multilocular cyst in the tail of pancreas.
Specimen adequacy: Satisfactory for evaluation.
Category: Pancreaticobiliary neoplasm, low-risk/grade (PaN-low).
Diagnosis: Low-grade neoplastic mucinous cyst. See comment.
Comment: The specimen is mildly cellular, showing mildly atypical mucinous epithelium, extracellular mucin, and histiocytes. The differential diagnosis includes low-grade intraductal papillary mucinous neoplasm and low-grade mucinous cystic neoplasm. Correlation with imaging is required.

Sample report 2

Nature of specimen: FNAB of a unilocular cyst in the head of pancreas.
Specimen adequacy: Evaluation is limited by absence of cyst-lining epithelium.
Category: Pancreaticobiliary neoplasm, low-risk/grade (PaN-low).
Diagnosis: Thick, colloid-like extracellular mucin consistent with a neoplastic mucinous cyst. See comment.
Comment: A mucinous etiology is based on the quality and quantity of extracellular mucin, which is inconsistent with gastrointestinal contamination. Grade is indeterminate because of the absence of neoplastic epithelium, but high-grade epithelial atypia is absent, as is background necrosis. Correlation with imaging features required.

Sample report 3

Nature of specimen: FNAB of a cyst in the body of the pancreas.
Specimen adequacy: Evaluation is limited by absence of cyst-lining epithelium.
Category: Pancreaticobiliary neoplasm, low-risk/grade (PaN-low).
Diagnosis: Neoplastic mucinous cyst, based on elevated cyst fluid CEA (568 ng/mL). See comment.
Comment: The specimen is acellular, showing thin extracellular mucin and elevated cyst fluid CEA (568 ng/mL), findings consistent with a neoplastic mucinous cyst. Amylase is 1034 U/L. Grade is indeterminate because of the absence of neoplastic epithelium, but high-grade epithelial atypia is absent, as is background necrosis. Correlation with imaging features required. Molecular analysis is pending and may be informative.

Sample report 4

Nature of specimen: FNAB of a cyst in the head of the pancreas.
Specimen adequacy: Evaluation is limited by scant cellularity.
Category: Pancreaticobiliary neoplasm, low-risk/grade (PaN-low).
Diagnosis: Low-grade neoplastic mucinous cyst. See comment.
Comment: The specimen is mildly cellular, showing bland mucinous glandular cells and thin, watery extracellular mucoid cyst fluid. Concurrent cyst fluid analysis shows an elevated CEA level (≥ 192 ng/mL). There is scant bland gastric-type epithelium with mild atypia, favoured to be cyst-lining epithelium in this transduodenal FNAB. High-grade epithelial atypia is not present, nor is background necrosis.

Sample report 5

Nature of specimen: FNAB of multicystic mass in head of pancreas.

Diagnostic summary:
Category: Pancreaticobiliary neoplasm, low-risk/grade (PaN-low).
Diagnosis: Low-grade neoplastic mucinous cyst. See microscopic description.

Microscopic description: The specimen is highly cellular, showing papillary tissue fragments of mild to moderately atypical mucinous epithelial cells and background extracellular mucin. Features of high-grade atypia are not identified, and background necrosis is absent. The findings support a low-grade (low- to intermediate-grade) intraductal papillary mucinous neoplasm.

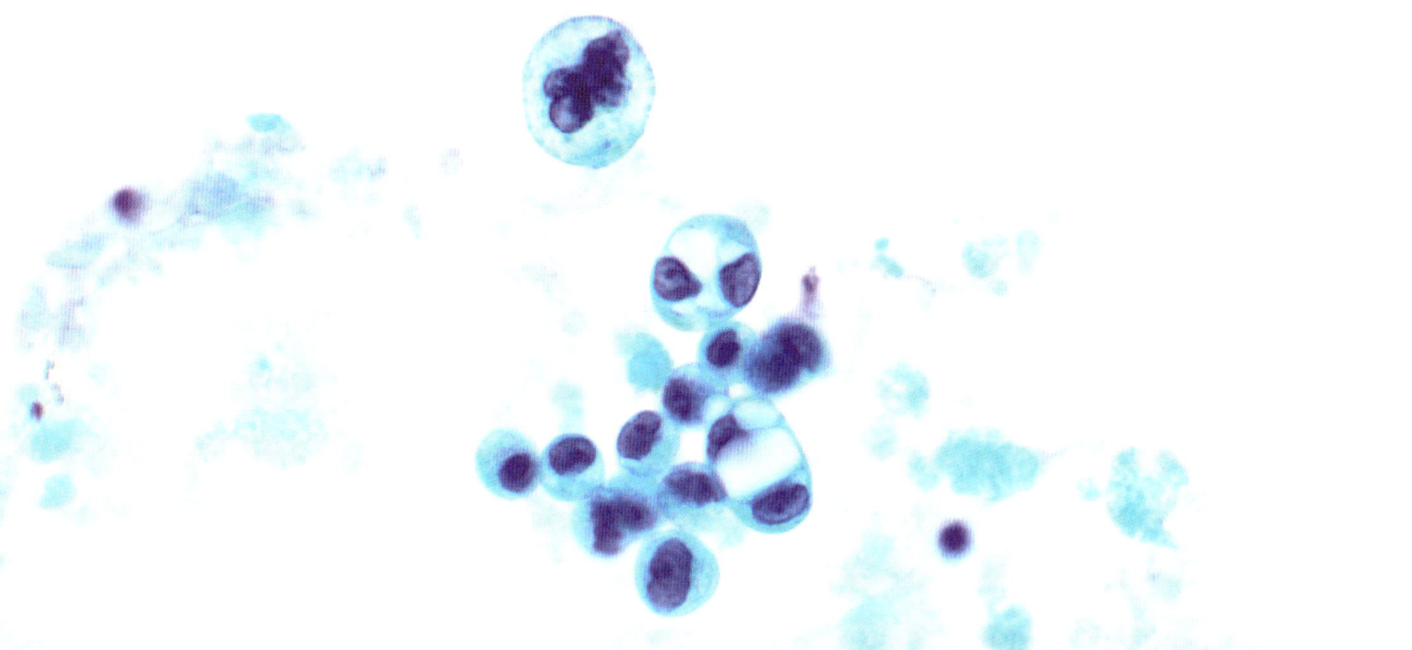

7

Diagnostic category: Pancreaticobiliary neoplasm, high-risk/grade

Edited by: Centeno BA, Reid MD

Introduction

Pitman MB
Centeno BA

The category "Pancreaticobiliary neoplasm, high-risk/grade (PaN-high)" has been extracted from the "Neoplastic: other" category of the Papanicolaou Society of Cytopathology (PSC) System for Reporting Pancreaticobiliary Cytology {642}, which included intraductal papillary mucinous neoplasm and mucinous cystic neoplasm, as well as the low-grade malignancies pancreatic neuroendocrine tumour (PanNET) and solid pseudopapillary neoplasm. Maintaining alignment with the WHO classification of tumours of the digestive system, this new category is now limited to intraductal and cystic neoplasms with high-grade epithelial atypia encompassing features of high-grade dysplasia, and it may include some cysts with invasive carcinoma. Because cytopathological atypia can be difficult to classify with great accuracy even among experts in the field {645}, and because the intermediate-grade dysplasia of intraductal and cystic lesions is histopathologically classified as "low-grade" and greatly overlaps morphologically with that of high-grade atypia {645}, using this category rather than "Suspicious for malignancy" for these lesions provides a more flexible and less anxious patient management paradigm than "Suspicious for malignancy", particularly when conservative patient management is recommended.

Definition

Pitman MB
Centeno BA

A specimen categorized as "Pancreaticobiliary neoplasm, high-risk/grade (PaN-high)" has features of an intraductal and/or cystic neoplasm with high-grade epithelial atypia.

Discussion and background

Pitman MB
Centeno BA
Klapman J

Cytopathology is the best test for the detection of invasive carcinoma, because CEA does not correlate with grade {140} and molecular analysis is not yet the standard of care in the evaluation of cyst fluids. Therefore, outside of high-risk imaging, it is the detection of high-grade epithelial atypia that signifies a cyst with a high risk of malignancy, harbouring either high-grade dysplasia or possibly invasive carcinoma.

High-grade epithelial atypia has a sensitivity of 89% and a specificity of 98% for detecting a high-risk cyst {308}. High-grade epithelial atypia is defined as a cell smaller than a 12 µm duodenal enterocyte with a high N:C ratio and abnormal chromatin, which can be hypochromatic or hyperchromatic, with or without a background of cellular necrosis. With these criteria, there is overall good interobserver variability in distinguishing low-risk/grade from high-risk/grade cysts {644,652,543,257,645}. However, with the addition of intermediate-grade dysplasia in the low-grade group, it is virtually impossible to accurately stratify cysts with intermediate-grade dysplasia into low- and high-risk groups, making the addition of genetic testing very important in accurately identifying high-risk cysts {257}.

Genetic analysis can contribute to the assessment of risk by detecting mutations, which occur late in the progression to malignancy, including the *TP53* mutation and deletions in *CDKN2A* (*P16*) and *SMAD4* {700,549,454,809}. Mutations in *PIK3CA* and *PTEN* equivalent to *KRAS* or *GNAS* are sensitive and specific for intraductal papillary mucinous neoplasm (IPMN) with either high-grade dysplasia or invasive carcinoma {787}. Low level of mutations of *PTEN*, *PIK3CA*, and *TP53* in low-grade IPMN may indicate a risk for transformation to high-grade {787}. Mutant allele frequencies of > 55% for *GNAS* correlate with high-grade IPMN {787}.

The differential diagnosis of high-grade epithelial atypia includes cyst fluid with small cyst-lining cells, singly or in tissue fragments, with a high N:C ratio and nuclear atypia that can be variable. The primary lesions in the differential diagnosis of a branch duct IPMN include a low-grade IPMN with intermediate-grade dysplasia {257}, cystic neuroendocrine tumour (NET) {562}, and cystic acinar cell cystadenoma with transformation {123}. Distinction between these lesions is reliant on cells in a cell block for ICC or fresh cyst fluid for genetic analysis (see *Pancreatic intraductal papillary mucinous neoplasm, high-grade*, p. 101, for additional information).

Risk of malignancy and management recommendations

Pitman MB
Centeno BA
Klapman J

The estimated risk of malignancy of the "Pancreaticobiliary neoplasm, high-risk/grade (PaN-high)" category is 60–95% {306, 792,307,824}. Surgically fit patients should be considered for surgical resection; however, conservative observation is a reasonable option where the risk of surgery is high and especially if the imaging features do not show high-risk features. Patient management decisions are based on the risk of malignancy relative to the risk of surgery. Current guidelines are largely based on imaging features {838,839,204,878,537}. High-risk imaging features include obstructive jaundice in a patient with a cyst in the pancreatic head and an enhancing solid component within a cyst or a main pancreatic duct > 10 mm. The presence of any of these high-risk features will lead to surgical intervention in a surgically fit patient without a preoperative diagnosis. Worrisome features warranting further evaluation with an EUS-FNAB include a cyst > 30 mm, thickened or enhanced cyst walls, a main pancreatic duct 5–9 mm, a non-enhancing mural nodule, or an abrupt change in the calibre of the pancreatic duct with distal pancreatic atrophy. A cytopathology report with a "PaN-high" categorization should also be considered a high-risk test result, warranting surgical resection {838,839,204,878,537}.

There is no current risk of malignancy for this category in bile duct brushings. The use of this category in bile duct brushing remains to be determined. The "Suspicious for malignancy" category will probably be used instead, given the lack of cytological criteria for intraductal lesions with high-grade dysplasia.

Pancreatic intraepithelial neoplasia, high-grade

HooKim K
Avadhani V
Fukushima N

Definition

High-grade pancreatic intraepithelial neoplasia (HG-PanIN) is defined as a < 5 mm, non-invasive, flat or micropapillary, mucinous epithelial neoplasia with severe atypia confined to the pancreatic ducts.

Clinical features and imaging

The prevalence of pancreatic intraepithelial neoplasia with severe dysplasia (HG-PanIN) is unknown, because patients are usually asymptomatic and lesions are not visible on imaging. Most studies on HG-PanIN represent case reports and small series {939,750,706}. Diagnosis is usually made on resection specimens. Imaging features predictive of progression include a solid mass, cyst, or duct changes {98}. An autopsy study suggested an association with cystic changes and fibrosis on ultrasound {528}.

Histopathology

HG-PanIN is a non–mass-forming microscopic pancreatic intraductal lesion that is by definition < 5 mm in diameter and is lined by flattened, tufted, papillary, micropapillary, or cribriform mucinous epithelium with severe cytoarchitectural atypia. This includes nuclear crowding, loss of polarity, high N:C ratio, nuclear pleomorphism, variable chromatin, and irregular nuclear membranes. Prominent nucleoli and abnormal mitotic figures may be seen {324}.

Key diagnostic cytopathological features

- Mildly to scantly cellular ductal component in a background of benign acinar tissue
- Compact ductal sheets and small, tight papillary tissue fragments without fibrovascular cores
- Cells are small with a high N:C ratio, dense cytoplasm, distinct cytoplasmic borders, and central nuclei
- Nuclear crowding with moderate nuclear atypia and small monomorphic nuclei (~10 μm), although rare cells with large nuclei measuring > 15 μm may be seen
- Focal nuclear membrane irregularity and hyperchromasia, but chromatin clearing may also be seen
- Occasional nucleoli
- Focal or no cellular discohesion
- Marked anisonucleosis and nuclear moulding are absent or limited to two or three tissue fragments per slide, i.e. < 12 fragments, or are absent on Pap-stained smears
- Clean background showing no significant necrosis, cystic change, cellular discohesion, pleomorphism, or abundant colloid-like mucin

Reference(s): {280,279,353}

Discussion and differential diagnosis

HG-PanIN has no distinctive diagnostic cytopathological features but instead shows features that overlap with those of reactive atypia, other high-risk precursor mucinous lesions, and pancreatic ductal adenocarcinoma (PDAC). The differential diagnoses include chronic pancreatitis, low-grade (including intermediate-grade) pancreatic intraepithelial neoplasia (LG-PanIN), intraductal papillary mucinous neoplasm with high-grade dysplasia, and PDAC.

In chronic pancreatitis, benign and reactive ductal cells and acini with a lymphoid predominant inflammatory infiltrate are seen. Ductal epithelium may show mild cytopathological atypia compatible with reactive change {68,353}. LG-PanIN with intermediate-grade dysplasia is flat or papillary with pseudostratified nuclei and moderate cytopathological atypia

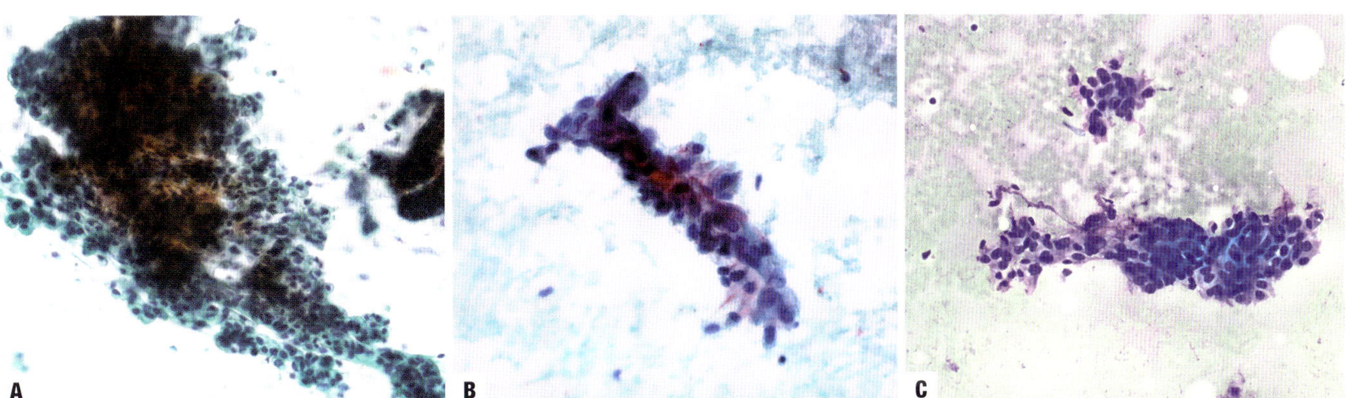

Fig. 7.01 Pancreatic intraepithelial neoplasia, high-grade. **A** Pancreatic juice cytology. Intact large and small groups of high-grade pancreatic intraepithelial neoplasia cells arranged as papillary-cohesive tissue fragments. The cytoplasm is dense to clear and there is mild anisonucleosis. The hyperchromatic nuclei are relatively centrally located and moderately overlapped (Pap). **B** Rare atypical crowded papillary tissue fragment without a fibrovascular core, with overlapping, hyperchromatic nuclei and mucinous cytoplasm (Pap). **C** Tissue fragments show architectural disorder with irregularly spaced cells with abundant cytoplasm that is columnar at the edges of the tissue fragments, focally distinct cell borders, and mildly atypical nuclei. There is mild to moderate nuclear enlargement and anisonucleosis (Giemsa).

{60}. Marked architectural alterations are absent and mitoses are rare {353}. Intraductal papillary mucinous neoplasms with high-grade dysplasia are recognizable on imaging, whereas HG-PanIN lesions are invisible or may rarely be associated with secondary peripheral pancreatic parenchymal atrophy {279,957}. It may be cytopathologically impossible to distinguish these two lesions, especially intraductal papillary mucinous neoplasm with intestinal or pancreaticobiliary phenotype {279}. The distinction of HG-PanIN from PDAC is difficult, particularly if HG-PanIN is extensive. Correlation with imaging is important because PDAC will show a mass on imaging. Generally, PDAC has more cellularity with more overt features of malignancy {279,353}.

Ancillary testing

Ancillary studies may aid the management of indeterminate cases {655}. Molecular aberrations and abnormal biomarker expression increase with PanIN grade. Studies also demonstrate a biological continuum between HG-PanIN and PDAC {210}. HG-PanIN is associated with accumulation of genetic alterations, starting from telomere shortening, *KRAS* mutations, and *CDKN2A* mutations (p16 loss), and later on *TP53* and *SMAD4* alterations {320,869, 567}. The presence of late mutations is specific for high-grade dysplasia or malignancy. Like PDAC, HG-PanIN may also show abnormal p53 protein expression (16–57%), complete loss of SMAD4 (28%), positivity for S100P (41–100%) and maspin (78%), loss of VHL protein, and increased Ki-67 staining {320,513,492, 23,189,508}. FISH studies on PanIN have also detected chromosomal copy-number losses and gains, *KRAS* point mutations, and telomere shortening {312,869}.

Biliary intraepithelial neoplasia, high-grade

Zen Y
Clayton A
Stelow EB

Definition

Biliary intraepithelial neoplasia, high-grade (BilIN-high) is defined as a non-invasive intraductal lesion with a flat or micropapillary architecture and severe cytopathological atypia.

Clinical features and imaging

BilIN-high typically develops in the large extrahepatic bile ducts and less frequently in the intrahepatic septal ducts, and it is uncommon in the interlobular bile ducts. It is usually found incidentally in surgical specimens resected for other reasons or in explanted livers. Most cases diagnosed in clinical practice have underlying chronic cholangiopathy such as primary sclerosing cholangitis, hepatolithiasis, liver fluke infestation, or a choledochal cyst {971,978,394}.

Because it is not mass-forming, BilIN-high cannot be identified by current imaging modalities. PET is negative in BilIN-high, but it may be weakly avid due to an underlying cholangiopathy {720}.

Histopathology

The biliary epithelium is arranged in a flat, micropapillary, or pseudopapillary architecture with foci of cellular and nuclear stratification {971}. The cells have overt dysplastic features including nuclear pleomorphism, hyperchromasia (or clearing), anisonucleosis, irregular nuclear membranes, and loss of cellular polarity. Mitotic figures including atypical forms may be identified. Intraepithelial extension into peribiliary glands is often observed and should not be mistaken for invasive malignancy. BilIN-high typically has a pancreaticobiliary-type morphology, but some cases show intestinal differentiation with brush borders and intervening goblet cells {977}.

Key diagnostic cytopathological features

- Relatively small sheets or tissue fragments of cholangiocytes, although large or 3D tissue fragments may coexist
- Tissue fragments are cohesive, and their cellularity is moderately increased with overlapping nuclei
- Nuclear enlargement, nuclear membrane irregularity, anisonucleosis, and hyperchromasia are common
- Bizarre single cells are uncommon
- Variably inflammatory background

Discussion and differential diagnosis

BilIN-high has been termed "severe biliary dysplasia", and the diagnostic term of "carcinoma in situ" is interchangeably used in some countries. A specific diagnosis of BilIN-high is not likely to be provided by cytopathology, and the categorization is usually "Atypical" or "Suspicious for malignancy". Given the fact that the difference between BilIN-high and cholangiocarcinoma depends on the presence or absence of histopathological stromal invasion, the discrimination between the two purely on the basis of cytopathological grounds is not possible, but both warrant surgical resection. Forceps biopsies that obtain subepithelial stroma may show invasive carcinoma, ruling out the diagnosis of BilIN-high. The presence of a mass lesion on imaging suggests cholangiocarcinoma rather than BilIN-high.

Significant regenerative or degenerative changes of cholangiocytes may be seen in chronic cholangiopathy, such as primary sclerosing cholangitis and hepatolithiasis, because of the inherent underlying inflammatory condition and the instrumentation from brushings and stents. The background features on brushing thus depend on the underlying cholangiopathy, and most cases have at least a focally inflammatory background, although intraepithelial neutrophils among dysplastic cells are

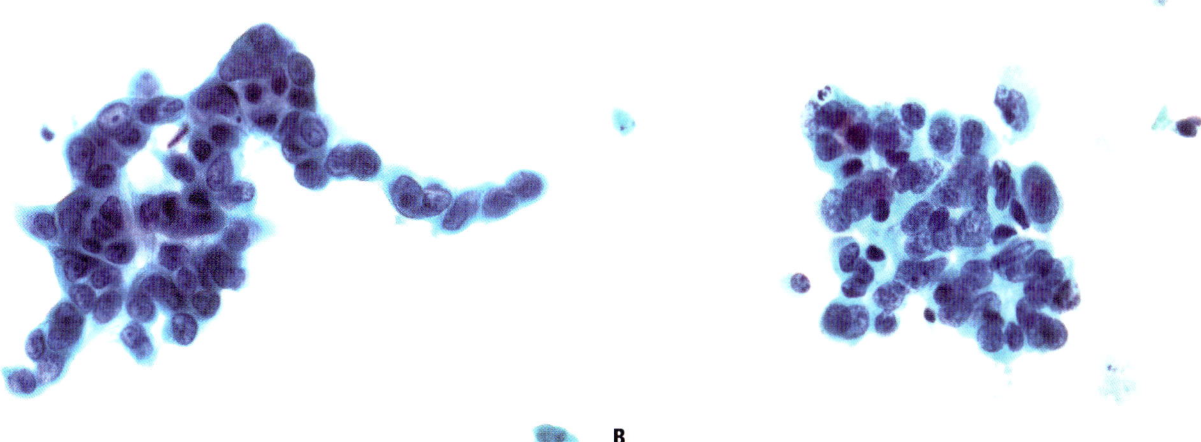

Fig. 7.02 Biliary intraepithelial neoplasia, high-grade. **A** This relatively cohesive tissue fragment shows irregularities in nuclear size and nuclear membrane (Pap). **B** This tissue fragment shows loss of polarity, crowding, irregular spacing, and high-grade nuclear atypia with high N:C ratio, coarse chromatin, and hyperchromasia (liquid-based cytopathology, Pap).

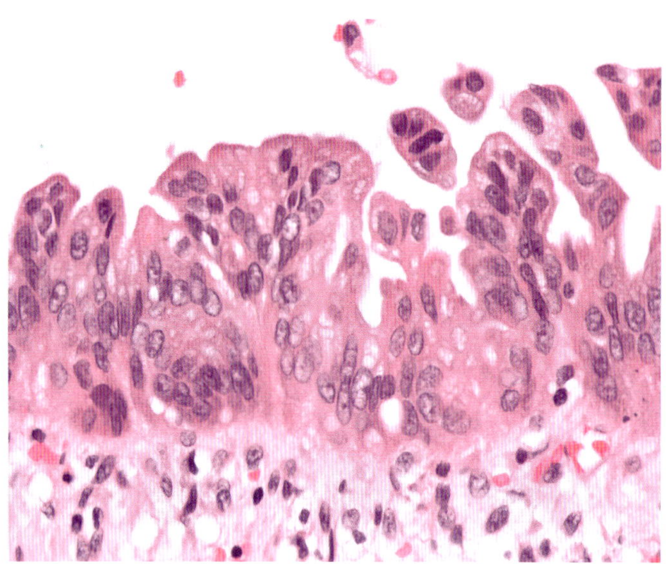

Fig. 7.03 Biliary intraepithelial neoplasia, high-grade. The cellular polarity is highly irregular, with pseudostratification and piled-up nuclei (formalin-fixed, paraffin-embedded tissue section; H&E).

less frequent than those in reactive cholangiocytes. Because of these underlying inflammatory and reactive/reparative conditions, a high threshold for the diagnosis of BilIN-high is warranted. Atypical cells with equivocal atypia often require repeat cytopathology and/or bile duct biopsy {514}.

Ancillary testing

ICC markers potentially useful for the diagnosis of BilIN-high include p53, S100P, and maspin {405}. Because diffuse p53 overexpression is seen in 10% of BilIN-high cases and 80% of invasive cholangiocarcinoma cases, diffuse p53 overexpression would favour cholangiocarcinoma {581}. S100 is usually negative or only weakly positive in reactive cholangiocytes, whereas it is overexpressed in low-grade BilIN (BilIN-low) (50%), BilIN-high (> 90%), and cholangiocarcinoma (> 90%) {19}. Likewise, maspin is negative in reactive epithelium and widely expressed in BilIN-low (30%), BilIN-high (50%), and cholangiocarcinoma (80%) {378}.

Detection of a *KRAS* mutation supports neoplasia, but mutations are identified in only 30% of BilIN-high and cholangiocarcinoma cases {330}. In patients with primary sclerosing cholangitis, FISH demonstrates aneuploidy in 10% of reactive cholangiocytes and in 80% of BilIN-high or cholangiocarcinoma cases {514}. In addition, loss of 9p21 (*CDKN2A* [*P16*]) using FISH has been identified as an additional abnormality in BilIN-high and cholangiocarcinoma from explanted livers in patients with primary sclerosing cholangitis {394}, lending support to the use of FISH for the early detection of neoplasia in the biliary tree.

Molecular testing with next-generation sequencing has been shown to be as good as FISH in detecting a high-risk stricture {192}. Routine incorporation of next-generation sequencing with bile duct brushing cytopathology improves the detection of malignancy {788}.

Pancreatic intraductal papillary mucinous neoplasm, high-grade

Pitman MB
Centeno BA
Rosenbaum MW

Definition

High-grade pancreatic intraductal papillary mucinous neoplasm (IPMN) is visible grossly on imaging and involves the main pancreatic duct and/or its branches.

Clinical features and imaging

High-grade IPMN shows increased incidence and prevalence in the elderly with increasing age and has a mean age of 62–67 years {116}. In Japan and the Republic of Korea, high-grade IPMN has a male predilection, whereas in the USA and Italy there is an almost equal sex distribution {340,743, 211}. Presenting symptoms include epigastric pain, chronic pancreatitis, weight loss, diabetes mellitus, and jaundice {423, 717,797,855,950}. Despite symptoms, high-grade IPMN is commonly detected incidentally, owing to the increased use of cross-sectional imaging, and it accounts for most incidental pancreatic cysts {116}. Imaging findings depend on whether the high-grade IPMN is of main duct type, branch duct type, or combined type. Features that may correspond to high-grade dysplasia or invasive carcinoma in any of these types include a main duct diameter > 10 mm or an enhancing mural nodule > 5 mm {839}. A main duct diameter between 5 and 9.9 mm or a cyst diameter > 40 mm are worrisome features warranting FNAB to evaluate for high-grade cytopathology {839,204}.

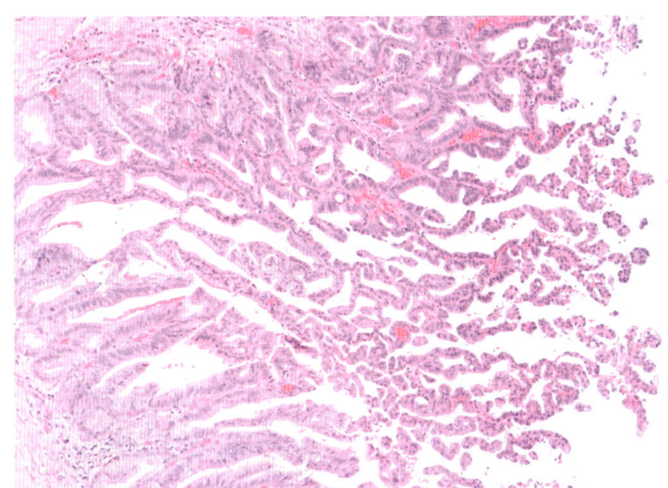

Fig. 7.04 Intraductal papillary mucinous neoplasm with high-grade dysplasia. The complex papillary fronds and buds of high-grade epithelium slough off into the cyst lumen and are aspirated with cyst fluid aspiration by FNAB (formalin-fixed, paraffin-embedded tissue section; H&E).

Histopathology

A two-tiered system for grading intraductal neoplasia has replaced the three-tiered system of low-, intermediate-, and high-grade dysplasia {324}. Intermediate-grade dysplasia is grouped with low-grade IPMN, leaving high-grade IPMN with high-grade dysplastic epithelium of pancreaticobiliary, intestinal, or gastric type lining the cystically dilated ducts {910}. Grading is based on the highest grade of epithelium present, which is determined by architectural complexity and cytopathological atypia. Pancreaticobiliary-type epithelium is high-grade, whereas intestinal-type epithelium is either low-grade (including intermediate-grade) or high-grade. Gastric-type epithelium can be any grade but is most often low-grade {60}. High-grade IPMN has epithelium with macropapillae and micropapillae with irregular, complex branching and budding, and cells showing severe cytopathological atypia with pseudostratification, loss of polarity, high N:C ratio, and sometimes prominent nucleoli. Cells sloughing off into the cyst fluid are often those seen in FNAB material when cysts are drained. Oncocytic IPMN is now recognized as a distinct entity.

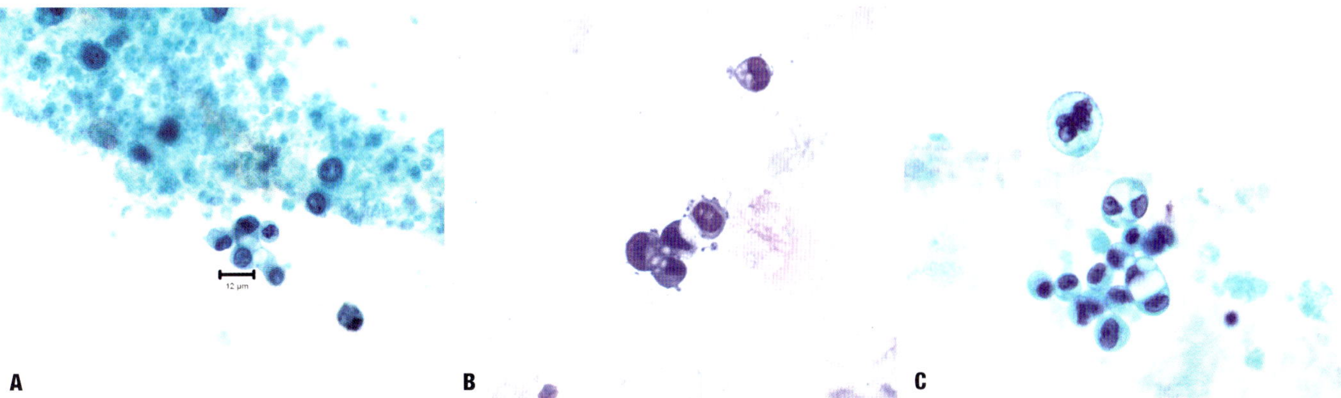

Fig. 7.05 Intraductal papillary mucinous neoplasm with high-grade dysplasia. **A** High-grade epithelial atypia defines a high-risk/grade cyst with at least high-grade dysplasia, characterized by small cells (similar in size to a 12 µm duodenal enterocyte), high N:C ratio, and abnormal chromatin. Cytoplasmic mucin vacuoles are variable. The background necrosis adds support to the diagnosis (Pap). **B** High-grade epithelial atypia has small cells with increased N:C ratios and variably irregular nuclear membranes (Giemsa). **C** Epithelial cells with high-grade epithelial atypia show variable amounts of cytoplasmic mucin, often less than in low-grade intraductal papillary mucinous neoplasms and even carcinomas (Pap).

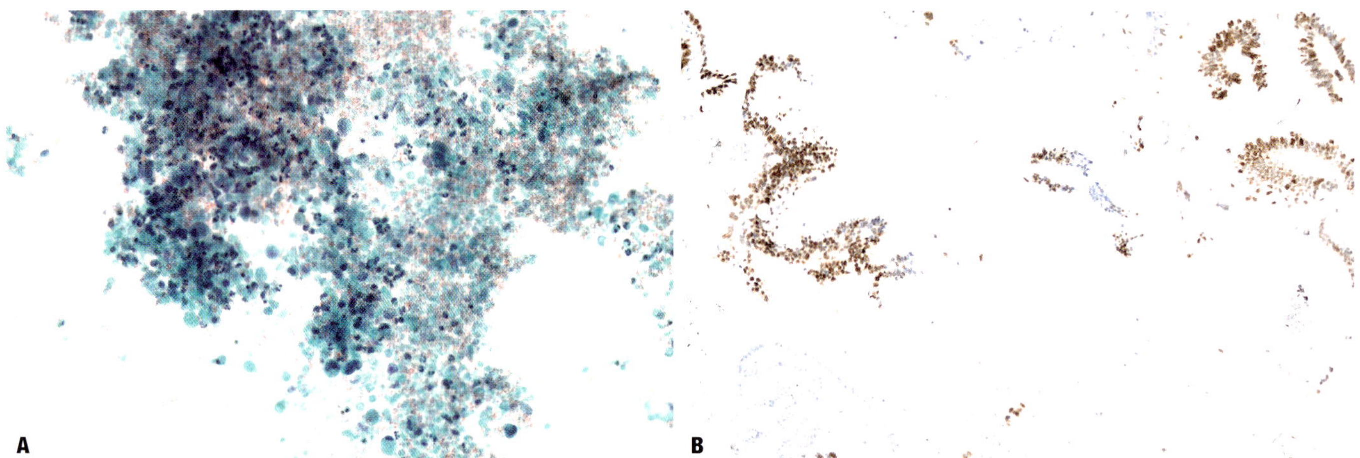

Fig. 7.06 Intraductal papillary mucinous neoplasm with high-grade dysplasia. **A** Background necrosis is commonly seen in high-grade intraductal papillary mucinous neoplasm but is not an accurate marker for distinguishing intraductal from invasive tumours. Oncotic (degenerate) cells are present, consistent with cyst contents (Pap). **B** Strong, diffuse nuclear p53 expression correlates with the genetic mutation and supports the diagnosis of a high-risk/grade cyst (ICC).

Key diagnostic cytopathological features

- Hypercellularity as compared with low-grade IPMN
- Small cells (smaller than a 12 μm duodenal enterocyte)
- Increased N:C ratio
- Nuclear envelope abnormalities
- Abnormal chromatin pattern, which can be hypochromatic or hyperchromatic
- Prominent nucleoli variable
- Residual cytoplasmic mucin variable
- Background necrosis in most cases
- Background inflammation variable

Reference(s): {644,543}

Discussion and differential diagnosis

Mucinous cysts with high-grade atypia (HGA) may represent a mucinous cystic neoplasm or IPMN with high-grade dysplasia or an associated invasive carcinoma. The high-grade IPMN diagnosis depends on finding epithelium characteristic of an IPMN, such as intestinal-type epithelium in papillary fronds, or on finding imaging correlation showing typical features of an IPMN. If only small tissue fragments of HGA or a solitary cystic mass without connection to the duct are present, it may be impossible to make a specific diagnosis of IPMN {309}. A generic diagnosis of a "mucinous cyst with HGA" is sufficient in these cases because resection is warranted regardless of the specific cyst type.

A secondarily cystic conventional ductal adenocarcinoma is in the differential diagnosis, but these tumours generally show overtly malignant cytopathology and solid and cystic imaging features.

Colloid carcinoma warrants consideration, given the presence of abundant extracellular mucin with floating tumour cells. Distinction requires correlation with imaging because colloid carcinoma presents as a solid mass usually associated with a main duct IPMN rather than a branch duct cyst {11,749,676,568}.

Cystic neuroendocrine tumours (NETs) produce cells with a high N:C ratio and sometimes nucleoli, but the cytoplasm will be non-mucinous in all of the cells, and the salt-and-pepper granular chromatin and round, smooth nuclear membranes of the cells from a NET will differentiate it from the HGA of an IPMN {562}.

Fig. 7.07 A Intraductal papillary mucinous neoplasm with high-grade dysplasia. This small, cohesive tissue fragment of crowded epithelium with high-grade atypia in intraductal papillary mucinous neoplasm with high-grade dysplasia is similar to those seen in mucinous cystic neoplasm with high-grade dysplasia (Pap). **B** Mucinous cystic neoplasm with high-grade dysplasia. This small, cohesive tissue fragment of epithelium with high-grade atypia in mucinous cystic neoplasm with high-grade dysplasia has features similar to those seen in intraductal papillary mucinous neoplasm with high-grade dysplasia (Pap).

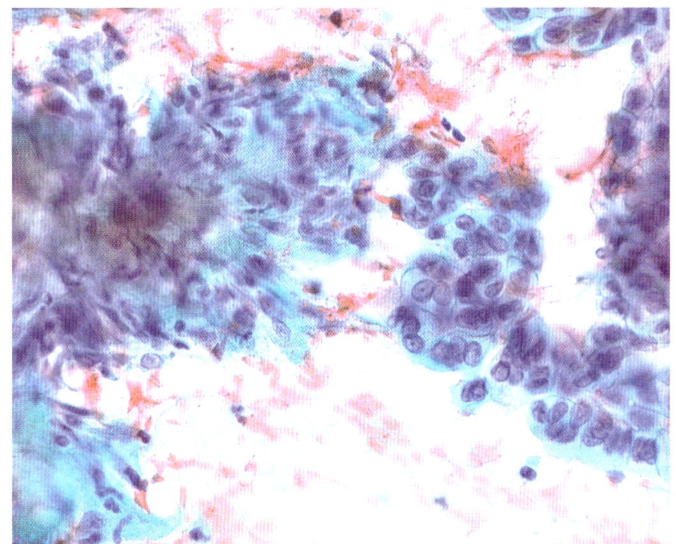

Fig. 7.08 Pancreatic ductal adenocarcinoma with cystic degeneration. Secondarily cystic pancreatic ductal adenocarcinoma can mimic intraductal papillary mucinous neoplasm on imaging. The cells typically are overtly malignant (Pap).

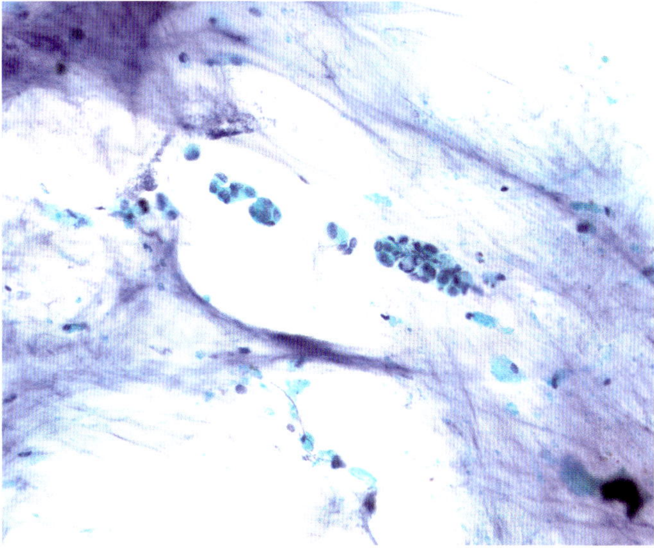

Fig. 7.09 Colloid carcinoma. Tumour cells floating in thick extracellular mucin are features of both high-grade intraductal papillary mucinous neoplasm and colloid carcinoma. The distinction is made by correlation with imaging, where colloid carcinoma is a solid mass and high-grade intraductal papillary mucinous neoplasm is a cyst (Pap).

Ancillary testing

Ancillary tests that support the high-risk/grade nature of the cyst include the detection of mutations known to be associated with adenocarcinoma and high-grade dysplasia. This can be achieved by molecular testing of cyst fluid or ICC stains on cell blocks. Late mutations in the adenoma–carcinoma progression include *TP53* {31,364,700,787}, *SMAD4* {31,364,700}, *CDKN2A* (*P16*) {364,700}, *PTEN* {787,239}, *PIK3CA* {787}, and aneuploidy / loss of heterozygosity in certain regions {809}. Mutant allelic frequency mutations in *PIK3CA*, *PTEN*, and *TP53* genes equivalent to *KRAS* or *GNAS* are sensitive and specific for IPMN with either high grade dysplasia or associated invasive carcinoma {787}. Low-level mutations of *PTEN*, *PIK3CA*, and *TP53* in low-grade IPMN may indicate a risk of transformation to high-grade IPMN {787}. Mutant allele frequencies of > 55% for *GNAS* correlate with high-grade IPMN {787}.

ICC results from cell blocks include p53 mutant expression, which is strong nuclear staining or the null pattern with no expression {753,401}, and loss of nuclear staining for SMAD4 {440,333} or p16 {3}. These stains can be challenging on scant specimens and should be interpreted with caution.

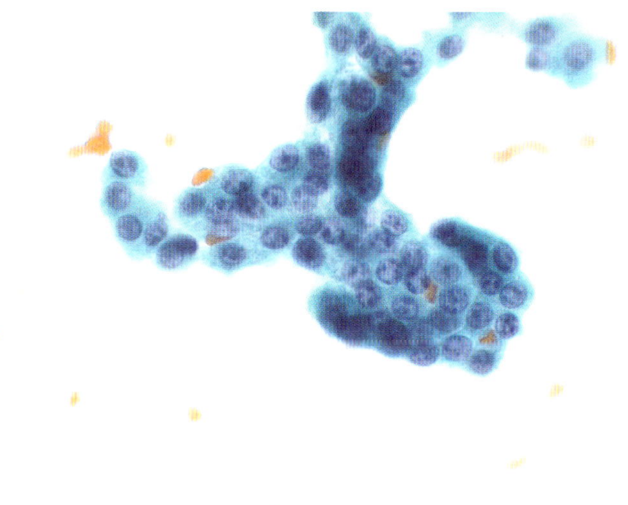

Fig. 7.10 Cystic neuroendocrine tumour (NET). Tissue fragment showing cells of a cystic NET that are distinguished from high-grade atypia by the coarse stippled chromatin and complete lack of cytoplasmic mucin (Pap).

Intraductal papillary neoplasm of the bile duct, high-grade

Zen Y
HooKim K

Definition

Intraductal papillary neoplasm of the bile duct (IPNB) with high-grade dysplasia is defined as a premalignant neoplasm of the biliary tree that is characterized by an intraductal papillary proliferation of dysplastic cells with severe cytoarchitectural atypia.

Clinical features and imaging

IPNB occurs anywhere along the biliary tree from the intrahepatic bile duct to the distal extrahepatic biliary tree {973}. Similar neoplasms in the gallbladder are termed "intracholecystic papillary neoplasm".

IPNB may occur in patients with hepatolithiasis and is infrequently associated with choledochal cyst and primary sclerosing cholangitis {978,977}.

Some patients present with abdominal symptoms, such as pain and discomfort, and other cases are incidentally found on imaging studies performed for other reasons. Obstructive jaundice is less common than in patients with cholangiocarcinoma.

Two characteristic imaging findings are an intraductal tumour and duct dilatation. Extensive duct dilatation with an appearance of a cystic tumour is often observed in intrahepatic IPNB, whereas an intraductal solid mass with upstream duct dilatation due to obstruction is commonly seen in extrahepatic IPNB {429, 972}. Endoscopy may identify mucus secretion from the orifice of the ampulla of Vater.

Histopathology

High-grade IPNB shows a high-grade papillary proliferation of neoplastic cells along thin fibrovascular stalks within the dilated bile ducts {972,229}. When there is a component of invasive carcinoma, the diagnosis is IPNB with an associated invasive carcinoma that is a cholangiocarcinoma. Abundant extracellular mucus may be present. On the basis of the morphology of tumour cells, IPNB is classified into pancreaticobiliary (40%), intestinal (30%), gastric (20%), and oncocytic (10%) types {972,229}. In the first three types, columnar tumour cells show enlarged nuclei, coarse chromatin, and moderate nuclear pleomorphism with intracytoplasmic mucin at least focally {973}. There is also architectural distortion. Low-grade components may be present, particularly in gastric-type IPNB {229}. Oncocytic-type IPNB, also referred to as intraductal oncocytic papillary neoplasm, contains oncocytic cells with abundant eosinophilic cytoplasm and central, round nuclei, arranged in arborizing papillae, cribriform glands, or solid nests. Different histopathological types may coexist in a single tumour. Associated invasive adenocarcinoma is observed in 50% of IPNB cases at the initial presentation. The invasive components consist of tubular adenocarcinoma, mucinous carcinoma, or a combination of the two {973}. IPNB is currently classified into types 1 and 2 on the basis of microscopic appearance, and the two types have distinct clinicopathological features.

Key diagnostic cytopathological features

- Direct biliary brushings are usually cellular
- Intrahepatic cystic IPNB may be less cellular, with variable mucin and debris
- Tissue fragments with a papillary architecture in a mucinous background are variable
- Small tissue fragments or 3D tissue fragments or large papillae with or without fibrovascular stalks
- Cells show severe atypia, with hyperchromatic, crowded, piled-up nuclei; irregular nuclear contours; and intracytoplasmic mucin
- Pseudostratification of elongated nuclei correlates with intestinal-type IPNB

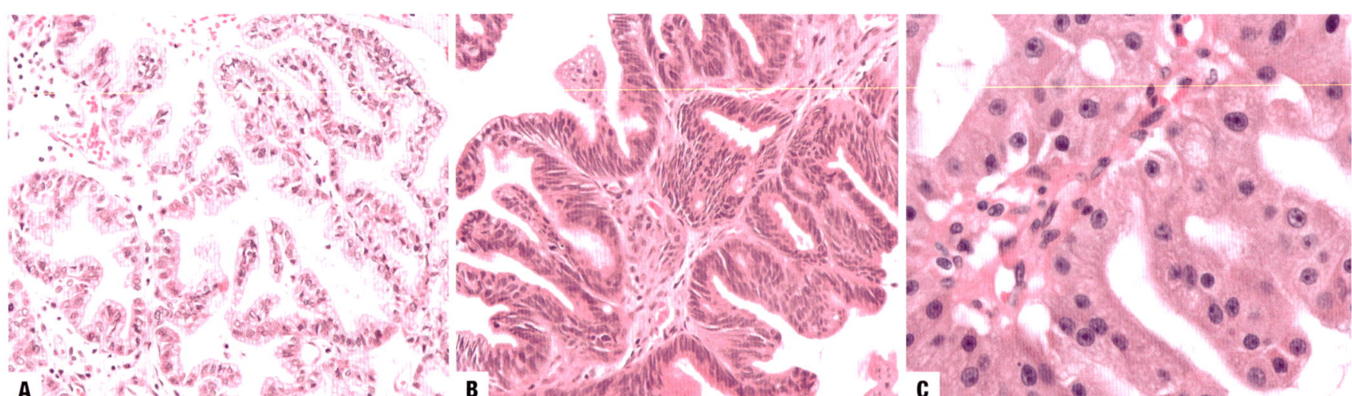

Fig. 7.11 Intraductal papillary neoplasm of the bile duct. **A** Intraductal papillary neoplasm of the bile duct with high-grade dysplasia. Gastric-type epithelium with high N:C ratio, irregular nuclei, and scant mucinous cytoplasm (formalin-fixed, paraffin-embedded tissue section; H&E). **B** Intraductal papillary neoplasm of the bile duct with high-grade dysplasia. Histology of pancreaticobiliary-type epithelium in micropapillary tufts (formalin-fixed, paraffin-embedded tissue section; H&E). **C** Intraductal papillary neoplasm of the bile duct, oncocytic type. The abundant granular cytoplasm of the tumour cells makes identification of the oncocytic type straightforward (formalin-fixed, paraffin-embedded tissue section; H&E).

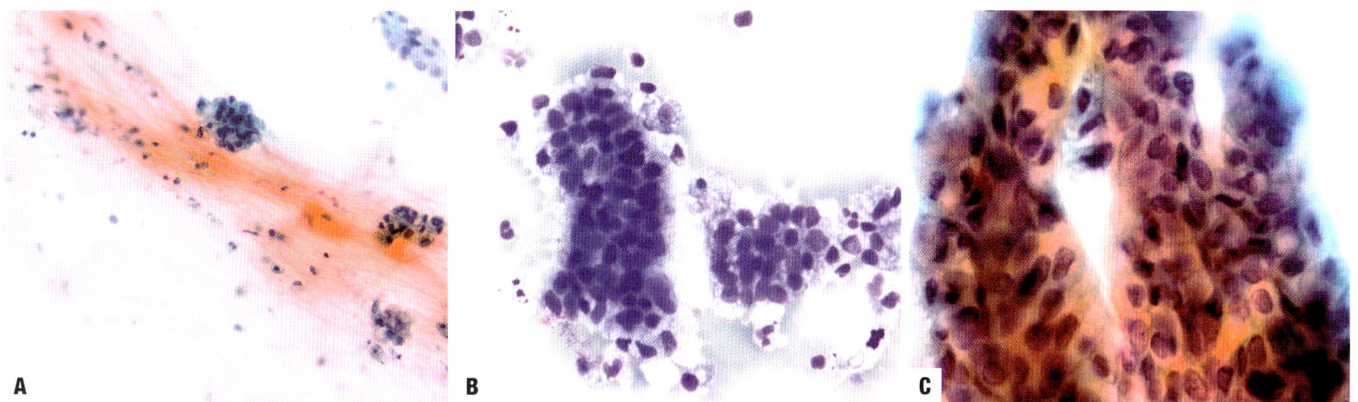

Fig. 7.12 Intraductal papillary neoplasm of the bile duct with high-grade dysplasia. **A** Small tissue fragments are also observed against a mucinous background (Pap). **B** The cells have enlarged nuclei, irregular nuclear membranes, intracytoplasmic mucus, and distinct nucleoli (Giemsa). **C** Cholangiocytes show cellular overlapping, nuclear enlargement, and irregular nuclear membranes (Pap).

- Dense eosinophilic cytoplasm and central nuclei are seen in oncocytic-type IPNB
- The background may contain abundant mucin
- Necrosis is uncommon

Discussion and differential diagnosis

Samples can be obtained by bile duct brushing, aspirated bile cytopathology, or FNAB of intrahepatic cystic masses.

The main differential diagnosis is cholangiocarcinoma. Papillary tissue fragments and abundant mucin favour IPNB, whereas discohesive dysplastic cells with a necrotic background suggest cholangiocarcinoma. However, cytopathology alone cannot distinguish between high-grade IPNB and cholangiocarcinoma, but this distinction is not essential because surgical resection is the treatment of choice for both. Clinicopathological correlation, particularly with imaging findings, may assist in the discrimination.

Ancillary testing

No ICC markers specific for IPNB are available. Unlike cholangiocarcinoma, approximately 50% of IPNBs harbour mutations in *APC*, *CTNNB1*, *GNAS*, or *STK11* {228,22,33}. Most cases of oncocytic-type IPNB have fusion genes involving *PRKACA* or *PRKACB* {790,892}. Sequencing of these genes is expected to be useful for the diagnosis {790}. Some cases also have mutations in *KRAS* and *TP53*, similarly to cholangiocarcinoma {228, 22,33}.

Mucinous cystic neoplasm, high-grade

Cai G
Stelow EB
Zhang ML

Definition

High-grade mucinous cystic neoplasm (MCN) is a cystic, mucin-producing epithelial neoplasm with distinctive subepithelial ovarian-type stroma and high-grade epithelial dysplasia or possible associated invasive carcinoma.

Clinical features and imaging

MCNs constitute 8% of cystic pancreatic lesions and < 5% of hepatobiliary cysts {433,116,171}. Almost all occur in middle-aged women. In the pancreas, > 90% arise in the body or tail. Imaging shows large, well-defined multiloculated cysts with thick walls and without connection to the pancreatic ducts {433,940}.

About 15% of MCNs have an associated invasive carcinoma component {724,940,351}. MCNs with invasive carcinoma are seen in patients who are 5–10 years older than those with MCN without invasive carcinoma {433}. Features suggestive of associated invasive carcinoma include large size (> 50 mm), irregular cyst wall thickening, mural nodules, papillary projections, and elevated serum CA19-9 levels (> 37 U/mL) {940,351}.

Histopathology

MCNs are lined by mucinous epithelium with underlying ovarian-type stroma. MCNs with high-grade dysplasia demonstrate high-grade architectural features including papillary structures with irregular branching and budding and nuclear stratification with loss of polarity. The tumour cells are pleomorphic with prominent nucleoli and frequent mitoses. The subepithelial ovarian-type stroma is usually composed of a dense proliferation of spindle cells but may become hypocellular, particularly around areas of high-grade dysplasia or invasive carcinoma {351}.

Key diagnostic cytopathological features

- Low to moderate cellularity
- Variable amounts of thick, colloid-like extracellular mucin

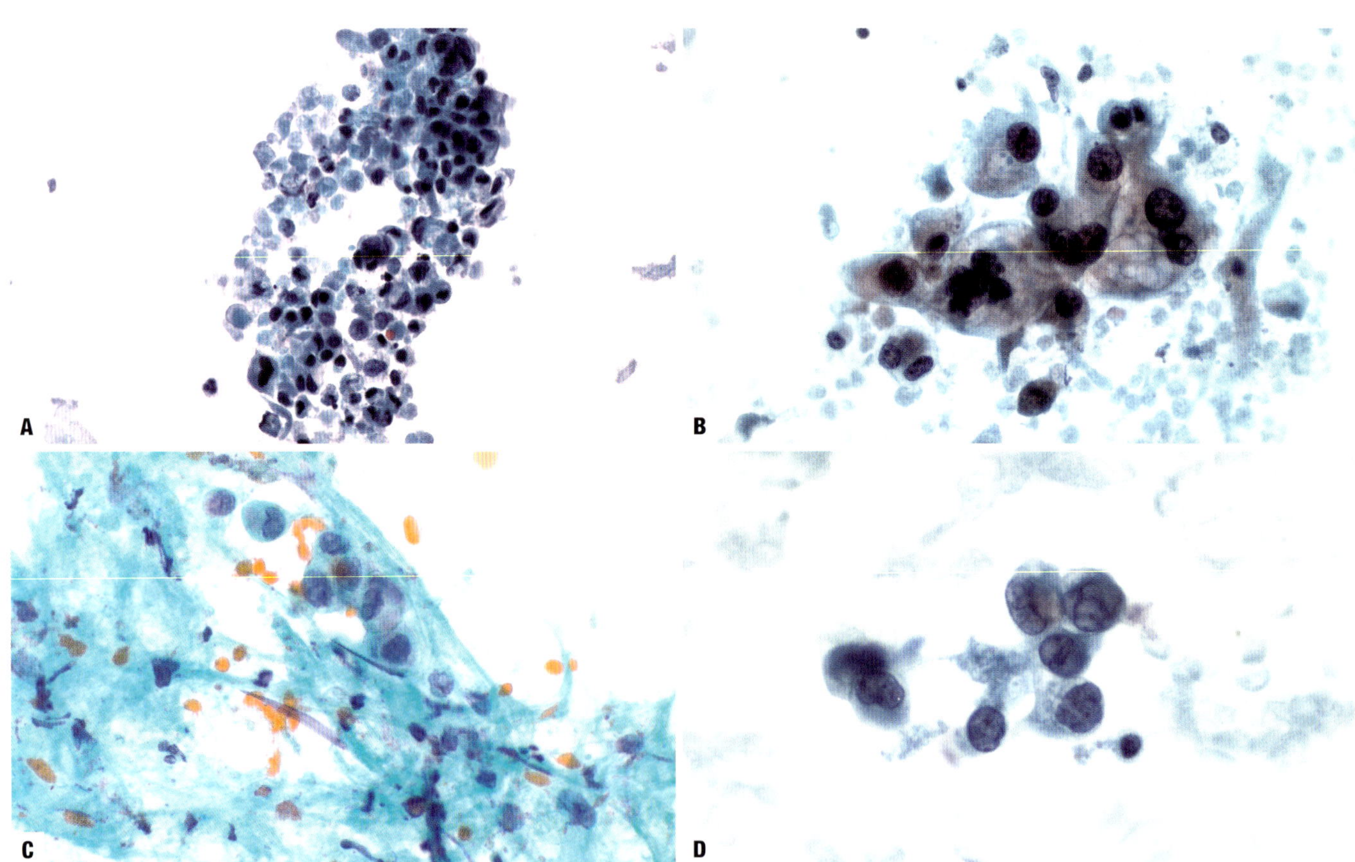

Fig. 7.13 Mucinous cystic neoplasm with high-grade epithelial atypia. **A** The cyst fluid contains markedly atypical epithelial cells with a high N:C ratio and hyperchromasia in a background of cellular necrosis (Pap). **B** Cyst FNAB shows a few markedly atypical epithelial cells associated with cellular necrosis (Pap). **C** Cyst FNAB shows a few markedly atypical epithelial cells associated with extracellular mucin (Pap). **D** Cyst FNAB shows a few markedly atypical epithelial cells with a high N:C ratio and hyperchromasia (Pap). **A–D** Because there is no biopsy showing the subepithelial ovarian-type stroma, this case would be diagnosed as a neoplastic mucinous cyst with high-grade epithelial atypia and placed in the "Pancreaticobiliary neoplasm, high-risk/grade (PaN-high)" category. Resection showed high-grade dysplasia (Pap).

- Atypical epithelial cells in crowded sheets, papillary tissue fragments, and as single cells
- Pleomorphic cells with a high N:C ratio that contain variable amounts of cytoplasmic mucin
- Nuclear enlargement, nuclear membrane irregularities, hypochromasia or hyperchromasia, and frequent mitotic figures
- Ovarian-type stroma is not likely to be seen on FNAB
- Background necrosis is frequently present

Reference(s): {748}

Discussion and differential diagnosis

Diagnosis of a mucinous cyst can be made on the basis of the presence of thick, colloid-like extracellular mucin, mucinous epithelial cells, and/or elevated CEA (> 192 ng/mL) {649,244}. Features of high-grade cytopathological atypia include background cellular necrosis and pleomorphic tumour cells with hypochromasia or hyperchromasia and nuclear membrane irregularities. A consistent cytopathological finding in high-grade tumours is the presence of small tumour cells (smaller than a typical 12 μm duodenal enterocyte) with a high N:C ratio {308,644}. Mitotic figures and background necrosis support a high-grade cyst.

The primary differential diagnosis is intraductal papillary mucinous neoplasm (IPMN). Main duct–type IPMN can usually be distinguished on imaging from MCN, because MCNs typically do not involve or communicate with the pancreatic duct system. However, differentiating branch duct–type IPMN can pose diagnostic difficulty. The only feature that is diagnostic of MCN is subepithelial ovarian-type stroma, which in most cases can only be evaluated on a fine-needle core or microforceps biopsy {982}. Other entities in the differential diagnosis include pseudocyst, serous cystadenoma, or secondarily cystic solid malignancies such as pancreatic neuroendocrine tumours (PanNETs) or ductal adenocarcinomas.

Ancillary testing

The neoplastic cells are positive for CK7, CK8, CK18, CK19, EMA (MUC1), CEA, and MUC5AC {754,231}. The invasive carcinoma component can show loss of nuclear SMAD4 expression and the presence of mutant-phenotype p53 expression as either overexpression or complete loss of expression. The ovarian-type stromal cells express desmin, SMA, inhibin, PR (60–90%), and ER (30%) {951,231,969}.

Cyst fluid CEA elevation > 192 ng/mL supports the diagnosis of a mucinous cyst but does not differentiate MCN from IPMN, nor does the CEA level correlate with grade {91,876,802,564, 757}. Not all MCNs have elevated cyst fluid CEA, so a low CEA does not exclude the diagnosis. Similarly, cyst fluid amylase levels cannot be used to distinguish MCN from IPMN {848,635}. Although the cyst fluid from most MCNs has low levels of amylase and most IPMNs have high levels of amylase, the opposite can happen.

Molecular studies may aid in the diagnosis of MCN. Although there are no known genetic mutations specific to MCN, *KRAS* mutations are found in 80% of high-grade MCNs {681,654,923}, and detection of a *GNAS* mutation supports the diagnosis of IPMN over MCN {926}. Late mutations in the progression to carcinoma, such as *TP53*, *CDKN2A* (*P16*), and *SMAD4*, have also been detected in high-grade MCN {923,700}.

Intraductal oncocytic papillary neoplasm

Reid MD
Zhang ML

Definition

Intraductal oncocytic papillary neoplasm (IOPN) is an intraductal epithelial neoplasm of the main and/or branch pancreatic ducts and bile ducts that comprises complex papillae lined by mitochondria-rich oncocytic epithelium that is mucin-depleted.

Clinical features and imaging

IOPNs account for 4.5% of all intraductal pancreatic neoplasms. They are most commonly found in the pancreatic head but can also be seen in the biliary tree {8,900}. Patients are typically aged 36–87 years (mean: 60 years), and there is an equal sex distribution {8,900}. Tumours may be discovered incidentally or during workup for abdominal pain or jaundice. By imaging, most lesions are entirely cystic, but some may be partly or completely solid {218}. Because of the high metabolic activity of mitochondria-rich oncocytes, IOPNs demonstrate high uptake on PET {218,385}.

Histopathology

On gross examination, IOPNs typically form tan-brown cystic masses with nodular papillary or solid projections within dilated ducts, and they are large (mean size: 55 mm). Histopathologically, oncocytic epithelium forms characteristically complex arborizing papillae with thin or broad oedematous fibrovascular cores {8,900}. Papillae are lined by two to five layers of cuboidal or columnar epithelium with round to oval nuclei, prominent nucleoli, and granular eosinophilic cytoplasm. Cribriform growth with scattered intercellular luminal spaces and occasional goblet cells may be seen. Fusion of papillae results in more solid growth. Single cell necrosis and nuclear atypia may be striking in some cases.

IOPNs are considered high-grade because of their architectural complexity and nuclear atypia. However, high-grade atypia does not necessarily correlate with the presence of invasive carcinoma {8,900,60}. Invasive carcinoma is seen in approximately 30% of cases and when present is often limited and tubular, although it may be oncocytic {8,900,547}. Even invasive cases exhibit relatively indolent behaviour with a favourable prognosis {547,523}.

Key diagnostic cytopathological features

- Hypercellular smears, with minimal or no thick background mucin
- Complex sheets and papillae with branching fibrovascular cores
- Polygonal cells, resembling oncocytic (Hürthle) cells of the thyroid
- Cells have well-defined borders, low N:C ratios, round to oval nuclei, and a distinctly granular magenta cytoplasm (Giemsa) or granular bluish-green cytoplasm (Pap)
- Intracellular mucin is minimal
- Oval to irregular, hyperchromatic or hypochromatic nuclei with large, slightly eccentric nucleoli that may touch the nuclear membrane
- Abnormal mitoses, degenerative atypia, apoptotic debris, and coagulative necrosis

Reference(s): {301,368,683,559}

Discussion and differential diagnosis

IOPN was formerly classified as a subtype of intraductal papillary mucinous neoplasm (IPMN). However, because of its distinctive histomorphology and its unique molecular profile and biology, it is now classified as a separate entity. The distinctive cytopathological features make definite diagnosis possible on cytopathology.

Because it forms complex masses, IOPN is often misdiagnosed as pancreatic ductal adenocarcinoma on imaging {8,

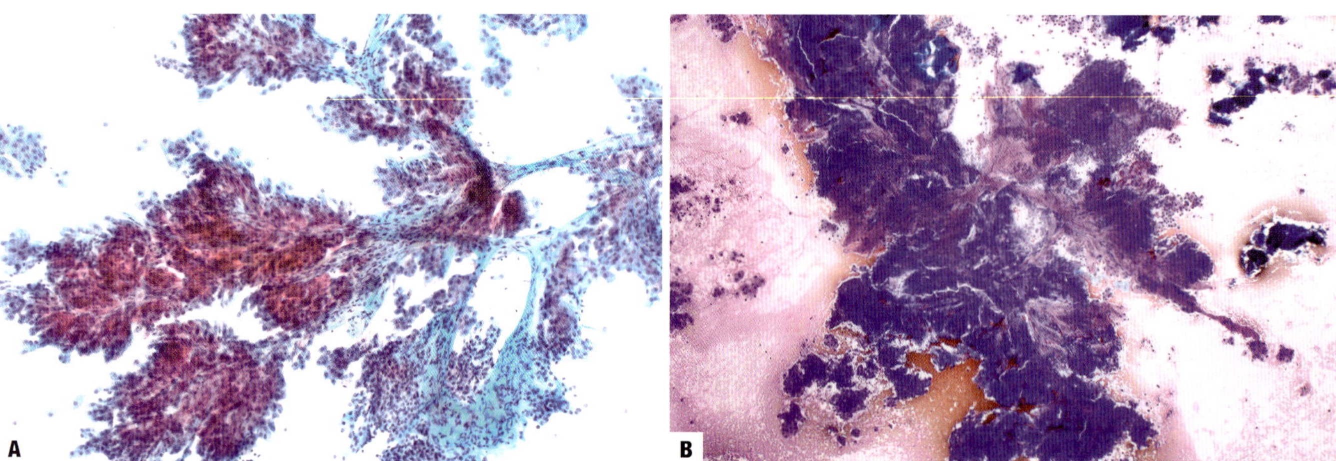

Fig. 7.14 Intraductal oncocytic papillary neoplasm. **A** Branching fibrovascular cores covered by oncocytic cells (Pap). **B** Hypercellular smear composed of complex tissue fragments with branching magenta-coloured fibrovascular cores and sheets (Giemsa).

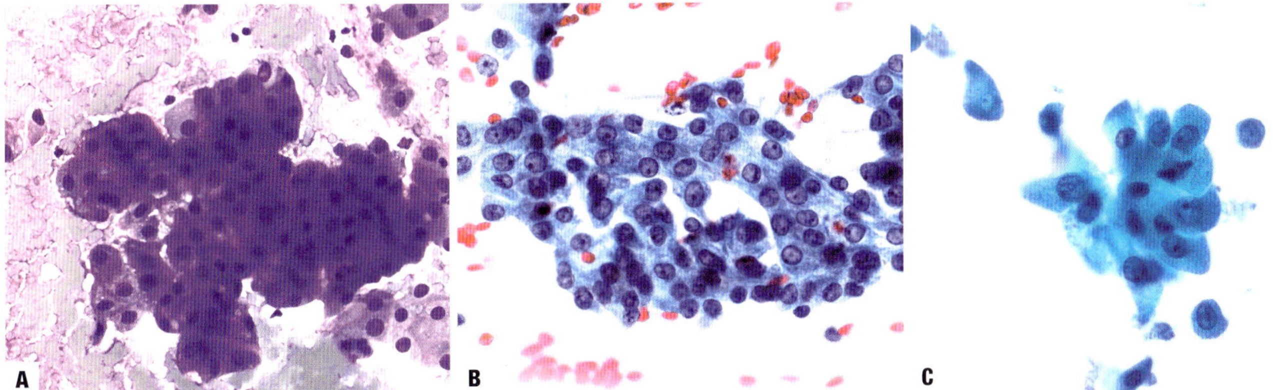

Fig. 7.15 Intraductal oncocytic papillary neoplasm. **A** Sheet of oncocytic cells with oval nuclei and abundant granular cytoplasm containing dense blue granules (Giemsa). **B** Oncocytic cells have dense granular cytoplasm and nuclei ranging from oval to irregular, with prominent, slightly eccentric nucleoli (Pap). **C** Small, cohesive tissue fragment of tall oncocytic cells with cytoplasmic granules, oval to round nuclei, prominent nucleoli, and an occasional intranuclear inclusion (liquid-based cytopathology, Pap).

683}. Another imaging and cytopathological differential is IPMN. The presence of thick extracellular mucin and abundant cytoplasmic mucin supports IPMN because these features are rare in IOPN {683}. Pancreatic ductal adenocarcinoma and pancreaticobiliary-type IPMN are both cytopathologically high-grade and less mucinous than gastric- or intestinal-type IPMN, and they can also be excluded cytopathologically.

The cytopathological features of IOPN are consistent with high-grade epithelial atypia {683,644,643}. Papillae may be seen on liquid-based cytopathology but are more easily discernible on direct FNAB smears and cell block preparations, where they are covered by pseudostratified, oncocytic epithelium with empty rounded intercellular spaces or occasional mucin-containing cells {683,301,559}. Invasive carcinoma arising in IOPN may show classic pancreaticobiliary-type features or be more oncocytic.

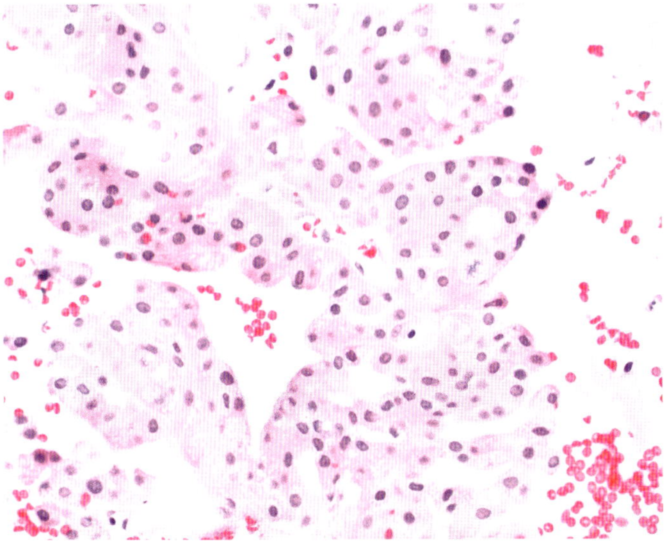

Fig. 7.16 Intraductal oncocytic papillary neoplasm. Cell block showing fused papillae with thin fibrovascular cores covered by pseudostratified oncocytic epithelium with intercellular spaces, mucin vacuoles, and occasional abnormal mitoses (H&E).

Other pancreatic lesions with solid-cystic growth should be considered in the differential diagnosis. These include the primary pancreatic neoplasms, acinar cell carcinoma and pancreatic neuroendocrine tumour (PanNET) with oncocytic features, as well as pancreatic metastases with oncocytic features, such as hepatocellular carcinoma and oncocytic (Hürthle) cell carcinoma {922,63}. Acinar cell carcinoma is often large like IOPN, may involve pancreatic ducts, and is also composed of cells with large nuclei, prominent nucleoli, and granular zymogen-rich cytoplasm, resembling IOPN {63,774,853}. Unlike IOPN, acinar cell carcinoma expresses the acinar cell markers trypsin, chymotrypsin, and BCL10, which are all negative in IOPN {774,321}. Oncocytic neuroendocrine tumour (NET) has plasmacytoid cells with eccentric granular cytoplasm and nuclei with prominent nucleoli, resembling IOPN, but unlike IOPN it expresses neuroendocrine ICC markers {931,129}.

Ancillary testing

By ICC, IOPNs are positive for mesothelin (88%), MUC6 (89%), and EMA (MUC1) (50%) {61,59}. Interspersed goblet cells may be positive for MUC2 and MUC5AC {59}. Tumour cells may show nuclear p53 overexpression (24%) or abnormal β-catenin expression (5%) {59}. HepPar1 can be positive in as many as 60% of IOPNs, but albumin FISH is negative {900,59}. Genetically, IOPNs are distinct from IPMNs. They have recurrent rearrangements in *PRKACA* and *PRKACB*, and they harbour mutations in *ARHGAP26*, *ASXL1*, *EPHA8*, and *ERBB4* (but not in *KRAS* or *GNAS*) {790,892}. Cyst fluid CEA levels are low (< 193 ng/mL) {959}.

Intraductal tubulopapillary neoplasm

Basturk O

Definition

Intraductal tubulopapillary neoplasm (ITPN) is an intraductal epithelial neoplasm of the pancreas and bile ducts with ductal differentiation and high-grade dysplasia, lacking overt mucin production.

Clinical features and imaging

ITPNs account for 3% of intraductal pancreatic neoplasms {936}. About half occur in the pancreatic head, and one third involve it diffusely {57}. There is a slight female predominance, and patients range in age from 25 to 84 years (mean: 55 years) {57}. Most present with nonspecific symptoms, such as abdominal pain, vomiting, weight loss, steatorrhea, and diabetes mellitus. Obstructive jaundice is uncommon {57}. The two-tone duct sign on CT and MRI and the cork-of-wine-bottle sign on magnetic resonance cholangiopancreatography and endoscopic retrograde cholangiopancreatography are indicators of intraductal tumour growth {569}.

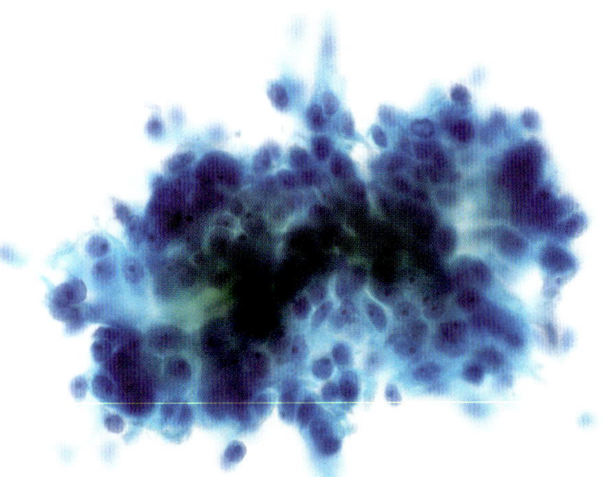

Fig. 7.17 Intraductal tubulopapillary neoplasm. Tissue fragments show an acinar tubular architecture, and the tumour cells have bluish-green cytoplasm and enlarged, eccentric nuclei with irregular nuclear membranes and prominent cherry-red nucleoli (liquid-based cytopathology, Pap).

Histopathology

On gross examination, ITPNs form fleshy to rubbery nodular masses, which are large (mean size: 45 mm), within dilated ducts, but the intraductal growth may be difficult to recognize {57,936}. Cyst formation is often less evident than in intraductal papillary mucinous neoplasms (IPMNs). Mucinous secretions are absent {305,821}.

Microscopically, ITPNs form cribriform nodules of back-to-back tubules with minimal papillae {57,736,936,832}. Tumour cells are predominantly cuboidal, with modest amounts of eosinophilic to amphophilic cytoplasm and undetectable cytoplasmic mucin {57, 15,936,431}. Tumour nuclei are uniform, round to oval, and atypical, with readily identifiable mitoses and foci of necrosis {936}.

ITPNs typically have a relatively homogeneous appearance and show high-grade dysplasia {936,832,833}. Invasive carcinoma is found in 70% of cases and is usually limited and composed of single cells or non-mucinous glands that extend away from the periphery of nodules into surrounding desmoplastic stroma {57,936,821}. Even invasive carcinomas exhibit relatively indolent behaviour, with a 5-year survival rate of 71% {57}.

Key diagnostic cytopathological features

- Hypercellular smears without thick background mucin
- Branching sheets or tissue fragments of overlapping cells with cribriform spaces representing tubules
- Tumour cells are enlarged cuboidal cells with anisonucleosis, high N:C ratios, and round to oval nuclei with irregular nuclear membranes and frequent prominent nucleoli

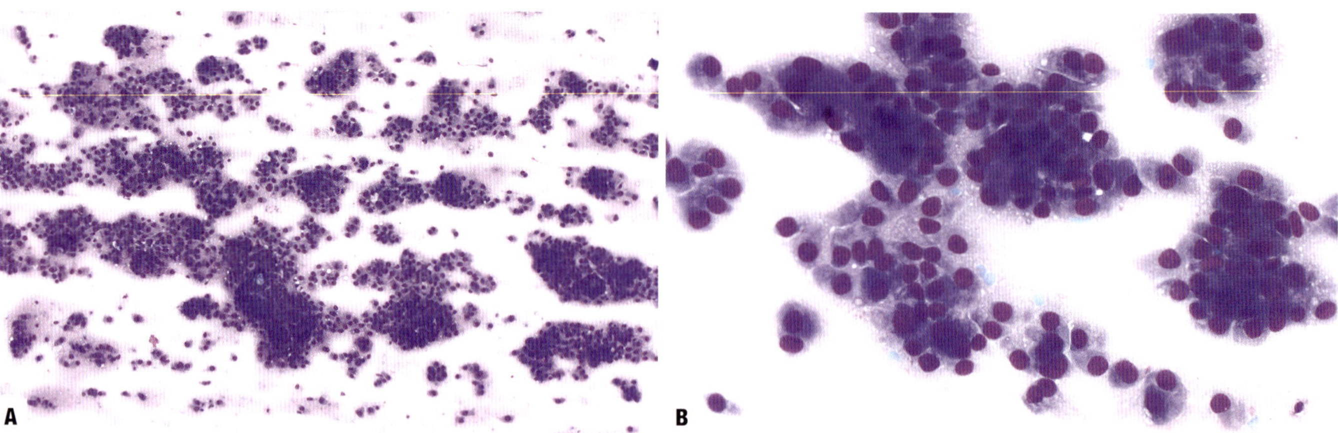

Fig. 7.18 Intraductal tubulopapillary neoplasm. **A** Hypercellular direct smear with complex tissue fragments and sheets of overlapping cells. Note the absence of thick background mucin (Giemsa). **B** Small tissue fragments of tumour cells have a vaguely acinar architecture and are cuboidal with enlarged, round to oval nuclei and visible to prominent nucleoli (Giemsa).

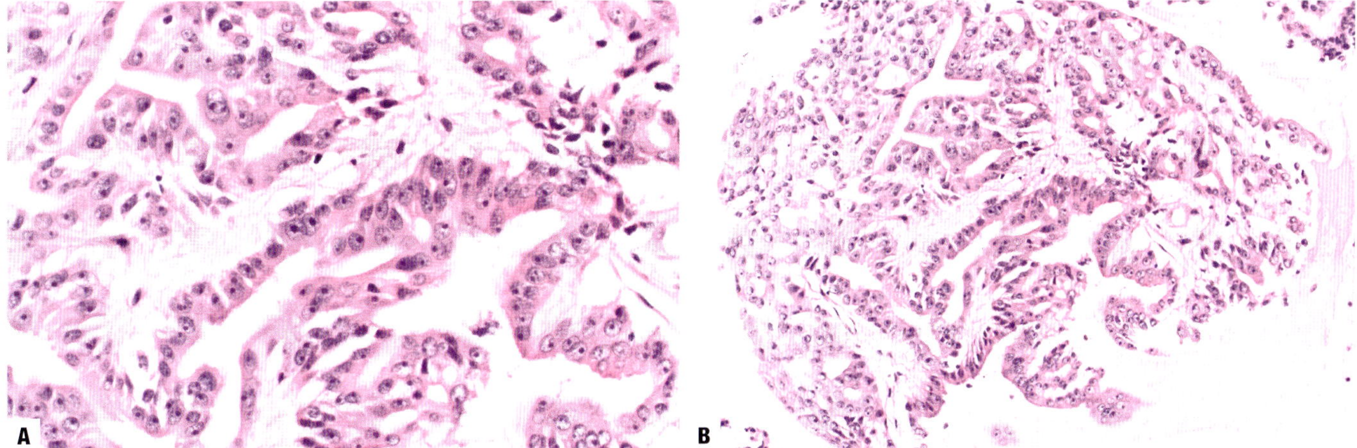

Fig. 7.19 Intraductal tubulopapillary neoplasm. **A** Cell block shows cuboidal tumour cells with a high N:C ratio, non-mucinous cytoplasm, and prominent nucleoli (H&E). **B** Tissue fragments in a cell block show the tubular and cribriform pattern typical of this neoplasm (H&E).

- Cytoplasm is bluish-green (Pap) and basophilic (Giemsa) and lacks cytoplasmic granules
- Goblet cells are absent
- Cell block shows tubules that often form cribriform units that are lined by mucin-depleted, cuboidal cells with high-grade cytopathological atypia
- High-grade cytopathological atypia in ITPN encompasses both high-grade dysplasia and invasive carcinoma, which are indistinguishable on cytopathology material alone

Reference(s): {728,831,983,233,263,40,675}

Discussion and differential diagnosis

In the current WHO Classification of Tumours, ITPN has been designated as a distinct entity among intraductal neoplasms that include IPMN, intraductal oncocytic papillary neoplasms, and high-grade pancreatic intraepithelial neoplasia.

Cytopathologically, the differential diagnoses include IPMN, acinar cell carcinoma, pancreatic neuroendocrine tumour (PanNET), and ductal adenocarcinoma.

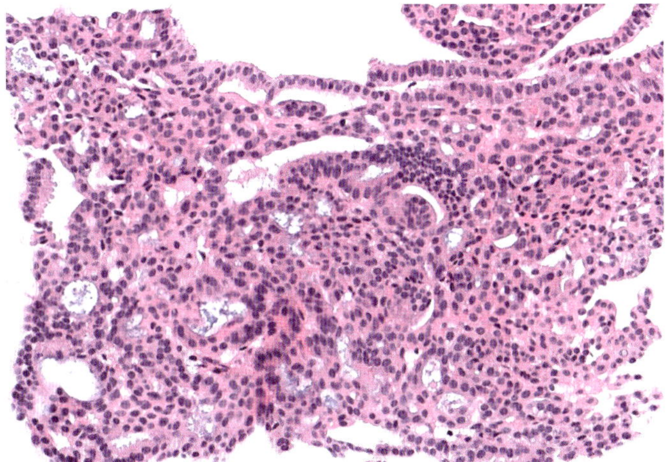

Fig. 7.20 Intraductal tubulopapillary neoplasm. Cell block shows that tumour cells are cuboidal with eosinophilic to amphophilic cytoplasm and enlarged nuclei. Although some tubules reveal wispy luminal mucin, no intracytoplasmic mucin or granules are present (core needle biopsy, H&E).

IPMN, especially pancreaticobiliary-type IPMN, is often difficult to distinguish from ITPN. Abundant background and cytoplasmic mucin, MUC5AC expression in the cell block material, and the presence of a spectrum of dysplasia favour pancreaticobiliary-type IPMN over ITPN {57,424,681,698}.

Acinar cell carcinoma may show intraductal growth and is composed of cells with large nuclei and prominent nucleoli, resembling ITPN {63}. However, acinar cell carcinoma often shows granular, zymogen-rich cytoplasm, and ICC labelling with the acinar markers trypsin, chymotrypsin, and BCL10 is essential to make the distinction {774,450}.

PanNET FNAB smears are generally cellular but, in contrast to ITPN, exhibit loosely cohesive tissue fragments and singly dispersed uniform plasmacytoid cells with salt-and-pepper granular chromatin and typically indistinct nucleoli. PanNET tumour cells are usually smaller and less pleomorphic than ITPN, and mitoses and necrosis are rare. Moreover, PanNETs are positive for chromogranin and synaptophysin, unlike ITPNs {931}.

In contrast to ITPN, ductal adenocarcinoma with cystic degeneration usually presents as a predominantly solid lesion with a focal cystic component. Tumour cells form tissue fragments that usually lack tubular, cribriform, or acinar structures. However, cytopathological distinction from ITPN is not reliable. When there is discordance between clinical presentation and cytopathological findings, it is wise to take a conservative approach by reporting markedly atypical cells and providing possible differentials.

Ancillary testing

By ICC, ITPNs are consistently positive for pancytokeratins (100%) and CK7 (100%) and commonly label for CK19 (89%). EMA (MUC1) (88%) and MUC6 (68%) are also expressed in most cases, but MUC2 and MUC5AC are almost never expressed {57,164,573,736}. Acinar and neuroendocrine markers are also negative. Genetically, the majority of the previously reported alterations related to ductal adenocarcinoma and IPMN are absent in ITPN {58,31,935,934,936}. However, certain chromatin-remodelling genes (*KMT2A* [*MLL1*], KTM2 [*MLL2*], *KMT2C* [*MLL3*], *BAP1*) and PI3K pathway genes (*PIK3CA*, *PTEN*) can be mutated {58}. A subset (18%) of ITPNs harbour *FGFR2* fusions {58}.

Sample reports: Pancreaticobiliary neoplasm, high-risk/grade

Basturk O
Rosenbaum MW
Zhang ML

Sample report 1

Clinical and imaging findings: Cystic mass with mural nodule in the head of the pancreas.
Specimen adequacy: Satisfactory for evaluation.
Category: Pancreaticobiliary neoplasm, high-risk/grade (PaN-high).
Diagnosis: Neoplastic mucinous cyst with at least high-grade dysplasia. See comment.
Comment: The endoscopic appearance of a cystic mass with an associated mural nodule is noted. The specimen shows mucinous epithelium in a background of thick extracellular mucin. Scattered epithelial groups demonstrate high-grade atypia with high N:C ratio, hyperchromasia, and nuclear membrane irregularities. The differential diagnosis includes intraductal papillary mucinous neoplasm and mucinous cystic neoplasm with high-grade dysplasia. Background cellular necrosis is seen, suggesting the possibility of an associated adenocarcinoma. Cyst fluid analysis shows markedly elevated CEA (3675 ng/mL) and amylase of 35 U/L, supporting a mucinous etiology.

Sample report 2

Clinical and imaging findings: Cystic lesion in body of pancreas in a 55-year-old woman.

Part A – Cyst contents, pancreatic head:
Specimen adequacy: Satisfactory for evaluation.
Category: Pancreaticobiliary neoplasm, high-risk/grade (PaN-high).
Diagnosis: Mucinous cyst with high-grade atypia. See comment.

Part B – Cyst wall, microforceps biopsy:
Diagnosis: Mucinous cystic neoplasm with high-grade dysplasia. See comment.

Comment: The cyst contents contain tissue fragments of mucinous epithelium with high-grade nuclear atypia. An elevated CEA level (758 ng/mL) is noted and is consistent with a mucinous etiology. The microforceps biopsy shows mucinous epithelium with areas of high-grade dysplasia and underlying cellular stroma. Immunoperoxidase stains reveal that the stromal cells are positive for ER and PR, consistent with the diagnosis of a mucinous cystic neoplasm. No necrosis or other features suspicious for adenocarcinoma are seen in this specimen.

Sample report 3

Clinical and imaging findings: Cystic mass in head of pancreas.
Specimen adequacy: Satisfactory for evaluation.
Category: Pancreaticobiliary neoplasm, high-risk/grade (PaN-high).
Diagnosis: Epithelial neoplasm with oncocytic features and high-grade atypia. See comment.
Comment: The FNAB shows large, flat sheets of intermediate-sized to large oncocytic cells with granular cytoplasm, round central nuclei, a high N:C ratio, and large peripherally located nucleoli. Necrotic debris is present in the background. The presence of a cystic mass on imaging is noted. The differential diagnosis predominantly includes intraductal oncocytic papillary neoplasm, neuroendocrine tumour (NET), and acinar cell carcinoma.

Sample report 4

Clinical and imaging findings: Dilated ducts with irregular filling defects.
Specimen adequacy: Satisfactory for evaluation.
Category: Pancreaticobiliary neoplasm, high-risk/grade (PaN-high).
Diagnosis: Papillary biliary epithelium with high-grade atypia. See comment.
Comment: Papillary tissue fragments are composed of small cells with high N:C ratios, irregular nuclei, and coarse chromatin. No mitotic figures are seen and no background necrosis is present. Immunoperoxidase stains of a cell block show diffuse, strong staining for p53 and loss of nuclear staining for SMAD4. These findings support at least high-grade dysplasia in consideration of the imaging findings of a dilated duct with filling defects, and suggest the diagnosis of high-grade intraductal papillary neoplasia of the bile duct. Invasive carcinoma cannot be excluded, however.

Sample report 5

Clinical and imaging findings: Dilated ducts in head of pancreas, sampled by bile duct brushing.

Diagnostic summary:
Category: Pancreaticobiliary neoplasm, high-risk/grade (PaN-high).
Diagnosis: Epithelial neoplasm with mucinous features and high-grade atypia. See microscopic description.

Microscopic description: These bile duct brushings are highly cellular and show papillary tissue fragments of mucinous epithelial cells and background mucin. Changes suggestive of high-grade nuclear atypia, including increased N:C ratio and nuclear hyperchromasia, are present.
Comment: The findings are consistent with an intraductal papillary neoplasm with at least high-grade dysplasia. Concurrent cyst fluid analysis shows an elevated CEA level of 1331 ng/mL, consistent with a mucinous etiology. Molecular analysis is pending and will be reported separately.

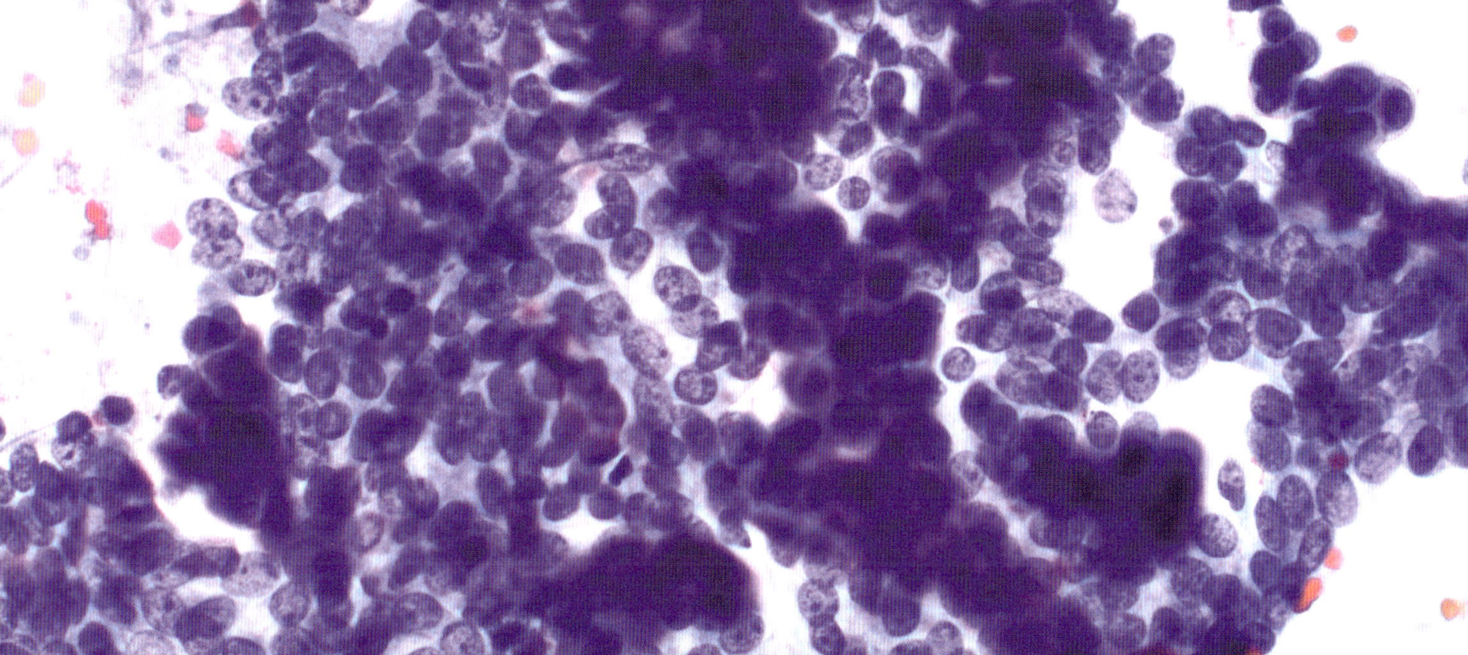

8

Diagnostic category: Suspicious for malignancy

Edited by: Layfield LJ

Introduction

Goyal A
Siddiqui MT

The cytopathological diagnosis of pancreaticobiliary malignancy is challenging, with clinical and imaging features overlapping between benign and malignant entities, difficulties in sampling, and the varying experience levels of endoscopists and cytopathologists {603,589,692,904,307}. Consequently, indeterminate cytopathological diagnoses are not uncommon. The "Suspicious for malignancy" category has been reported to account for 4.7–16% of all cytopathological diagnoses in the pancreaticobiliary tract {965,111,752,134}.

This category implies that the findings are highly concerning for but not diagnostic of malignancy. A definitive diagnosis of malignancy may be limited by scant cellularity, or the tumour cytomorphology may pose diagnostic difficulties, and there is insufficient tissue for ancillary studies. Confounding factors such as concurrent pancreatitis, particularly for pancreatic mass FNAB, and previous stent placement or primary sclerosing cholangitis for biliary brushings also lead to a high threshold for a diagnosis of malignancy {770,232,258,307}. A "Suspicious for malignancy" categorization does not provide a diagnosis of malignancy, which is required for neoadjuvant therapy, and it therefore poses a management dilemma for the patient care team.

Subclinical premalignant lesions of the pancreas, i.e. high-grade pancreatic intraepithelial neoplasia, may be inadvertently sampled by FNAB and can lead to a "Suspicious for malignancy" interpretation. Bile ducts with high-grade biliary intraepithelial neoplasia also typically lead to a "Suspicious for malignancy" categorization because the criteria for a specific diagnosis for these intraductal lesions are not defined.

Definition

Goyal A
Siddiqui MT

A specimen categorized as "Suspicious for malignancy" demonstrates some cytopathological features suggestive of malignancy, but with features insufficient in either number or quality to make an unequivocal diagnosis of malignancy.

Discussion and background

Siddiqui MT
Goyal A
Heymann JJ

A "Suspicious for malignancy" categorization in pancreaticobiliary cytopathology is most commonly used in the setting of a scant specimen of a well-differentiated adenocarcinoma or for cases with rare ductal cells with marked cytopathological atypia, especially when the mass is not distinct on imaging. The aim is to avoid false positive diagnoses, including the inadvertent sampling of high-grade pancreatic intraepithelial neoplasia {353,68}. A "Suspicious for malignancy" categorization is common for bile duct brushings where the architectural and cytological atypia is difficult to distinguish from reactive and reparative atypia due to indwelling stents, stones, or underlying inflammatory conditions including primary sclerosing cholangitis.

Wherever possible, a "Suspicious for malignancy" report should state the malignancy suspected or a differential diagnosis based initially on the cytopathological findings, which determine the selection of ICC and other ancillary testing. The ancillary testing may lead to a change in the category and a specific diagnosis of a carcinoma or other malignancy and should be presented in an integrated final report.

Well-differentiated adenocarcinoma becomes a challenging diagnosis when all cytopathological criteria are not present and/or a limited number of lesional cells are identified. Diagnostic criteria for well-differentiated adenocarcinoma include architectural disorder with moderate to marked nuclear crowding and overlapping, loss of polarity, anisonucleosis to the extent of ≥ 4× variation in individual cell nuclei within tissue fragments, nuclear enlargement, increased N:C ratio, nuclear membrane irregularities, and parachromatin clearing. Other features including coarse or clumped chromatin, prominent nucleoli, and dispersed single malignant cells, which become more common with increasing grades of malignancy {493, 141,956,68,646}. Most diagnostic features should be readily

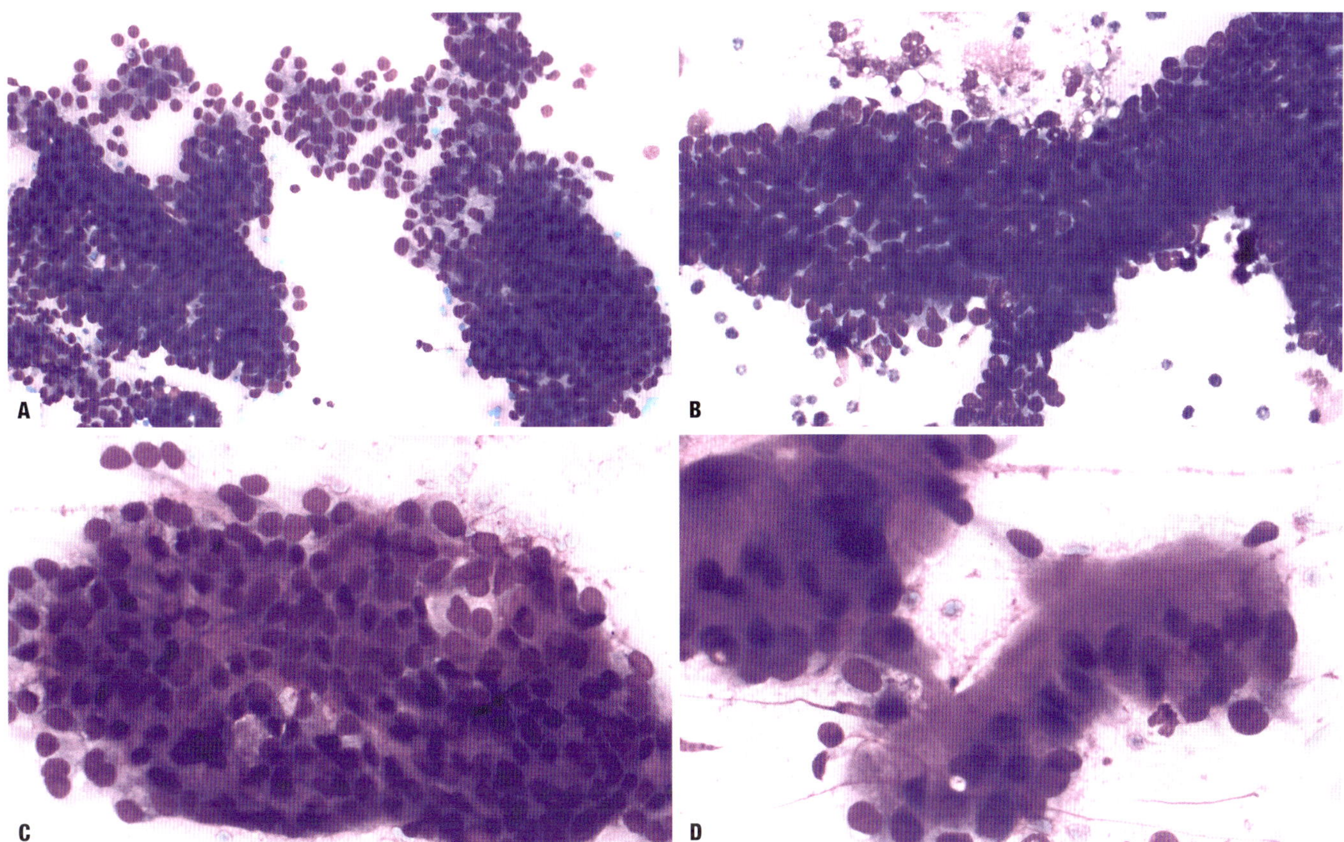

Fig. 8.01 Diagnostic category: "Suspicious for malignancy". **A** Suspicious for acinar cell carcinoma. This solid mass FNAB shows 3D tissue fragments of uniform polygonal cells with granular cytoplasm, suspicious for acinar cell carcinoma without a cell block for confirmatory ancillary testing (Giemsa). **B** Suspicious for pancreatic ductal adenocarcinoma. Although this tissue fragment of ductal epithelium shows marked nuclear crowding and overlap, it lacks nuclear membrane irregularities, abnormal chromatin, and anisonucleosis of 4:1 for definitive diagnosis as malignant (Giemsa). **C** Suspicious for pancreatic ductal adenocarcinoma. Well-differentiated pancreatic ductal adenocarcinoma is bland and difficult to diagnose as malignant. The tissue fragment shows architectural disorganization (drunken-honeycomb pattern) but lacks significant anisonucleosis and visible cytoplasmic mucin for a definitive diagnosis as malignant (Giemsa). **D** Suspicious for pancreatic ductal adenocarcinoma. This tissue fragment of ductal cells is pseudostratified, with mild anisonucleosis and loss of polarity (Giemsa).

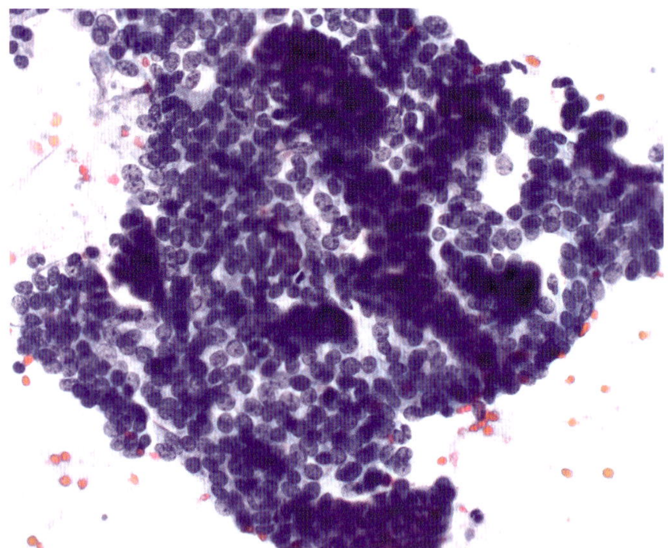

Fig. 8.02 Pancreatic ductal adenocarcinoma. Well-differentiated pancreatic ductal adenocarcinoma with nuclear crowding, parachromatin clearing, and small nucleoli. Such specimens are often assigned to the "Suspicious for malignancy" category (Pap).

identifiable in several tissue fragments for a definitive diagnosis of malignancy. If they are only partially present or seen focally, a "Suspicious for malignancy" categorization is more appropriate. Utilization of this category in this situation will prevent misinterpretation of reactive atypia associated with pancreatitis or contaminant gastrointestinal epithelium with reactive changes as malignant. Reactive atypia is usually seen in a limited number of tissue fragments with lesser degrees of architectural crowding and anisonucleosis, a low N:C ratio, and smooth to minimally irregular nuclear membranes {353}.

Cytopathological diagnosis of adenocarcinoma is challenging in bile duct brushings. Most of the malignancies that are confidently diagnosed on bile duct brushing cytopathology are high-grade carcinomas {268,258}. A majority of the criteria should be satisfied in a sufficiently cellular sample for a "Malignant" categorization to be made. In the presence of a stone, an indwelling stent, or a history of primary sclerosing cholangitis, caution should be exercised because of the presence of coexisting reactive changes. A definitive diagnosis of malignancy should only be rendered when the cytopathological features are very pronounced {268,258,232}.

Neoplastic mucinous cysts can be placed in this category when FNAB from a cyst with high-risk imaging features demonstrates high-grade epithelial atypia in a background of coagulative-type necrosis and high-risk imaging features, findings that raise concern for but are not diagnostic of invasive carcinoma. Another consideration for a "Suspicious for malignancy" categorization is when there is a lack of adequate material for confirmatory ancillary studies for the characterization of malignancies such as neuroendocrine tumour (NET) or acinar cell carcinoma {643}. Other examples of diagnostic difficulties may include insufficient tissue for the confirmation of a possible metastasis, lymphoma, or poorly differentiated neuroendocrine carcinoma (NEC).

In the Papanicolaou Society of Cytopathology (PSC) reporting system {650}, pancreatic NETs (PanNETs) and solid pseudopapillary neoplasms were included in the "Neoplastic: other" category, and so FNABs that were suggestive but not diagnostic of these neoplasms were placed in the "Atypical" category. In this WHO Reporting System, PanNET and solid pseudopapillary neoplasm are categorized as malignant neoplasms per the fifth-edition WHO classification of digestive system tumours {910}. Therefore, an indeterminate FNAB that is suggestive of one of these neoplasms should be interpreted as "Suspicious for malignancy".

Given the difficulties associated with the diagnosis of a pancreaticobiliary malignancy, a "Suspicious for malignancy" cytopathological categorization may be unavoidable and most appropriate. However, when encountering such a scenario, obtaining consultation intradepartmentally or from an expert or recommending additional tissue sampling, particularly at the time of rapid onsite evaluation (ROSE), may result in a more definitive diagnosis. In a study of 1225 pancreatic solid lesion FNABs, Virk and colleagues reported a reduction in indeterminate diagnoses from 11.55% to 7.88% after the institution of departmental consensus review {883}. Ancillary studies such as next-generation sequencing or FISH may provide additional information for establishing a malignant diagnosis in specimens otherwise categorized as "Suspicious for malignancy" {226,192, 79,247,370,700,787}.

Risk of malignancy and management recommendations

Goyal A
Klapman J
Siddiqui MT

The fundamental role of a standardized system for cytopathological diagnoses is the stratification of the risk of malignancy associated with the different diagnostic categories, which aids patient management. As a result, it is important to distinguish between the "Atypical" category and the "Suspicious for malignancy" category, because they are associated with different risks of malignancy and may be managed differently. The risk of malignancy for the "Suspicious for malignancy" category varies with the specimen type and the site of sampling, ranging from 80% to 100% for EUS-FNAB of the pancreas {792,307,824,306} and from 74% to 100% for bile duct brushings {875,111,192,952, 658,468,595}.

Management of a "Suspicious for malignancy" categorization is highly dependent on the correlation of the cytopathology with the clinical and imaging findings and the results of contributory ancillary tests such as ICC and molecular pathology analysis. Depending on the combination of findings, it may prompt surgical intervention or further investigation. It is important to note that a "Suspicious for malignancy" cytopathological categorization by itself is not an indication for surgery or for neoadjuvant therapy.

Sample reports: Suspicious for malignancy

Goyal A
Siddiqui MT

Sample report 1

Clinical and imaging findings: Solid tumour in head of pancreas.
Specimen adequacy: Satisfactory for evaluation.
Category: Suspicious for malignancy.
Diagnosis: Few markedly atypical ductal cells suspicious for adenocarcinoma. See comment.
Comment: The FNAB reveals rare groups of markedly atypical epithelial cells that are quantitatively insufficient for a diagnosis of adenocarcinoma.

Sample report 2

Clinical and imaging findings: Cystic mass with mural nodule in body of pancreas.
Specimen adequacy: Satisfactory for evaluation.
Category: Suspicious for malignancy.
Diagnosis: Mucinous cyst with high-grade epithelial atypia in a background of coagulative necrosis, suspicious for invasive adenocarcinoma. See comment.
Comment: The endoscopic appearance of a cystic mass with an associated mural nodule coupled with the markedly atypical but few epithelial cells in the cyst fluid is suspicious for invasive carcinoma.

Sample report 3

Clinical and imaging findings: Solid tumour in head of pancreas.

Diagnostic summary:
Category: Suspicious for malignancy.
Diagnosis: Suspicious for acinar cell carcinoma. See microscopic description.

Microscopic description: These highly cellular smears show cytopathological findings suspicious for acinar cell carcinoma. The cell block has insufficient material for confirmatory ancillary testing.

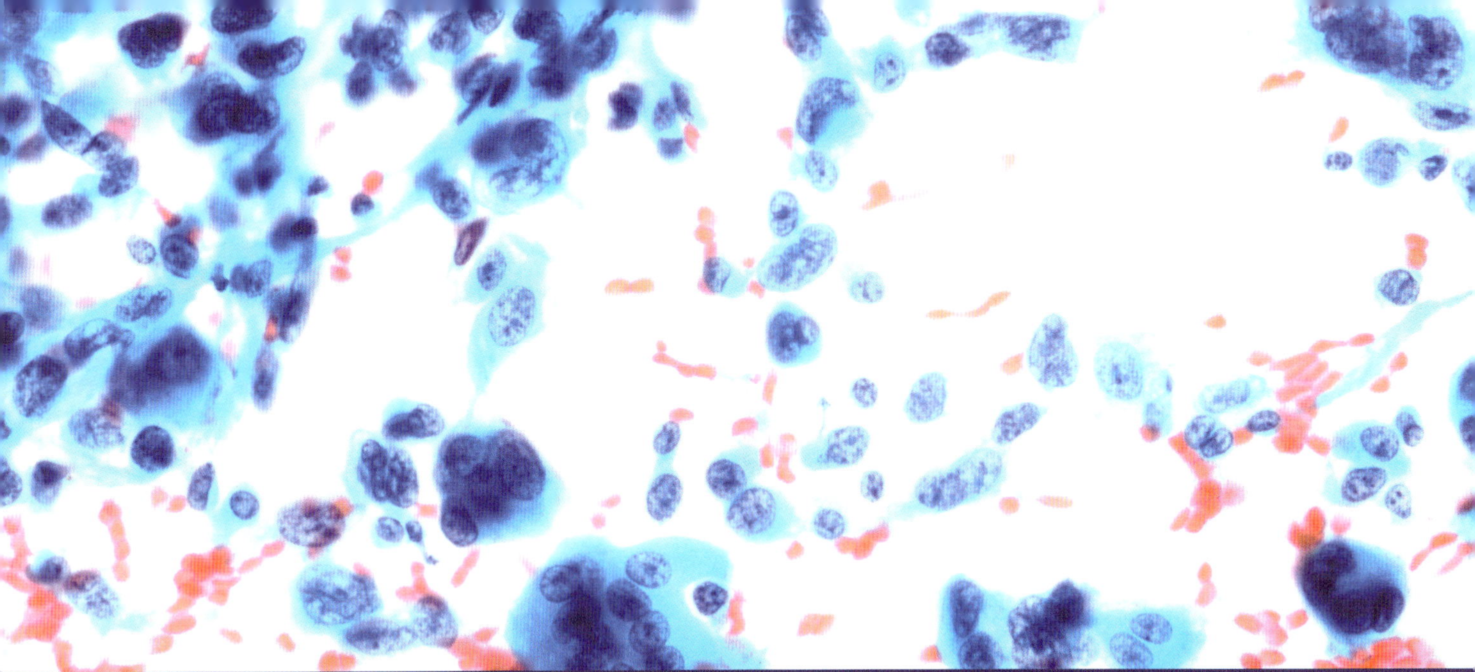

9

Diagnostic category: Malignant

Edited by: Centeno BA, Fukushima N

Introduction

Chhieng DC
Dhillon J

The majority of primary pancreatic malignant neoplasms in adults are pancreatic ductal adenocarcinoma or one of its subtypes, accounting for > 90% of all pancreatic malignancies {416, 910}. Cholangiocarcinoma, arising from the distal common bile duct, often presents as a pancreatic mass because of frequent extension into the pancreas and duodenum. It is morphologically indistinguishable from pancreatic ductal adenocarcinoma. More often, it is identified on bile duct brushings of bile duct strictures, rather than by FNAB, which is used to diagnose most pancreatic masses.

Unlike in the Papanicolaou Society of Cytopathology (PSC) System for Reporting Pancreaticobiliary Cytology {643}, and in keeping with the WHO classification of pancreatic tumours {910}, well-differentiated neuroendocrine tumours (NETs) (G1–G3) and solid pseudopapillary neoplasms are included in the "Malignant" category (rather than the "Neoplastic: other" category of the PSC system).

Other primary pancreatic malignant tumours are rare and include acinar cell carcinoma, poorly differentiated neuroendocrine carcinomas (NECs), primary non-Hodgkin lymphoma, and pancreatoblastoma, which is the most common primary pancreatic malignancy of infancy and early childhood {910}. In addition, the pancreas is the site of metastases and direct secondary involvement by other malignancies. Spindle cell malignancies, including gastrointestinal stromal tumours, may involve the pancreaticobiliary tract as either primary or secondary malignancies.

Definition

Chhieng DC
Dhillon J

A specimen categorized as "Malignant" demonstrates unequivocal cytopathological features of malignancy.

Discussion and background

Chhieng DC
Klapman J
Pitman MB

The diagnosis of pancreatic ductal adenocarcinoma (PDAC) is usually straightforward when sufficient cellular material is present, and with the use of next-generation biopsy needles for EUS-FNAB, potentially fewer biopsies are likely to be indeterminate {619}. Because many patients are referred to neoadjuvant therapy before surgical intervention, and adjuvant therapy alone within clinical trials is used in unresectable cases, a definite diagnosis of malignancy is required before the clinical team will begin treatment. In cases that are indeterminate, ancillary studies may help to provide a diagnosis of malignancy. Ancillary studies are essential in patients with a history of previous malignancy and possible metastases to the pancreaticobiliary tract, undifferentiated malignancies, or neoplasms with cytopathological features of a non-ductal neoplasm.

When assessing a pancreatic FNAB, it is advisable to have a low threshold for ordering ancillary studies to diagnose neuroendocrine neoplasms, acinar cell carcinoma, and metastases, particularly renal cell carcinoma, because these may have features overlapping with those of PDAC. Also, although management may not change for most subtypes of PDAC, patients with squamous differentiation may have platinum-based drugs added to their regimen {177}. Therefore, it is advisable to assess each case for evidence of adenosquamous carcinoma and for squamous differentiation in poorly differentiated PDAC.

Interpretation of the cytopathological and small biopsy findings should ideally occur with a multimodal approach, taking into account the clinical presentation and imaging features of the lesion {963}. For example, patients with hypoglycaemia may have a functioning neuroendocrine tumour (NET), and patients with lipase hypersecretion and subcutaneous fat necrosis may have acinar cell carcinoma. Imaging showing a double-duct sign, where the distal common bile duct and main pancreatic duct are both constricted in the pancreatic head with downstream dilatation, certainly should be regarded as PDAC till proved otherwise {540}. A round, well-circumscribed mass is more likely a NET than PDAC. Discussing the limitations of the biopsy samples with the clinical care team can help guide patient management and may suggest additional workup or beneficial ancillary studies for the pathologist.

Risk of malignancy and management recommendations

Chhieng DC
Klapman J
Pitman MB

Based on the Papanicolaou Society of Cytopathology (PSC) System for Reporting Pancreaticobiliary Cytology, the "Positive (for malignancy)" rates in pancreatic FNAB are relatively high and range widely (28–52%), with a mean of 40% {71, 124,307,461,824,924} (see Table 9.01). The data from all 6 studies were from various academic practices located in the USA (*n* = 4) {71,307,824,461}, United Kingdom (1) {924}, and China (1) {824}. In contrast, the risk of malignancy of a positive pancreatic FNAB varies little (99–100%) {792,307, 824,306}.

The "Positive (for malignancy)" rates of bile duct brushings based on the PSC System for Reporting Pancreaticobiliary Cytology have not been studied as much as those of pancreatic FNAB, with only 2 studies to date {631,468}. However, inclusion of older studies with these 2 studies shows that the rates of reporting "Positive (for malignancy)" in biliary tract exfoliative cytology range widely (12–51.5%). The data are from various locations, including the USA (*n* = 5) {498,256,890,111,468}, Asia (2) {538,241}, and Europe (1) {631} (see Table 9.02). The risk of malignancy of a positive biliary tract cytology varies from 96% to 100%{875,111,192,952,658,468,595}. Integrating either FISH or next-generation sequencing to biliary tract cytology improves the sensitivity of detection of malignant bile duct lesions {192,788}.

These observations imply that a positive cytological diagnosis of a pancreatic or biliary tract malignancy is highly specific; therefore, patients with cytopathologically confirmed unresectable pancreatic ductal carcinoma or cholangiocarcinoma can be treated with neoadjuvant treatment without requiring histological confirmation. False positive diagnoses of pancreatic FNABs are rare. Most false positive diagnoses are attributed to interpretation errors as a result of overinterpretation of florid reactive atypia in chronic pancreatitis, especially autoimmune pancreatitis {746,770}. There are also rare reports of high-grade pancreatic intraepithelial neoplasia (HG-PanIN) misdiagnosed cytopathologically as adenocarcinoma {353}. The most common cause of false positive biliary tract cytology is reactive atypia in the background of primary sclerosing cholangitis {241}.

A cytological diagnosis of pancreatic neuroendocrine tumour (PanNET) demonstrates excellent specificity, with a risk of malignancy ranging from 98% to 100% {71,128,313}. Histological follow-up of cases with a false positive cytological diagnosis of PanNET reveals chronic pancreatitis with or without nesidioblastosis {71,128}.

Surgical resection is currently the only means to achieve long-term survival in patients with biopsy-proven pancreatic ductal adenocarcinoma {532}. Unfortunately, only 15–20% of patients present with resectable disease that is amenable to surgery {532}. The increasing use of neoadjuvant therapies and advances in surgical techniques have broadened the pool of patients, especially those with borderline resectable disease, who are eligible for surgical resection {397}. For those with locally advanced and/or metastatic disease, systemic therapy with or without radiation is indicated {532}. Eligible candidates can also enrol into clinical trials.

Recent gains in the molecular understanding of pancreatic ductal carcinoma have led to the increased use of personalized therapy. One such example would be microsatellite instability (MSI), although it is only detected in approximately 1% of patients with the disease {328}. However, 40% of patients who have MSI respond to immune checkpoint inhibition and derive improved survival from this therapy {469,470}. Therefore, it is important for patients with unresectable and metastatic disease to be tested for MSI. MSI and other genetic mutations can be readily analysed on FNAB cell blocks and residual needle rinses.

Surgical resection is recommended for all functioning PanNETs and localized non-functioning PanNETs (without widespread metastasis), and the surgical options include simple enucleation, central pancreatectomy, distal pancreatectomy with or without splenectomy, and pancreaticoduodenectomy, depending on tumour location {756}. Although some authors recommend conservative observation (watch and wait) for patients with non-functioning PanNETs measuring < 20 mm {208}, it remains controversial {527,714,215,759}.

Surgical management is usually the first line of treatment for less common primary malignancies in the pancreas. If the

Table 9.01 Rate of "Malignant" category and associated risk of malignancy for FNAB of pancreatic masses

Series	City	Country	Rate of "Malignant" category	Risk of malignancy
Layfield et al., 2014 {461}	Columbia, MO	USA	44%	98.58%
Bergeron et al., 2015 {71}	Charleston, SC	USA	52%	97.37%
Chen et al., 2017 {124}	Beijing	China	43%	100.00%
Hoda et al., 2019 {307}	Boston, MA	USA	28%	100.00%
Sung et al., 2020 {824}	New York, NY	USA	29%	99.61%
Hoda et al., 2021 {306}	Boston, MA	USA	34%	100.00%

Table 9.02 Rate of "Malignant" category and associated risk of malignancy for biliary tract exfoliative cytopathology specimens

Series	City	Country	Rate of "Malignant" category	Risk of malignancy
Logrono et al., 2000 {498}	Galveston, TX	USA	13%	88%
Govil et al., 2002 {256}	Chicago, IL	USA	12%	100%
Volmar et al., 2006 {890}	Chapel Hill, NC	USA	16%	99%
Chadwick et al., 2014 {111}	Salt Lake City, UT	USA	12%	100%
Mehmood et al., 2016 {538}	Lahore	Pakistan	52%	100%
Yeo et al., 2017 {952}	Daejeon	Republic of Korea	32%	96%
Geramizadeh et al., 2018 {241}	Shiraz	Islamic Republic of Iran	21%	94%
Pereira et al., 2020 {631}	Porto	Portugal	34%	98%
Layfield et al., 2022 {468}	Columbia, MO	USA	19%	91%

disease is not resectable, the patient is treated with adjuvant chemotherapy with or without radiation therapy.

Complete surgical resection is the only treatment to afford a chance of cure for cholangiocarcinoma {186}. Unfortunately, most tumours are inoperable at the time of presentation. Additional treatment modalities may include stenting, targeted radiation therapy, and systemic chemotherapy {186}.

Cholangiocarcinoma

Layfield LJ
Naito Y
Sigel C

Definition

Cholangiocarcinoma is a primary malignant epithelial neoplasm arising from bile duct epithelium.

Clinical features and imaging

For the purposes of this discussion of the clinical and imaging features, the focus here is on large duct biliary adenocarcinoma involving ducts most accessible to biliary brushing, including the large intrahepatic ducts near the hepatic hilum, which are proximal to the right and left hepatic ducts, and the extrahepatic bile ducts, which include the common bile duct between the cystic duct and ampulla. However, the cytopathological features, discussion, and ancillary testing are also applicable to the diagnosis of intrahepatic and perihilar cholangiocarcinoma.

The incidence of large duct cholangiocarcinoma is generally rare, at 1 case per 100 000 person-years, but there is significant geographical variation. The disease develops mostly in the sixth to seventh decade of life, with almost equal sex distribution, and jaundice accounts for most clinical presentations. Other symptoms are malaise, abdominal pain, and weight loss. Elevated serum CA19-9 (> 129 U/mL) is helpful in detecting carcinoma {481}. Risk factors include primary sclerosing cholangitis, bile duct cysts, hepatolithiasis, Caroli disease, and biliary flukes, but in many patients there is no identifiable etiology {862}. The prognosis is very poor, with a 1% 5-year survival rate.

Upon presentation, most patients are first evaluated by transabdominal ultrasound, which detects biliary dilatation. Imaging features of large duct cholangiocarcinoma include biliary stricture, wall thickening, dilatation, and filling defects. CT and magnetic resonance cholangiopancreatography are non-invasive means of assessing tumour extent and local staging {358,981}. With few exceptions, definitive pathological diagnosis must be obtained before treatment, and tumour sampling is usually done via endoscopic retrograde cholangiopancreatography, during which bile fluid, brushings, FNAB, and small tissue biopsies can be obtained {46}.

Histopathology

Large duct cholangiocarcinoma precursors include biliary intraepithelial neoplasia, intraductal papillary neoplasm, and intraductal tubular neoplasm {727,735,736,20}. Infiltrating cholangiocarcinomas form tubules and glands of columnar cells interspersed with desmoplastic stroma and have good, moderate, or poor differentiation {910}. Because the origin is most commonly large-calibre bile ducts or peribiliary ducts, the most common patterns of differentiation are ductal, intestinal, or gastric foveolar; other (rare) appearances include squamous, adenosquamous, mucinous, signet-ring cell, clear cell, undifferentiated, and sarcomatoid. Extrahepatic cholangiocarcinomas tend to infiltrate along the bile duct with conspicuous lymphovascular and perineural invasion.

Key diagnostic cytopathological features

- Loss of honeycomb pattern (drunken honeycomb)
- 3D architecture
- Hypercellularity with two-cell population
- Hypochromasia/hyperchromasia
- Nuclear pleomorphism
- Anisonucleosis (threefold to fourfold variability, or greater, in nuclear size in a single cell group)
- Increased N:C ratio (≥ 0.6)
- Cytoplasmic mucin
- Cellular discohesion with atypical single cells

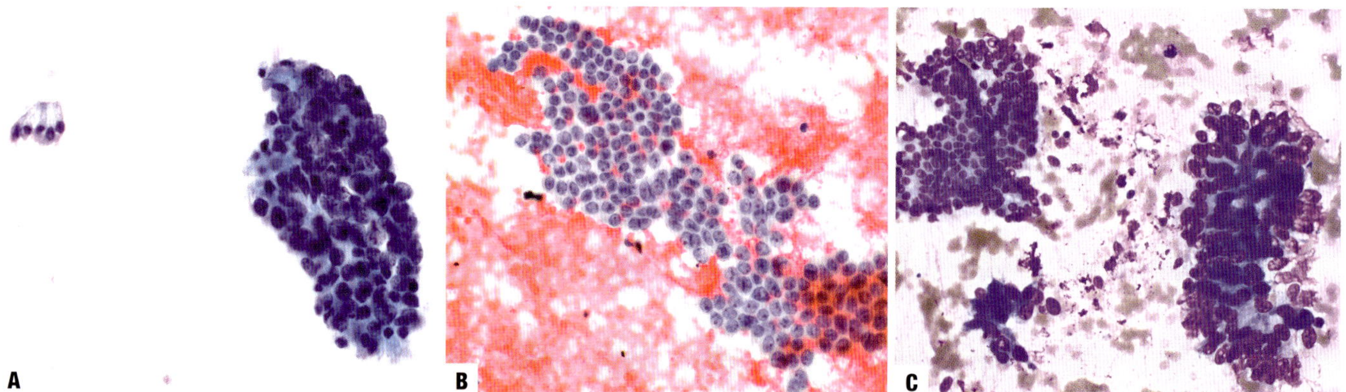

Fig. 9.01 Cholangiocarcinoma. **A** Moderately to poorly differentiated cholangiocarcinoma. This hyperchromatic crowded tissue fragment of glandular cells shows loss of polarity, high N:C ratio, marked crowding and anisonucleosis, enlarged pleomorphic hyperchromatic nuclei, and nuclear membrane irregularities (Pap). **B** Well-differentiated cholangiocarcinoma. Direct smear showing a mildly disordered and crowded sheet of glandular cells with a moderate degree of nuclear membrane abnormalities, angular nuclei, and prominent nucleoli (Pap). **C** Moderately differentiated cholangiocarcinoma. Tissue fragment showing marked nuclear crowding and loss of polarity, moderate anisonucleosis, and increased N:C ratio. A benign tissue fragment is on the left for comparison (Giemsa).

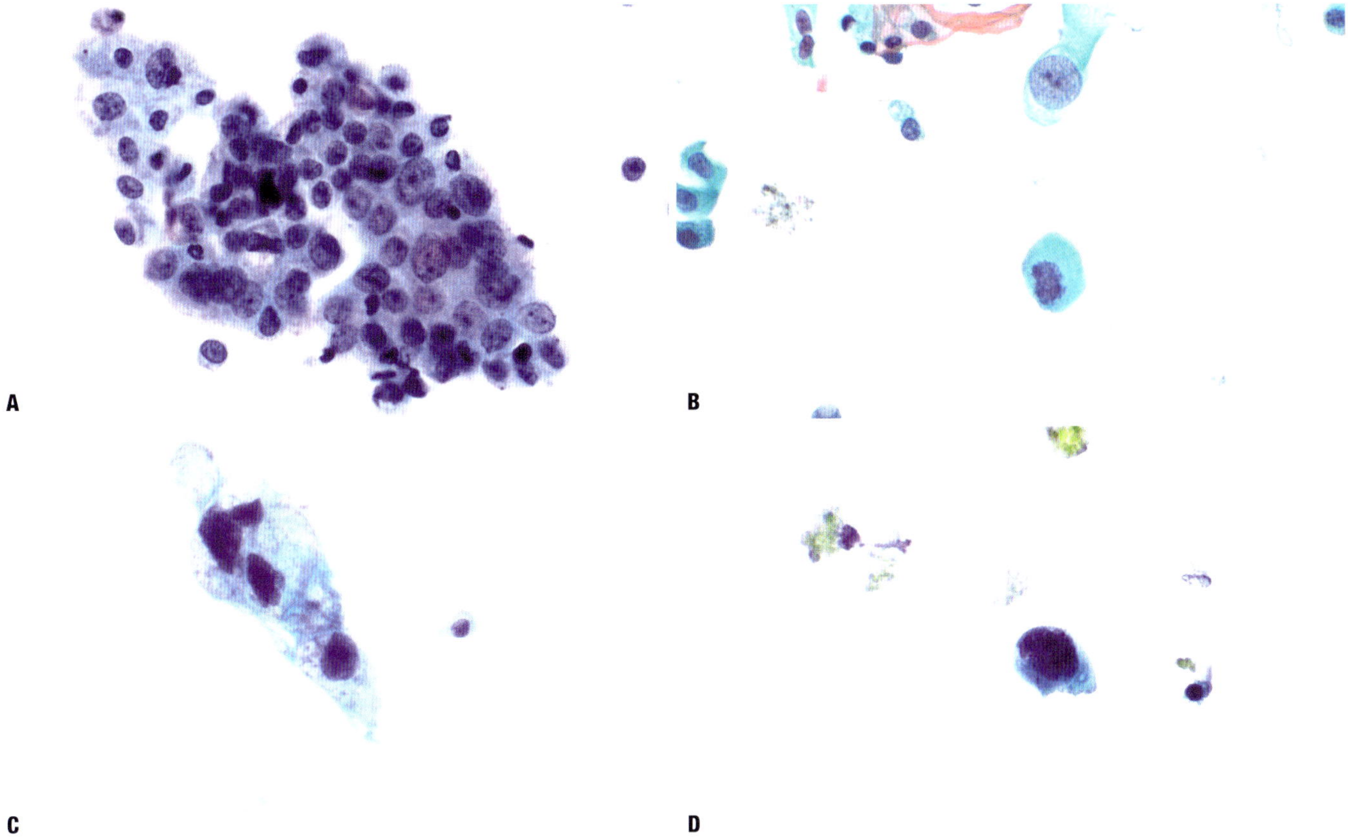

Fig. 9.02 Cholangiocarcinoma. **A** Tissue fragment showing nuclear crowding and overlapping and marked anisonucleosis with increased N:C ratio. Individual nuclei show chromatin clearing, prominent nucleoli, and nuclear membrane irregularities (Pap). **B** Bile duct brushing with single dispersed atypical cells showing cytomegaly and large nuclei with a mitotic figure, supporting a "Malignant" interpretation (note: for comparison, small benign columnar cells in the background) (liquid-based cytopathology, Pap). **C** Bile duct brushing showing a small tissue fragment of malignant cells with anisonucleosis, irregular nuclear membranes, hyperchromasia, and lacy mucinous cytoplasm (liquid-based cytopathology, Pap). **D** Bile duct brushing with a single atypical cell with intact eccentric cytoplasm, large hyperchromatic nucleus, and irregular nuclear membrane, supporting a "Malignant" interpretation (liquid-based cytopathology, Pap).

- Prominent nucleoli
- Enlarged nuclei
- Loss of polarity
- Bloody background
- Flat nuclei
- Cell-in-cell arrangement
- Nuclear moulding
- Chromatin clumping

Reference(s): {142,579,685,715,44}

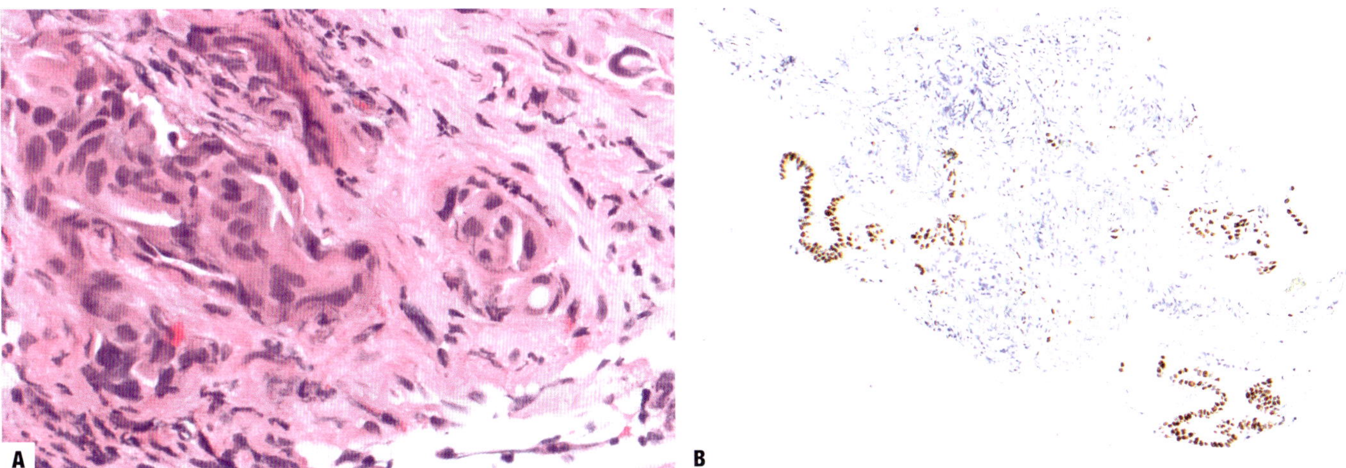

Fig. 9.03 Cholangiocarcinoma. **A** Forceps biopsy shows invasive glands, small strands, and single cells with intracytoplasmic vacuoles invading the stroma (H&E). **B** ICC for p53 shows strong nuclear staining in the neoplastic epithelium, supporting malignancy.

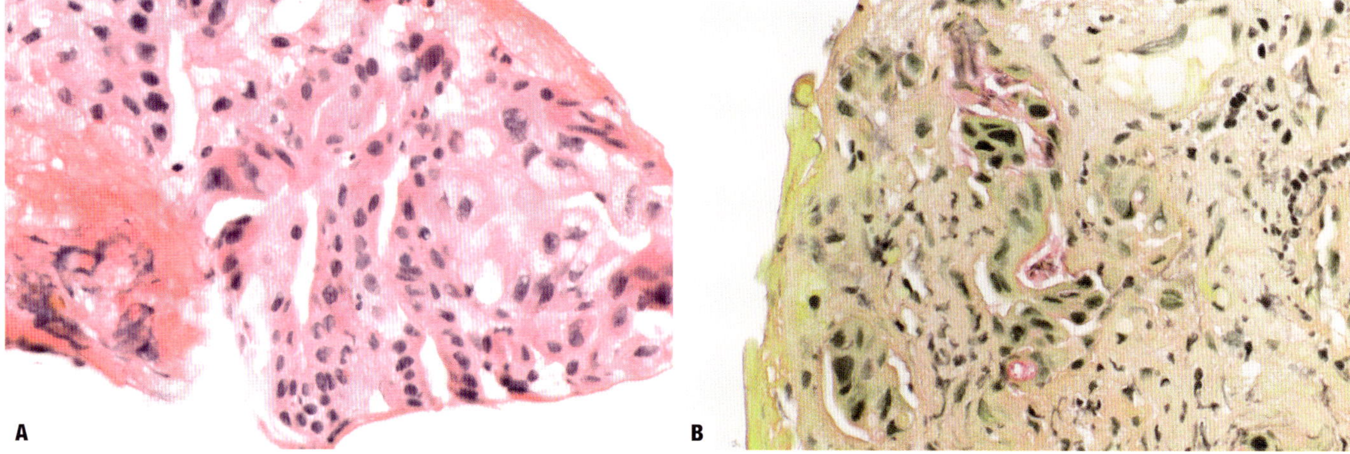

Fig. 9.04 Cholangiocarcinoma. **A** Forceps biopsy shows a tissue fragment of glandular cells showing a partial cribriform architecture with anisonucleosis, irregular nuclei, and lacy mucinous cytoplasm, which imparts a deceptively low N:C ratio (H&E). **B** Forceps biopsy stained by mucicarmine demonstrates extracellular and intracellular mucin within small glands and strands of malignant epithelium (mucicarmine).

Discussion and differential diagnosis

Cholangiocarcinoma requires distinction from reactive atypia of bile ducts due to inflammation, stones, and stents. Primary sclerosing cholangitis also represents a differential diagnostic challenge because of reactive atypia associated with primary sclerosing cholangitis.

Bile duct brushing cytology has a low sensitivity for the detection of carcinoma {467,142,685,256}. An indeterminate categorization of "Atypical" or "Suspicious for malignancy" is common, because of the high threshold for a definitive "Malignant" categorization by morphology alone {685}. A high threshold for a "Malignant" categorization is warranted because of the underlying injury and reactive/reparative changes that result from indwelling stents, stones, and inflammation from conditions such as primary sclerosing cholangitis.

Multivariate regression analysis has documented cytological features useful in the recognition of cholangiocarcinoma {579, 142,685,715,44}, and other studies have focused on cytological features useful for the diagnosis of cholangiocarcinoma in the setting of stent placements {258,290}. Cytological features of adenocarcinoma include 3D groups, nuclear enlargement (> 3× normal), pleomorphism, two-cell population, chromatin pattern changes (hypochromasia/hyperchromasia), high N:C ratio, cytoplasmic vacuoles, nuclear irregularity, cellular dyscohesion, hypercellularity, nuclear moulding, prominent nucleoli, single vacuolated cells, and anisonucleosis (≥ 1:6) {579,142,685,715,44,258,290}. The presence of a minimum of three criteria is recommended for definitive diagnosis {579,44}. The overall gestalt may be just as effective as systematically using criteria {685}.

Ancillary studies including ICC stains and molecular testing can aid in the differential diagnosis of cholangiocarcinoma from reactive processes, hepatocellular carcinoma, and a variety of metastatic malignancies of the biliary system (see ancillary testing).

Ancillary testing

When cytomorphological features supportive of adenocarcinoma are encountered in bile duct brushing or fine-needle aspiration, immunocytochemical techniques are rarely necessary

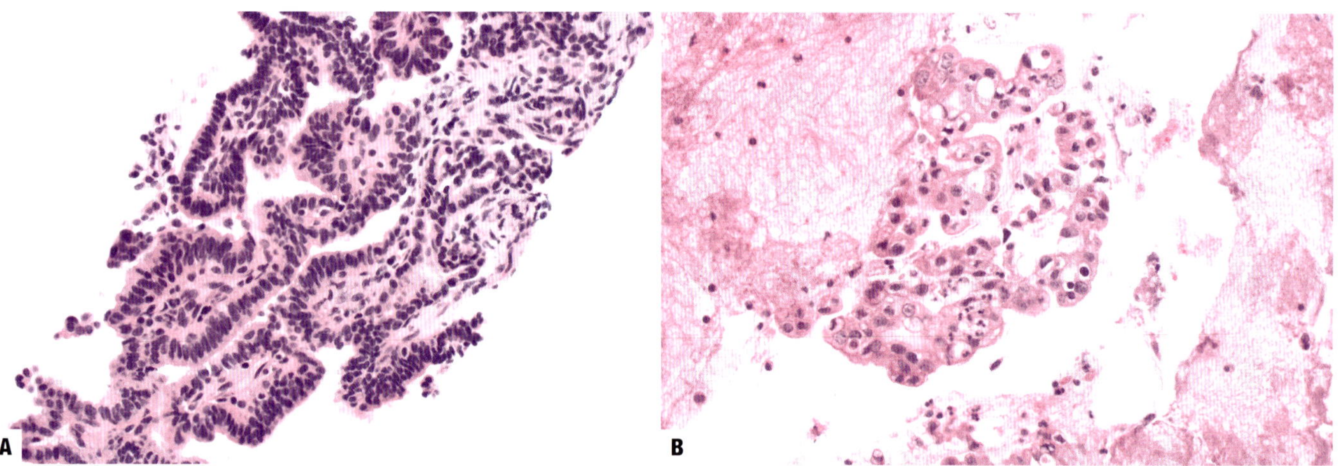

Fig. 9.05 Cholangiocarcinoma. **A** Well-differentiated cholangiocarcinoma. The cell block demonstrates glandular epithelium showing high-grade dysplasia with loss of nuclear polarity, nuclear enlargement and hyperchromasia, increased N:C ratio, and a focus in the upper-right corner with small glands and single cells in stroma, suggestive of invasion (H&E). **B** Cell block showing cords and nests of cells with loss of polarity, nuclear hyperchromasia, and nuclear membrane irregularities (H&E).

for clarification unless the morphology and/or clinical history raises concern for a neoplasm of non-pancreaticobiliary glandular differentiation (e.g. neuroendocrine carcinoma [NEC], mesenchymal neoplasm) or metastasis. ICC study aids in the separation of cholangiocarcinoma from hepatocellular carcinoma and a variety of metastatic malignancies to the pancreas and peripancreatic tissues. A caveat is that antibodies to distinguish pancreatic ductal adenocarcinoma from extrahepatic cholangiocarcinoma are lacking.

However, because of background reactive changes and low tumour proportion in brushing samples, ancillary techniques to aid in the detection of cholangiocarcinoma from reactive changes are often desired.

If the atypical cells of interest are present in a cell block, ICC for p53 (overexpression or absence) and/or SMAD4 (loss of expression) may be of value because these stains are abnormal in roughly half of large duct cholangiocarcinomas {136,36}. Other panels that have been studied to distinguish benign from malignant biliary brushings include S100, VHL protein, IMP3, and maspin {126,482}.

FISH is the most relevant ancillary technique used to detect polysomies associated with cholangiocarcinoma. When FISH is combined with biliary brushings, the sensitivity of detecting cholangiocarcinoma is increased (from 20% to 43%) {226}. A pancreaticobiliary-specific probe set that detects both cholangiocarcinoma and pancreatic ductal adenocarcinoma increased the rate of cancer detection by 19%, as compared with the probes in the UroVysion kit (Abbott Molecular, Abbott Park, Illinois, USA) {54}.

Recent studies have shown that next-generation sequencing performs comparably to FISH {192}, with a sensitivity and specificity when combined with cytology of 85% and 96%, respectively. Next-generation sequencing has several advantages over FISH, including decreasing costs, the ability to batch multiple specimens in a single run, and solid tumour genotyping with the identification of targetable mutations {192,788}.

Pancreatic ductal adenocarcinoma

Weynand B
Cocker R
Dhillon J
Goyal A
Jhala N
Kumarasinghe MP
Pitman MB
Reid MD

Definition

Pancreatic ductal adenocarcinoma (PDAC) is an invasive pancreatic epithelial neoplasm with glandular, ductal differentiation.

Clinical features and imaging

Patients with PDAC present with weight loss, abdominal pain, and jaundice. The carcinoma is often in a locally advanced or even metastatic stage at diagnosis. High serum levels of CA19-9 are a characteristic feature. The majority of PDACs arise in the head of the pancreas. The imaging features of solid masses in the pancreas begin the differential diagnosis process. On CT, PDAC appears as an irregularly shaped, poorly defined solid mass, often with an associated double-duct sign due to upstream pancreatic and biliary duct dilatation, which is considered a pathognomonic feature. On EUS, PDAC is an irregular, poorly defined, hypoechoic and hypovascular mass, which can be secondarily cystic if the tumour is largely necrotic {532,816, 963}. In contrast, the non-ductal solid primary malignancies of the pancreas, including neuroendocrine tumour (NET), acinar cell carcinoma, solid pseudopapillary neoplasm (SPN), and pancreatoblastoma, and metastases present as round, well-circumscribed, and well-defined masses.

Histopathology

PDAC is composed of invasive glands usually demonstrating luminal and/or intracellular mucin production, without a substantial component of any other histopathological type, in a desmoplastic stroma. Depending on the degree of differentiation, glandular structures are variably identifiable, but intratumoural heterogeneity is common. Malignant glands are irregular in shape and infiltrate the pancreatic parenchyma in a disorganized fashion, entrapping normal structures. Haemorrhage, extensive necrosis, and cystic degeneration can occur {910}.

Key diagnostic cytopathological features

- Usually highly cellular smears with mostly tissue fragments
- Loosely cohesive or crowded tissue fragments with or without isolated tumour cells
- Irregular nuclear spacing and loss of polarity in sheets (drunken honeycomb architecture)
- Clean background in well-differentiated PDAC, varying to abundant necrosis in high-grade PDAC
- Mucinous cytoplasm, sometimes finely vacuolated and lacy, resulting in a deceptively low N:C ratio
- Hypochromatic nuclei with parachromatin clearing, varying to hyperchromatic nuclei with irregular nuclear contours
- Nucleoli may be present and prominent
- Atypical mitotic figures
- Background necrosis often present, but not always

Discussion and differential diagnosis

PDAC is the most frequent diagnosis seen on FNAB of a solid pancreatic mass. The cytopathological material is commonly highly cellular, but it can be paucicellular if the stroma is very sclerotic. For high-grade cases with obvious malignant nuclear features, diagnosis is usually straightforward, indicated by characteristic cells with abundant, often clear, mucin-containing cytoplasm and well-defined cell borders. The carcinoma forms

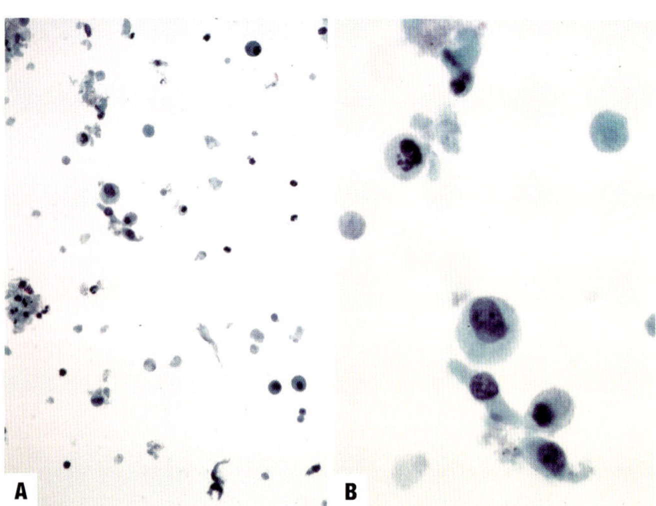

Fig. 9.06 Ductal adenocarcinoma. **A** Necrotic background with abundant cell debris, few histiocytes, and isolated histiocyte-like tumour cells, better recognized on higher magnification (liquid-based cytopathology, Pap). **B** Necrotic background with abundant cell debris and isolated single intact cells with irregular, hyperchromatic nuclei (liquid-based cytopathology, Pap).

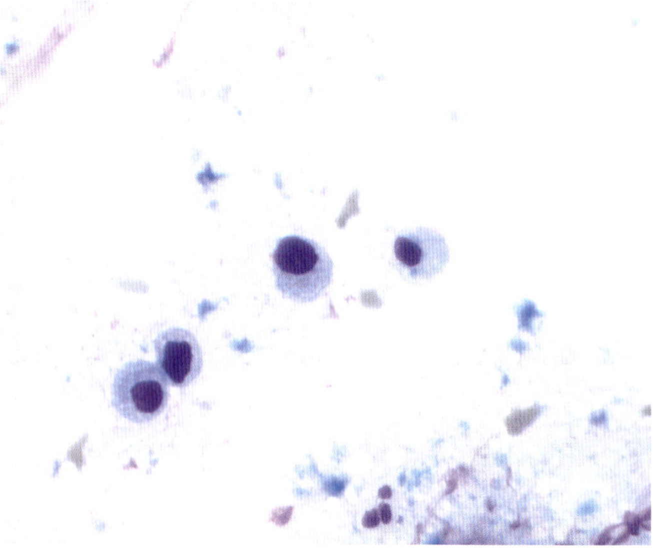

Fig. 9.07 Ductal adenocarcinoma. Single malignant cells with atypical nuclei and intact, eccentric, finely foamy cytoplasm add support to a "Malignant" interpretation (Giemsa).

Table 9.03 Immunocytochemistry (ICC) that helps to differentiate pancreatic adenocarcinoma from chronic pancreatitis

Marker	ICC in adenocarcinoma		
	Nucleus	Cytoplasm	Membrane
Clusterin	Negative	Positive	Negative
p16	Positive	Positive	Negative
Mesothelin	Negative	Positive	Positive
SMAD4	Positive or negative[a]	Negative	Negative
S100P	Positive	Positive	Negative
EMA (MUC1)	Negative	Positive	Negative
MUC2 (arising in IPMN)	Negative	Positive	Negative
MUC4	Negative	Positive	Negative
p53	Positive or negative[b]	Negative	Negative
Maspin	Positive	Positive	Negative
IMP3	Negative	Positive	Negative
Survivin	Negative	Positive	Negative

IPMN, intraductal papillary mucinous neoplasm.
[a]SMAD4, when present in ICC, will show nuclear positivity in benign cells and a subset of pancreatic ductal adenocarcinomas. [b]p53 is either diffuse and strongly positive or absent (null pattern).

hyperchromatic crowded tissue fragments, which vary in size from a few cells to large tissue fragments showing complex, cribriform architecture. In particular, the presence of single dispersed carcinoma cells is an important criterion for malignancy, because reactive changes in ductal epithelium can mimic adenocarcinoma but are not associated with isolated intact, atypical cells. Highly necrotic PDAC can be a diagnostic challenge because the necrotic cell debris may obscure the rare viable tumour cells, which are histiocyte-like with abundant, sometimes microvacuolated eccentric cytoplasm and hyperchromatic, irregular nuclei. In well-differentiated PDAC, it is important to recognize the predominance of glandular structures showing slight but significant nuclear irregularities, nuclear overlap and hypochromasia, and the drunken-honeycomb architecture {493}. Usually, there are a few high-grade ductal structures present, facilitating the diagnosis. When small tissue fragments are present in a cell block, they show a desmoplastic background infiltrated by single tumour cells, small groups, or large glands with a complex, cribriform architecture, and perineural or lymphatic vessel invasion can be recognized.

The foamy gland pattern is characterized by cells with an abundant lacy, microvesicular cytoplasm and an apical brush border–like zone, which stains with mucicarmine. The nuclei of these tumour cells are small, hyperchromatic, and eccentrically located {814,13}. The main differential diagnosis for this pattern includes benign, reactive mucinous ducts, and it also needs to be distinguished from the clear cell pattern in PDAC. In the clear

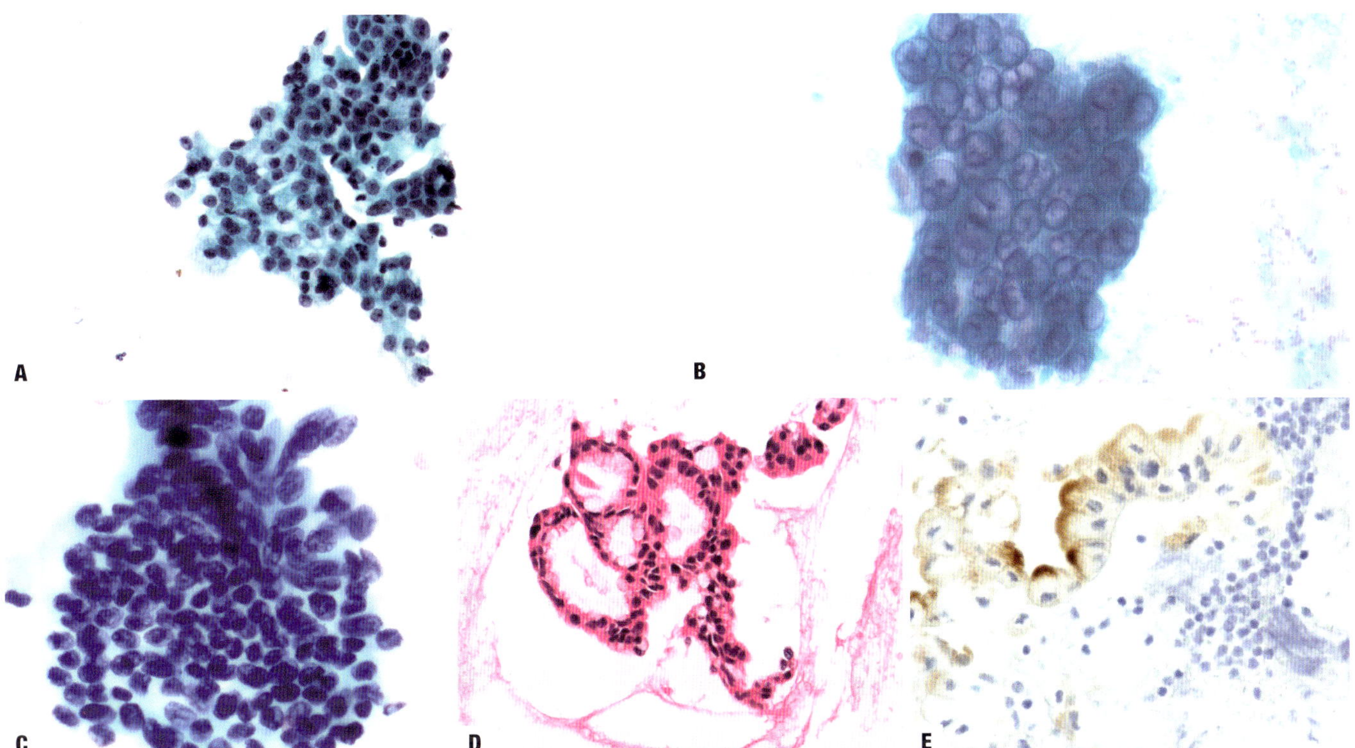

Fig. 9.08 **A** Ductal adenocarcinoma, well-differentiated. This glandular tissue fragment shows irregular nuclear spacing due to the variation in mucinous cytoplasm, yielding the drunken-honeycomb pattern typical of adenocarcinoma. Note the deceptively low N:C ratio, angulated nuclei, and hyperchromasia (Pap). **B** Ductal adenocarcinoma, well-differentiated. Parachromatin clearing producing pale nuclei rather than hyperchromasia is a common feature of pancreatic ductal adenocarcinoma and is best appreciated on the Pap. The nuclei are enlarged with marked indentations and grooves, and there is a high N:C ratio. **C** Well-differentiated adenocarcinoma. An example with focally unevenly spaced and overlapping nuclei of the drunken-honeycomb pattern, with mild anisonucleosis and nuclear indentations and occasional grooves (Pap). **D** Ductal adenocarcinoma. Cell block showing a tissue fragment with a cribriform architecture and composed of atypical cells with hyperchromatic nuclei, loss of polarity, and high N:C ratio (H&E). **E** Ductal adenocarcinoma. Cell block showing a glandular fragment showing positive cytoplasmic mesothelin expression in pancreatic adenocarcinoma (ICC).

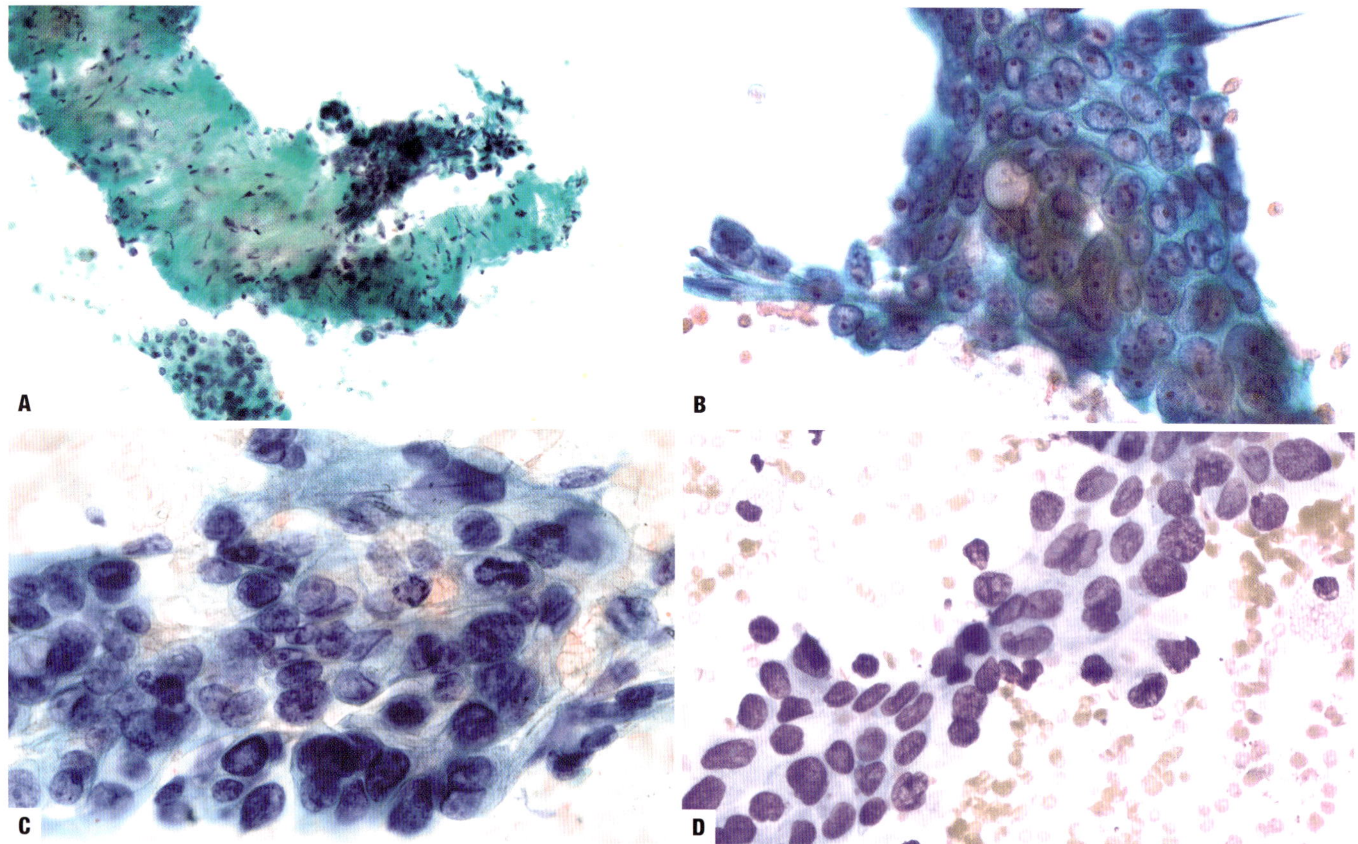

Fig. 9.09 Ductal adenocarcinoma, high-grade. **A** Hyperchromatic crowded tissue fragments of adenocarcinoma are present at the edge of a fragment of desmoplastic stroma (Pap). **B** This crowded tissue fragment of adenocarcinoma consists of cells with pleomorphic hyperchromatic nuclei and contains a single intracytoplasmic vacuole of mucin rather than the abundant mucinous cytoplasm seen in many carcinomas (Pap). **C** Tissue fragment consisting of large cells with marked anisonucleosis, hyperchromasia, irregular nuclear membranes, and nuclear overlap, providing diagnostic features for a straightforward diagnosis of high-grade ductal adenocarcinoma (Pap). **D** This tissue fragment shows a disordered arrangement of nuclei (drunken-honeycomb pattern), which are enlarged with irregular nuclear membranes (Giemsa).

cell pattern, areas of tumour cells with clear cytoplasm containing mucin are present, but the vacuoles are usually larger than those in reactive mucinous duct epithelium and the nuclear atypia makes the diagnosis straightforward. The main morphological differential diagnosis with clear cell PDAC is renal cell carcinoma {669}.

The cytopathological diagnosis of PDAC can be problematic when the cellularity is limited and when the tumour is well differentiated {68}. Pancreatitis, whether acute or chronic, or autoimmune, can be associated with reactive ductal atypia that can mimic PDAC. Usually the reactive ductal groups are few in number, with low cellularity, and are associated with a lesser degree of both architectural and cytopathological atypia. The cellular crowding tends to be mild to moderate and the cytoplasm is non-mucinous. Typically, reactive nuclei are enlarged with fine or coarse chromatin and the degree of anisonucleosis is less remarkable and < 1:4, with smooth, minimally irregular nuclear membranes. The background of pancreatitis can be necrotic but often shows autolysed or saponified tissue or inflammatory cells {465}. Cellular stromal tissue fragments representing inflamed stroma are suggestive of autoimmune pancreatitis {175}.

High-grade pancreatic intraepithelial neoplasia (HG-PanIN) is another entity that can be associated with pronounced architectural and cytopathological changes, including nuclear overlapping, hyperchromasia, anisonucleosis to the extent of 1:4 or greater at times, irregular nuclear membranes, and mucinous cytoplasm, and, therefore, can be difficult to distinguish from PDAC. However, in this scenario, the

Fig. 9.10 Poorly differentiated ductal adenocarcinoma. Crowded atypical glandular tissue fragment consisting of pleomorphic cells with a high N:C ratio and irregular, hyperchromatic nuclei varying in size, with eccentric mucinous cytoplasm (Pap).

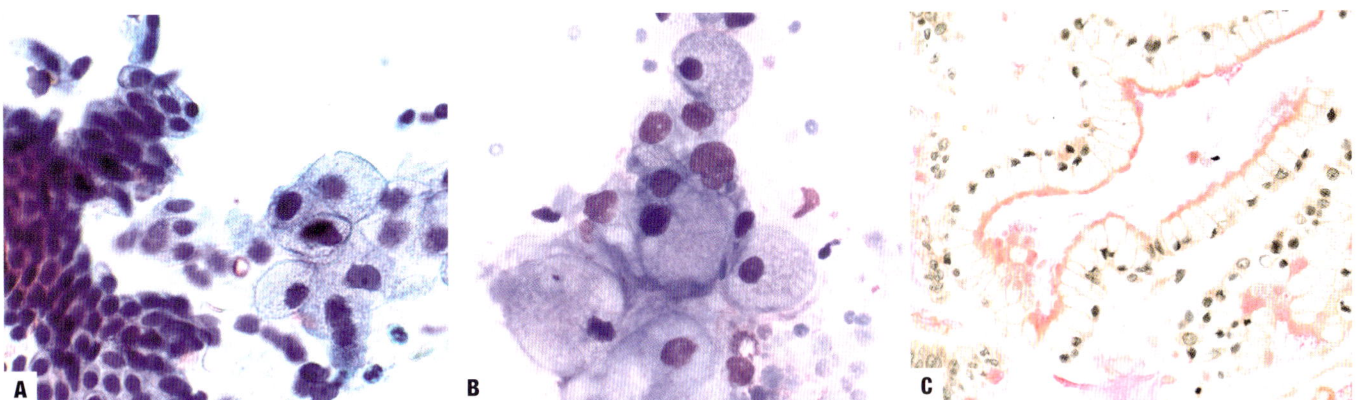

Fig. 9.11 Foamy gland pattern of ductal adenocarcinoma. **A** A minute sheet of deceptively bland tumour cells (centre) with abundant foamy, lacy cytoplasm yielding a low N:C ratio, adjacent to normal ductal epithelium (left) (Pap). **B** Tumour cells with a foamy gland pattern with abundant, often eccentric foamy cytoplasm can mimic histiocytes (Giemsa). **C** A mucicarmine stain of a cell block highlights the apical brush border–like luminal edge of the tumour cells.

abnormal cells are limited to a few cohesive tissue fragments with rare, if any, single cells {353}. Furthermore, HG-PanIN is a subclinical lesion not visible on imaging, whereas PDAC is an irregular, hypoechoic mass. Considering the above two mimics, caution should be exercised in making a definitive cytopathological diagnosis of PDAC on limited specimens {68,353,71}. The quantitative criteria necessary for a definitive diagnosis of PDAC have not been strictly defined, although some authors have proposed a minimum of six tissue fragments for this diagnosis {691}. Correlation with clinical history and imaging findings is also crucial in avoiding a false positive diagnosis {68,465,353}.

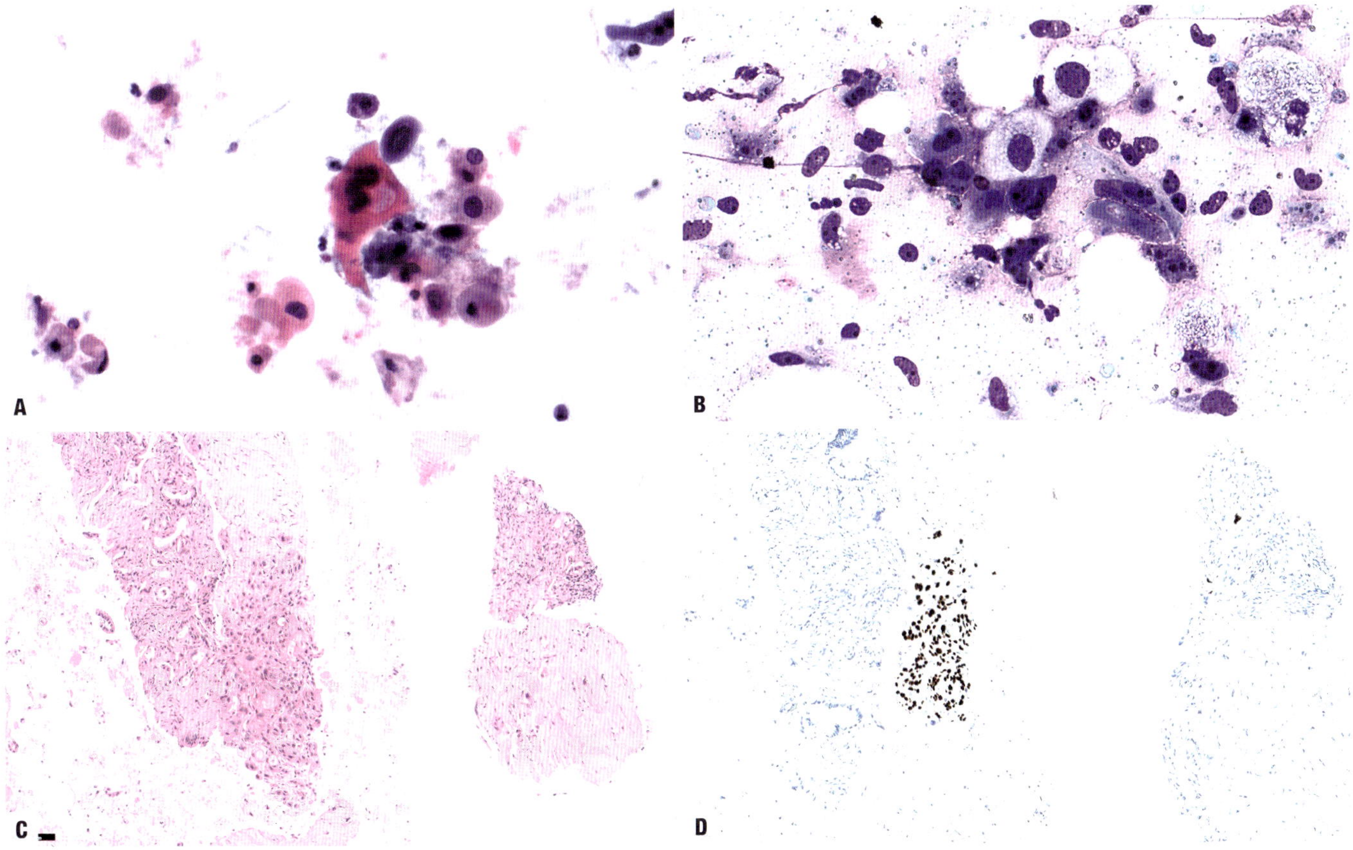

Fig. 9.12 Adenosquamous carcinoma. **A** Single polygonal squamous cells and a rare tadpole cell with pulled-out dense cytoplasm have pleomorphic, hyperchromatic, and often pyknotic nuclei. The dense cytoplasm of the smaller cells contains degenerative vacuoles (Pap). **B** Scattered single polygonal epithelial cells with enlarged, hyperchromatic, atypical nuclei, some showing the presence of cytoplasmic mucin, are present with an occasional goblet cell. Several cells with abundant eccentric cytoplasm containing particulate debris are present, along with cellular debris (Giemsa). **C** Thin core needle biopsy shows tissue fragments of neoplastic glandular and squamous components of adenosquamous carcinoma side by side with desmoplastic stroma and necrosis (H&E). **D** ICC for p40 in the tissue fragments obtained by thin core needle biopsy identifies the nuclei of the squamous component (ICC, p40).

Table 9.04 Key diagnostic features, ICC, and differential diagnosis of pancreatic ductal adenocarcinoma subtypes

Adenocarcinoma subtype	Key diagnostic cytopathological features	ICC	Differential diagnosis
Adenosquamous carcinoma	Squamous component: tissue fragments or single keratinized squamous cells with central atypical nuclei, anisonucleosis, distinct cell borders, dense cytoplasm, necrotic background, tumour cell necrosis, occasional tadpole cells (+/−), focal pearl formation; non-keratinized squamous cells in sheets with intercellular bridges Glandular component: rare, honeycombed sheets or vacuolated single cells with or without mucin	Squamous component: p40+, CK5/6+, p63+	Primary pancreatic or metastatic squamous cell carcinoma Radiation-induced squamous metaplasia
Colloid carcinoma	Abundant thick extracellular mucin Scant cellularity Scattered tumour cells, in 3D tissue fragments, strips, and singly, within the extracellular mucin Low-grade nuclear atypia Single cells with large solitary intracytoplasmic vacuoles consistent with mucin +/− Dysplastic intestinal-type epithelium, if an IPMN is sampled Degenerated and inflammatory cells admixed with abundant mucinous material that may represent cyst contents	CDX2+, MUC2+, CK20+, CK7−	Intestinal-type IPMN Metastatic mucinous or colloid carcinoma
Undifferentiated carcinoma, anaplastic type	Discohesive, single large pleomorphic tumour cells with abundant cytoplasm and sometimes rhabdoid features Multinucleated tumour giant cells with typically < 10 hyperchromatic nuclei with irregular nuclear membranes Inflammatory background composed of neutrophils and macrophages Emperipolesis of tumour cells, red blood cells, and/or inflammatory cells Mucin may be present in the anaplastic tumour cells	Loss of E-cadherin Giant cells express pancytokeratin Loss of SMARCB1 (INI1) in tumour cells with rhabdoid features	Metastatic anaplastic carcinoma from other organs such as lung and thyroid Melanoma Choriocarcinoma Poorly differentiated hepatocellular carcinoma Hodgkin lymphoma Anaplastic large cell lymphoma Epithelioid sarcoma
Undifferentiated carcinoma, sarcomatoid type	Pleomorphic spindle cells with a high N:C ratio Elongated eosinophilic or clear cytoplasm Frequent mitotic figures with or without necrosis	Loss of E-cadherin	Leiomyosarcoma, primary or metastatic Malignant peripheral nerve sheath tumour
Undifferentiated carcinoma with OGCs	Three distinct cell types: (1) benign macrophage-like OGCs; (2) malignant tumour giant cells, which are large, pleomorphic, and irregular with variable chromatin distribution; and (3) small spindled or histiocytoid tumour cells Usually, single dispersed OGCs with dense cytoplasm and numerous centrally clustered round to oval overlapping nuclei on Giemsa; their cytoplasm is dense and blue-grey, and it contains round to oval or irregular overlapping nuclei, some with prominent nucleoli on Pap staining Often PDAC component present	CD68, CD163, and CD45 (LCA) expression in the OGCs No expression of pancytokeratin, EMA, or p53 in the OGCs	PDAC Undifferentiated carcinoma with rhabdoid morphology NET and SPN with multinucleated giant cells

IPMN, intraductal papillary mucinous neoplasm; NET, neuroendocrine tumour; OGC, osteoclast-like giant cell; PDAC, pancreatic ductal adenocarcinoma; SPN, solid pseudopapillary neoplasm.

Another diagnostic pitfall can be the misinterpretation of contaminating gastric and duodenal epithelium as a well-differentiated PDAC. The contaminant epithelium is characteristically in the form of monolayered sheets and lacks the architectural and cytopathological features of PDAC, thereby aiding in the distinction {465}.

Subtypes

Adenosquamous carcinoma

Adenosquamous carcinomas have both glandular and squamous components, with ≥ 30% being squamous. The prognosis is very poor {413,381}. Cytomorphological patterns may include either the presence of both the glandular and squamous components, or the predominance of a keratinizing squamous cell carcinoma with or without a rare malignant glandular component {425,661}. This subtype is not easily distinguishable from PDAC on imaging, although the presence of central necrosis in the setting of a large infiltrative mass is regarded as a telltale sign by some authors {661,574}. The squamous component may be represented by keratinized nests of pleomorphic to polygonal cells with dense cytoplasm and squamous pearls or sheets of non-keratinized small cells with well-defined intercellular bridges. The glandular component may consist of sparse goblet cells or cuboidal to columnar epithelial cells with intracytoplasmic or extracellular mucin. The two components may be adjacent or in separate regions of the carcinoma.

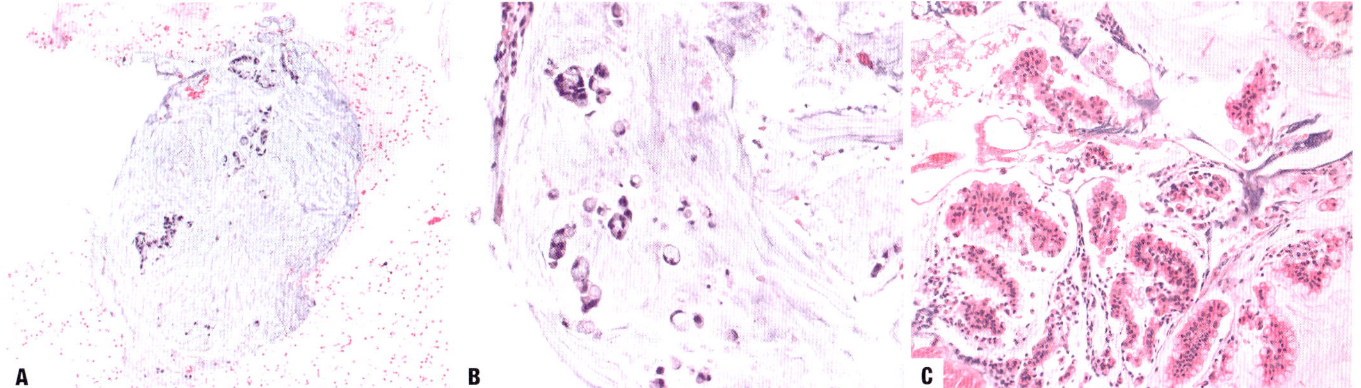

Fig. 9.13 Colloid carcinoma. **A** Tumour cells are seen floating in pools of thick extracellular mucin (H&E). **B** Cell block shows a mass of thick extracellular mucin in which tumour cells float. The tumour cells vary in the degree of nuclear atypia and range from bland to signet-ring cells (H&E). **C** Cell block shows tissue fragments, which are strips and 3D tissue fragments, and single cells with abundant intracytoplasmic mucin including goblet cells in a thick, mucinous background. Note the mild to moderate nuclear atypia (H&E). These cells are strongly positive for CDX2, MUC2, and CK20 by ICC.

Adenosquamous carcinoma should be distinguished from a metastatic squamous cell carcinoma, especially in the setting of a prior history or a concurrent primary tumour that has not yet been sampled, such as in the lung, oesophagus, or cervix. Complete absence of mucin or glandular morphology suggests a metastatic squamous cell carcinoma {611}. Primary squamous cell carcinoma of the pancreas associated with familial atypical mole–malignant melanoma syndrome is exceedingly rare {611}. Another consideration is radiation-induced squamous metaplasia that can arise in the setting of a treated PDAC {661}.

Colloid carcinoma

Colloid carcinoma of the pancreas is an adenocarcinoma in which > 80% of the neoplastic epithelium is suspended in extracellular mucin pools. These carcinomas tend to be large and well demarcated, and most arise in association with intestinal-type intraductal papillary mucinous neoplasms (IPMNs) {11,749}. Correlation of the imaging findings with FNAB material dominated by thick, colloid-like extracellular mucin containing a few low-grade glandular cells is suggestive of the diagnosis. Imaging features can be challenging, in that it is not uncommon to find a heterogeneous or low PET-avid mass on imaging {615}. Cytopathological features of colloid carcinoma may overlap with those of intestinal-type IPMN, and distinction from IPMN requires correlation with the EUS features. A cytopathological diagnosis of IPMN naturally raises the possibility of associated colloid carcinoma, especially if a solid mass or a mural nodule is identified by imaging or at EUS examination. The other important differential diagnosis is metastatic mucinous or colloid carcinoma of non-pancreatic origin. Distinction needs clinicopathological correlation. The cytopathological features accompanied by those of more typical PDAC should raise the possibility of PDAC with a mucinous component {11, 749,676,568}.

Undifferentiated carcinoma

Undifferentiated carcinoma is defined as a malignant epithelial neoplasm in which a substantial component of the neoplasm does not show definitive differentiation.

Undifferentiated carcinoma, anaplastic subtype

This subtype is more likely to be cystic than typical PDAC {319}. Many cases are associated with a dilated main pancreatic duct

Chapter 9

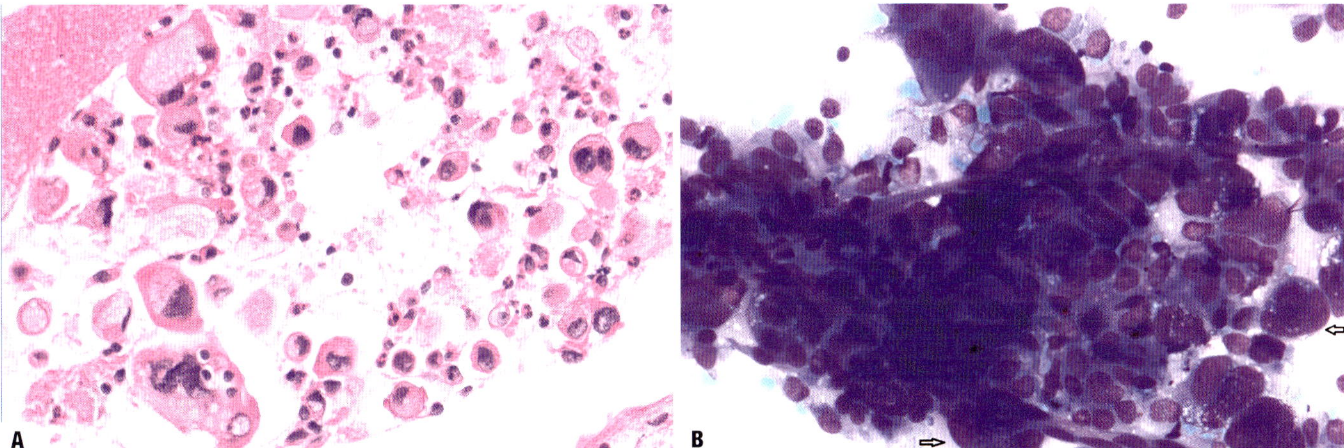

Fig. 9.14 Undifferentiated carcinoma, anaplastic type. **A** Cell block showing discohesive, single, large pleomorphic tumour cells with abundant cytoplasm and multinucleated tumour giant cells with typically < 10 highly pleomorphic nuclei. Note the emperipolesis of inflammatory cells by the tumour giant cells (H&E). **B** Crowded, disorganized tissue fragment of pleomorphic tumour cells with multinucleated tumour giant cells (Giemsa).

Table 9.05 Immunocytochemical differential diagnosis for the most common metastases to the pancreas

Tumour type	Stain
Pancreatic ductal adenocarcinoma	Positive: CK7, CK19, mesothelin, SMAD4
Renal cell carcinoma	Positive: PAX8, CD10, RCCm
Lung carcinoma	Positive: CK7, TTF1, napsin A Negative: CK20
Breast carcinoma	Positive: CK7, CK20, mammaglobin, GATA3
Colon carcinoma	Positive: CK20, CDX2, SATB2 Negative: CK7
Melanoma	Positive: S100, melan-A (MART1), HMB45, SOX10 Negative: cytokeratins

TTF1, thyroid transcription factor 1.

and may mimic IPMN on imaging {389}. This tumour comprises ≥ 80% of solid sheets lacking gland formation and is composed of pleomorphic mononuclear cells admixed with bizarre-appearing giant cells {820,910}. The carcinoma cells are poorly cohesive, with little intervening stroma. A neutrophilic infiltrate is present within the tumour. Emperipolesis by malignant giant cells of other tumour cells (cannibalism), inflammatory cells, and/or red blood cells is characteristic, and multinucleated histiocytic giant cells can also contain these cells {620}. Cytopathological smears are highly cellular and composed of cohesive tissue fragments with dispersed single, large, bizarre tumour cells. Carcinoma giant cells have abundant eosinophilic cytoplasm and multiple (usually < 10) centrally placed atypical pleomorphic nuclei. A neutrophilic infiltrate and necrosis are present in the background. Mitotic figures are frequent. Rare cases with rhabdoid cells that show loss of nuclear expression of SMARCB1 (INI1) have been described {608,722}. The differential diagnosis includes metastatic anaplastic carcinoma from other organs (e.g. lung, kidney, and thyroid), metastatic melanoma, choriocarcinoma, poorly differentiated hepatocellular carcinoma, Hodgkin lymphoma, anaplastic large cell lymphoma, and epithelioid sarcoma, because all these entities may exhibit large, pleomorphic tumour cells {620,198}. Tumours with rhabdoid features must be differentiated from malignant rhabdoid tumour, renal cell carcinoma with rhabdoid change, and epithelioid sarcoma. Tumour giant cells must be distinguished from foreign body giant cells and reactive macrophages.

Undifferentiated carcinoma, sarcomatoid subtype

This subtype is characterized by malignant spindle cells that demonstrate epithelial derivation but no light microscopic, ultrastructural, or immunocytochemical evidence of a specific line of mesenchymal differentiation {375}. At least 80% of the carcinoma displays spindle cell morphology. The spindle cells are arranged in a storiform or fascicular pattern {986} and form highly cellular nodules, which may be intermingled with scattered foci of a minor adenocarcinoma component {375,910}. Cytopathological smears are predominantly composed of pleomorphic oval to spindle cells that are present in tissue fragments and as single cells. These cells have a high N:C ratio. Frequent mitotic figures and necrosis are present. Rare foci of high-grade PDAC may be admixed. The differential diagnosis includes a primary pancreatic undifferentiated pleomorphic sarcoma, which is an extremely rare entity and is a diagnosis of exclusion {953}. Other metastatic and primary sarcomas of the pancreas, such as leiomyosarcoma and malignant peripheral nerve sheath tumour, should be considered in the differential.

Undifferentiated carcinoma with osteoclast-like giant cells

Undifferentiated carcinoma with osteoclast-like giant cells (UCOGC) is a carcinoma composed of malignant carcinoma cells admixed with benign, multinucleated, osteoclast-like giant cells (OGCs). Smears range from paucicellular to moderately cellular with necrotic debris or acute inflammation {682}. There are three distinct cell types in UCOGC and all are recognizable on cytopathology: firstly, benign macrophage-like osteoclast-like giant cells; secondly, malignant tumour giant cells with large, pleomorphic and irregular nuclei with variable chromatin distribution; and thirdly, small spindle or histiocytoid carcinoma cells {572,238,570,776,897,682,804,908}. Depending on the number of nuclei, OGCs range from 50 to 500 µm, and they may be overlooked when admixed with malignant tumour giant cells. By Giemsa, OGCs have dense cytoplasm and numerous centrally clustered round to oval overlapping nuclei. By Pap, OGC cytoplasm is dense and blue-grey, and it contains similar round to oval or irregular overlapping nuclei, some with

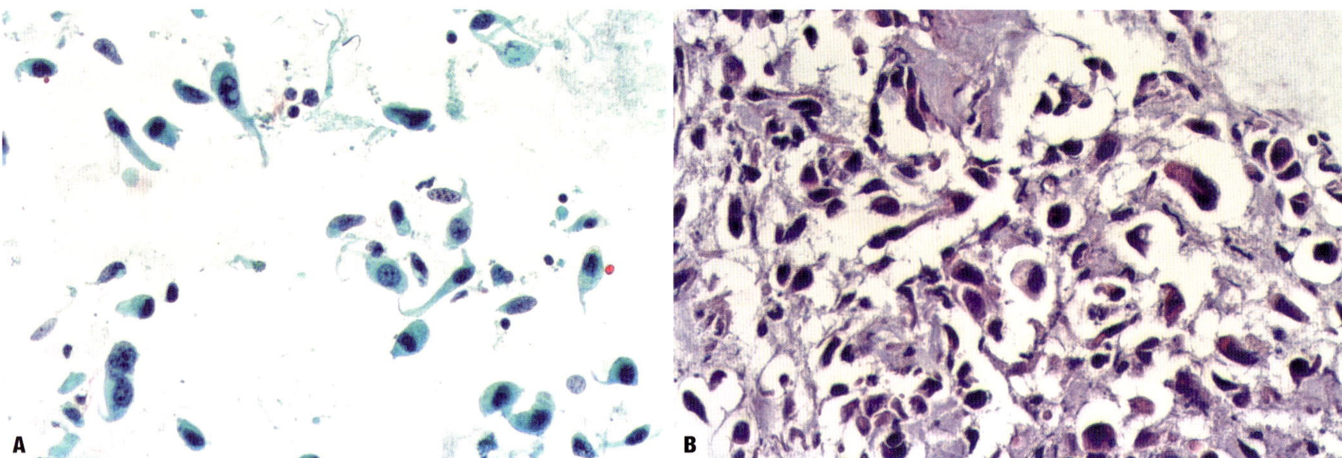

Fig. 9.15 Undifferentiated carcinoma, sarcomatoid type. **A** Single intact cells are discohesive, pleomorphic spindle cells, with large hyperchromatic and pleomorphic nuclei, resembling a sarcoma (Pap). **B** Cell block showing discohesive spindle cells with hyperchromatic pleomorphic nuclei present in a fibrotic stroma, resembling a sarcoma (H&E).

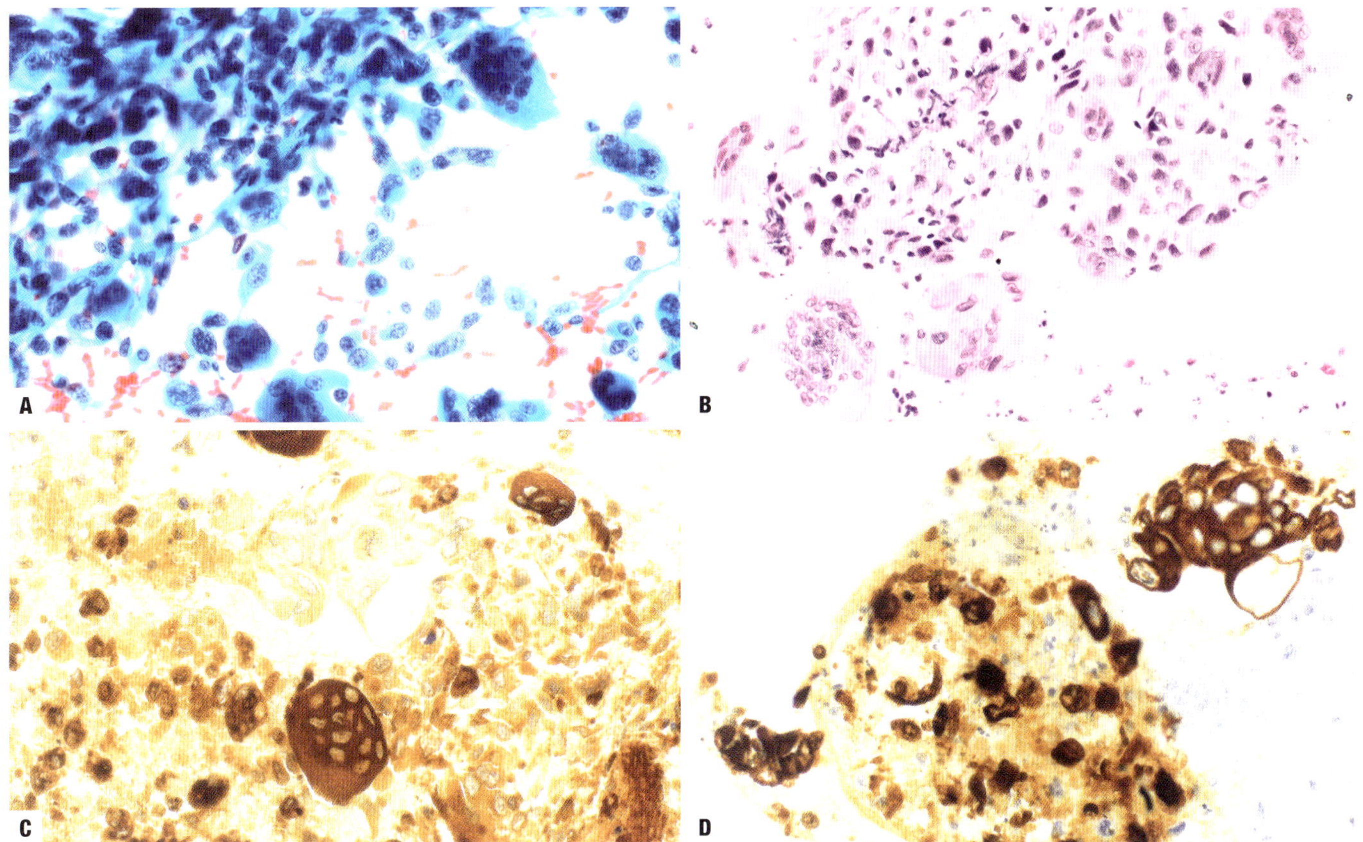

Fig. 9.16 Undifferentiated carcinoma with osteoclast-like giant cells. **A** The benign multinucleated osteoclast-like giant cells are adjacent to the malignant mononuclear hyperchromatic epithelial cells (Pap). **B** Cell block showing multiple osteoclast-like giant cells with pleomorphic nuclei, tumour cells with eccentric cytoplasm and highly pleomorphic nuclei, and considerable necrotic debris (H&E). **C** The benign osteoclast-like giant cells are positive for CD68 (ICC). **D** Pleomorphic tumour cells are positive for pancytokeratin, whereas adjacent osteoclast-like giant cells are negative (ICC).

prominent nucleoli. Carcinoma giant cells are cytopathologically malignant, with high N:C ratios and irregular, pleomorphic, single-lobed or polylobated nuclei with hypochromasia or hyperchromasia, macronucleoli, and abnormal mitoses. Spindle or histiocytoid carcinoma cells are variable in number, smaller than OGCs, and often present in 3D or syncytial tissue fragments with surrounding fibrotic stroma or debris. These cells have either elongated, tapered nuclei or are more epithelioid or histiocyte-like with cytoplasmic microvesicles. An adenocarcinoma component is present in the majority of cases and shows classic PDAC cytopathological features {682,776,804}. Cell blocks often contain easily recognizable OGCs even if the carcinoma giant cells or spindle or histiocytoid cells are limited.

The OGCs in UCOGC represent histiocytes, which are probably recruited by the malignant component {908,181}. The differential diagnosis of UCOGC includes typical PDAC, which does not have multiple OGCs. Seeing an acute inflammatory infiltrate, debris, and giant cells should raise the consideration of acute or chronic pancreatitis, but these giant cells lack the frankly malignant nuclei of the giant cells seen in UCOGC. Another differential is undifferentiated carcinoma with rhabdoid morphology, which shows *KRAS* mutation or SMARCB1 (INI1) loss. Malignant cells in UCOGC show retained SMARCB1 (INI1) staining {682}. Multinucleated giant cells may be seen in pancreatic NET or SPN, where they are known as multinucleated degenerating cercariform cells {718}. Pancreatic NET and SPN have distinctive cytomorphology, with plasmacytoid cells with salt-and-pepper chromatin in NET, and branching papillae covered by cells with vesicular chromatin and longitudinal nuclear grooves in SPN, and their immunoprofiles should facilitate distinction.

Ancillary testing

Since their initial introduction, EUS-FNAB and recent innovations with new fine-gauge core biopsy needles have changed the diagnostic cytopathology landscape, facilitating diagnostic samples from small pancreatic lesions. Adequate tissue can now be obtained that allows ancillary testing to be performed for refining the diagnosis and personalizing the care of patients with pancreatic tumours.

Differentiating chronic pancreatitis with reactive ductal atypia from PDAC is often a challenge. Studies continue to explore ICC stains that could distinguish them (see Table 9.03, p. 131). Expression or loss of ICC markers in conjunction with cytomorphology may support the diagnosis of PDAC {130,355,347,184,26,462,829}. Practical, useful markers include mesothelin, p53, and SMAD4. Strong nuclear staining or total loss of staining (the null pattern) with p53 supports malignancy, as does the loss of nuclear staining for SMAD4. The diagnosis of cytopathological variants of pancreatic carcinoma may also be supported by stains, as listed in Table 9.04 (p. 134) {549}.

FISH has been shown to improve diagnostic sensitivity as well as specificity in distinguishing chronic pancreatitis from PDAC

{297,300}. A commonly used cocktail of FISH probes contains centromere probes for chromosomes 3, 7, and 17 (CEP3, CEP7, CEP17), and a locus-specific probe against 9p21 (*CDKN2A* [*P16*]). Polysomy in CEP3, CEP7 (which includes the locus for *EGFR*), and CEP17 (which includes loci for *TP53* and *BRCA2*) is more frequently associated with PDAC. Occasional loss may also be noted. Deletion of 9p21 is another common deletion associated with PDAC. A FISH probe set including 1q21 for the *MCL1* locus, 7p12 (which includes the *EGFR* locus), 8q24 (which includes the *MYC* locus), and a locus-specific probe against 9p21 (*CDKN2A* [*P16*]) is also used to differentiate chronic pancreatitis from PDAC {54}. Polysomy or deletion of these probes have been associated with PDAC.

Metastases to the pancreas are not as common as those to the lung and liver. Some tumours may mimic a pancreatic carcinoma, especially when they present as a single nodule, and this is typical of metastatic renal cell carcinoma, a tumour that is notorious for metastasizing decades after nephrectomy. ICC may further aid in differentiating pancreatic carcinoma from metastatic tumours (see Table 9.05, p. 136).

Next-generation sequencing or techniques that analyse the whole genome may be useful for diagnosis and therapeutic decision-making {893,593}. These tests can detect disruption of genes in PDAC (*KRAS*, *TP53*, *SMAD4*, *CDKN2A*, *ARID1A*, and *ROBO2*) and driver mutations of carcinogenesis (*KDM6A* and *PREX2*). These tests may also demonstrate focal amplifications of specific oncogenes (*ERBB2*, *MET*, *FGFR1*, *CDK6*, *PIK3R3*, and *PIK3CA*) that could be targeted to develop personalized therapies. Germline mutations and inactivation of DNA maintenance genes (*BRCA1*, *BRCA2*, or *PALB2*) may be detected {662,161}. PDAC may also demonstrate deficiency in mismatch repair genes {662,161,16}. PDACs that are microsatellite-unstable or express granulocyte–macrophage colony–stimulating factor are associated with an increase in neoantigens and promote recruitment of immune cells and inflammatory factors {65,328}. Tumours with a high level of microsatellite instability are associated with a favourable prognosis and are responsive to immunotherapies that can affect survival {242,328}. Mismatch repair can be analysed using ICC, PCR, or next-generation sequencing {328,242}. With limited sampling on cytopathology, assessment using PCR-based or next-generation sequencing testing may provide more precise information.

Pancreatic acinar cell carcinoma

Sigel C
Stelow EB

Definition

Pancreatic acinar cell carcinoma is a malignant pancreatic epithelial neoplasm with acinar cell differentiation.

Clinical features and imaging

Acinar cell carcinoma accounts for 1% of adult pancreatic carcinomas, with a reported increasing incidence {194}. Half of patients present at an advanced stage {194}. The mean age at presentation is in the sixth decade of life (range: 9–87 years) with a bimodal peak in childhood and advanced adulthood. There is a male predominance (70%) {194}. Clinical presentation is abdominal pain and weight loss {917}. On CT and MRI, acinar cell carcinoma is circumscribed and bulky, with a persisting enhancing pattern {849,327}. Location in the pancreatic head is slightly more common. Cystic degeneration and intraductal growth can occur. Serum tumour markers CEA and CA19-9 are not associated with acinar cell carcinoma, and although lipase may have mild elevations, the lipase hypersecretion syndrome encompassing fever, subcutaneous fat necrosis, eosinophilia, and polyarthritis, which is a clinical clue to the diagnosis, is very rare.

Histopathology

Histopathologically, acinar cell carcinoma shows confluent cellularity and minimal stroma. There are acinar, trabecular, and solid architectural patterns {419}. Eosinophilic cytoplasm, reflecting the zymogen granules, is distinctive, but other morphologies include oncocytic, signet-ring cell, spindle cell, and hypogranular {418}. The nuclei usually have a single prominent nucleolus, but nucleoli are not universally present. There is no grading system, but poor differentiation, including solid architecture and nuclear pleomorphism, probably has prognostic significance {737}.

Key diagnostic cytopathological features

- Hypercellular smears with dense 3D tissue fragments and single cells
- Tissue fragments show lobulated, trabecular, and small acinar architecture
- Pyramidal and epithelioid tumour cells
- Large nuclei compared with those of benign acinar cells, with coarsely clumped chromatin, variable anisonucleosis, and prominent nucleoli, which are characteristic but not universally present
- Eccentric, finely granular blue (Giemsa), aqua (Pap), or eosinophilic (H&E) granular cytoplasm with indistinct cytoplasmic membranes; minute clear vacuoles representing negative images of zymogen granules are seen in the Giemsa
- Variable cytoplasmic volume, which varies from abundant to very scant
- Granular background in smears due to the spilled zymogen granules from the disrupted cytoplasm, particularly on the Giemsa and H&E
- Intact tissue fragments in the cell block show solid and acinar architectural patterns

Reference(s): {812,774}

Discussion and differential diagnosis

The differential diagnosis includes sampling of non-neoplastic pancreas and other cellular, monomorphic epithelial neoplasms of the pancreas. Relative to acinar cell carcinoma, non-neoplastic acinar tissue is more cohesive and FNAB smears show large, grape-like tissue fragments consisting of acini with variable degrees of fibrosis due to chronic pancreatitis {811}.

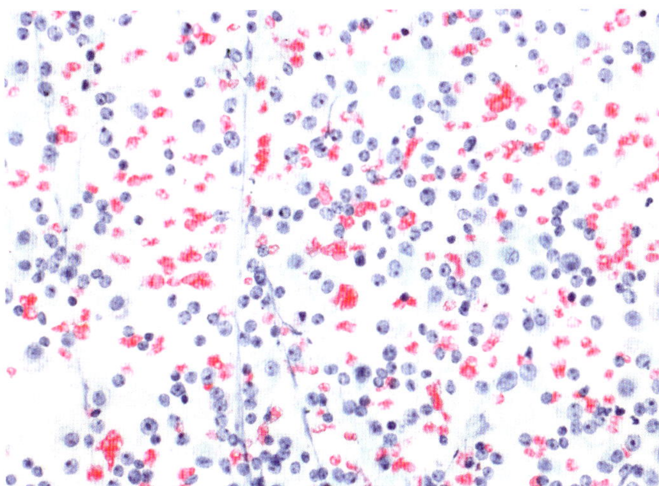

Fig. 9.17 Acinar cell carcinoma. Highly cellular direct smear of single dispersed neoplastic cells with delicate pale cytoplasm that is often stripped, leaving naked nuclei (Pap).

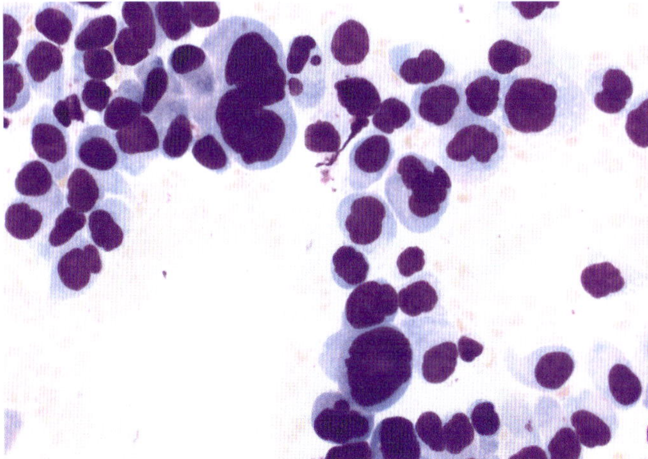

Fig. 9.18 Acinar cell carcinoma. Anisonucleosis, nuclear pleomorphism, and hyperchromasia are prominent in this poorly differentiated acinar cell carcinoma. Note the absence of mucinous cytoplasm. Granularity of the eccentric cytoplasm presents as fine vacuoles that represent negative images of zymogen granules, and is subtle (Giemsa).

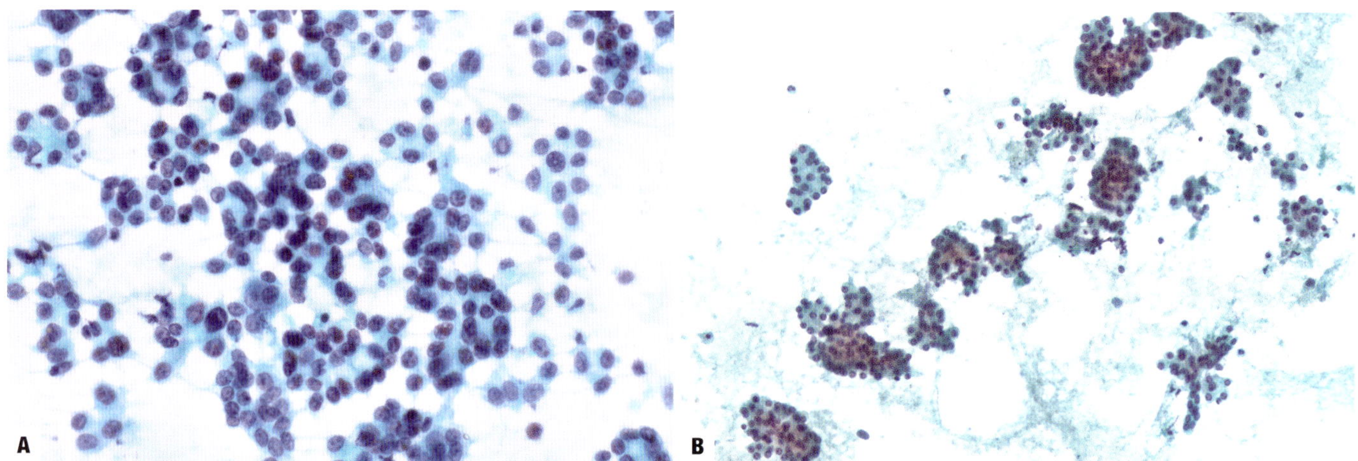

Fig. 9.19 A Acinar cell carcinoma. Small acinar tissue fragments resemble normal pancreatic acini, but note the discohesion and high N:C ratio. Nucleoli are not prominent in this tumour, which adds to its resemblance to normal tissue (Pap). **B** Benign pancreatic acini. Normal acinar tissue maintains small, grape-like acinar tissue fragments with few or no single intact cells or stripped naked nuclei (Pap).

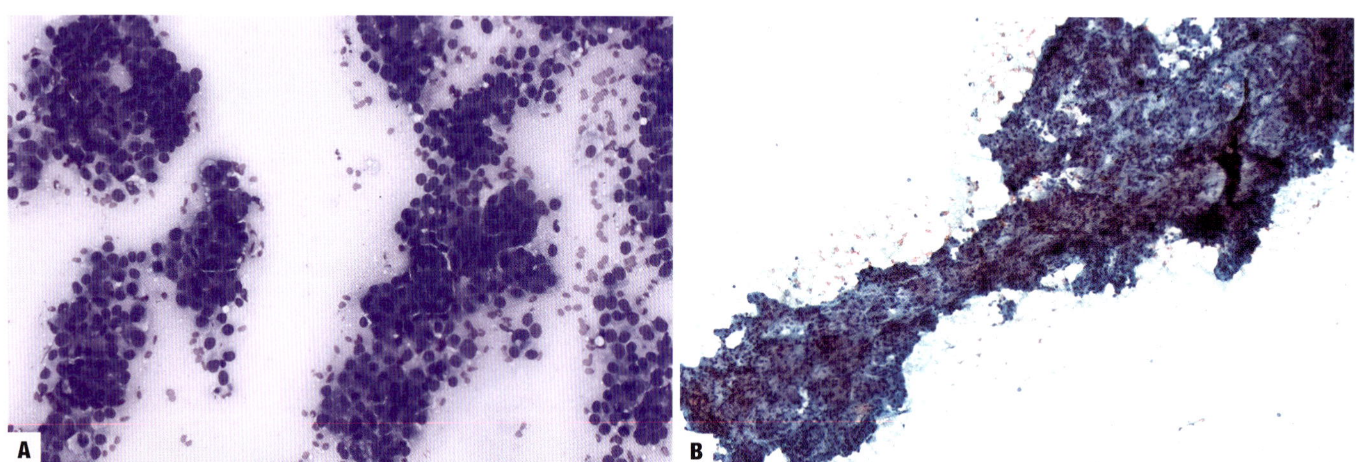

Fig. 9.20 A Acinar cell carcinoma. In contrast to normal pancreatic parenchyma, acinar cell carcinoma typically produces highly cellular smears composed of 3D crowded tissue fragments rather than the small, grape-like tissue fragments of benign acinar cells loosely connected to stromal strands (Giemsa). **B** Benign acinar pancreas. Benign acini of exocrine pancreas produce very cellular smears composed of organoid groups of small, grape-like acini attached to loose connective tissue (Pap).

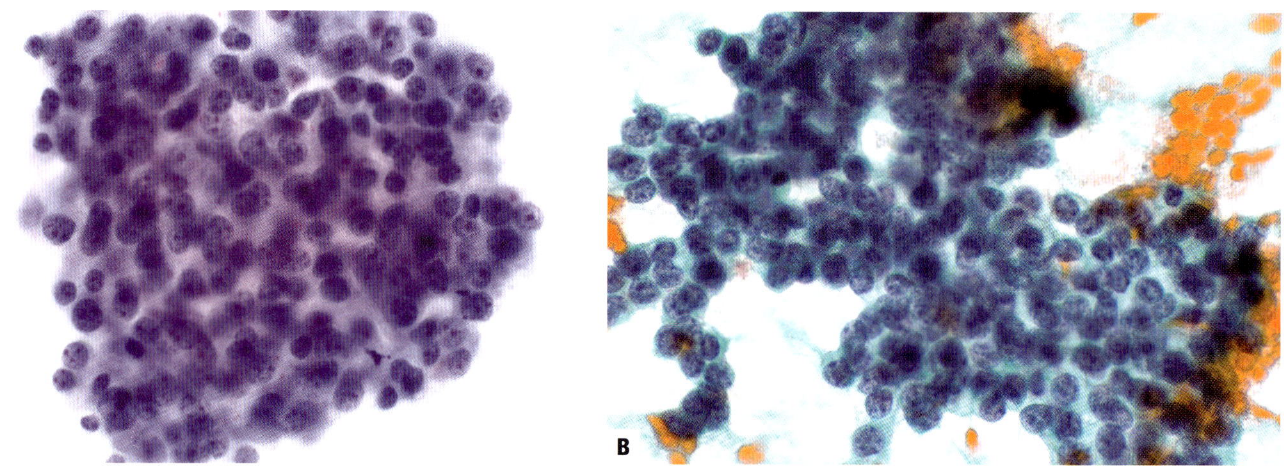

Fig. 9.21 A Acinar cell carcinoma. Liquid-based cytopathology rounds up the tissue fragments, making assessment of the granular cytoplasm difficult. Note the round, monomorphic nuclei with coarse chromatin, a feature that puts acinar cell carcinoma and neuroendocrine tumour (NET) at the top of the differential diagnosis for this tissue fragment, rather than adenocarcinoma (liquid-based cytopathology, Pap). **B** Well-differentiated NET. The primary differential diagnosis of acinar cell carcinoma is pancreatic NET (PanNET). Both tumours are composed of polygonal cells with round nuclei and coarse chromatin with or without nucleoli (Pap). Confirmation of a specific diagnosis is made by ICC.

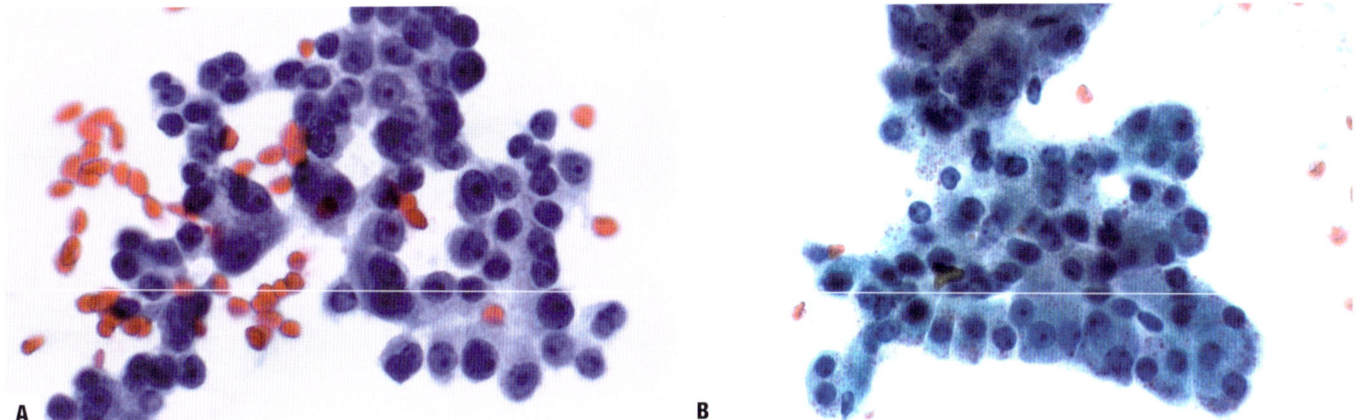

Fig. 9.22 **A** Acinar cell carcinoma. Most, but not all, acinar cell carcinomas have tumour cells with prominent nucleoli. Neuroendocrine tumours (NETs) can also have prominent nucleoli, so differentiation of these two tumours requires assessment of a constellation of features rather than the presence or absence of nucleoli (Pap). **B** Benign acinar pancreas. Benign acinar cells are polygonal with round nuclei, small nucleoli, and granular eccentric cytoplasm. Note the intercalated cells with slightly elongated nuclei within the acinus on the right of the image, a feature that supports a benign acinus (Pap).

However, FNAB of non-neoplastic acinar pancreas can produce numerous discrete acini and single cells, although benign acinar cells show minimal cytopathological nuclear atypia and small, inconspicuous nucleoli.

Other primary pancreatic neoplasms in the differential diagnosis include both well-differentiated neuroendocrine tumours (NETs) and poorly differentiated neuroendocrine carcinomas (NECs), solid pseudopapillary neoplasms, intraductal tubulopapillary neoplasm, and pancreatoblastomas {909,812}. These entities are cellular with loosely cohesive tissue fragments and single epithelioid neoplastic cells but exhibit subtle differences from acinar cell carcinoma. For example, NET typically has less-coarse chromatin and less-cohesive tissue fragments, as compared with the clumped chromatin and dense 3D tissue fragments of acinar cell carcinoma. Pancreatic NEC, which is poorly differentiated by definition, has more mitotic activity and apoptosis than acinar cell carcinoma. Solid pseudopapillary neoplasms have variable cytopathology, but in contrast to acinar cell carcinoma, the smears show intracellular and extracellular hyaline material, there are tissue fragments of arborizing capillaries with clinging neoplastic cells, and there is no acinar arrangement. The tumour cells show scant wispy tags of cytoplasm, with no prominent nucleoli or mitoses. Intraductal tubulopapillary neoplasm, like acinar cell carcinoma, has acinar-like tubular arrangements of polygonal cells and can have both intraductal and invasive components. Pancreatoblastomas are nearly identical to acinar cell carcinoma except for the defining telltale squamous nests.

Ancillary testing

ICC can support a definitive diagnosis of acinar cell carcinoma. Trypsin, chymotrypsin, and BCL10 are sensitive markers, particularly when two are used {450}. Ki-67 indexes are typically between 10% and 50%. Scattered cells express synaptophysin and chromogranin, whereas diffuse expression indicates a diagnosis of NET, NEC, or a mixed acinar–neuroendocrine carcinoma {774}. Nuclear β-catenin expression can be seen in a patchy distribution in acinar cell carcinoma, reflecting occasional *CTNNB1* and *APC* mutations, but strong, diffuse nuclear staining supports the diagnosis of a solid pseudopapillary neoplasm {6}. *BRAF* or *RAF1* fusions occur in 25% of cases and can be detected by FISH {898,72}.

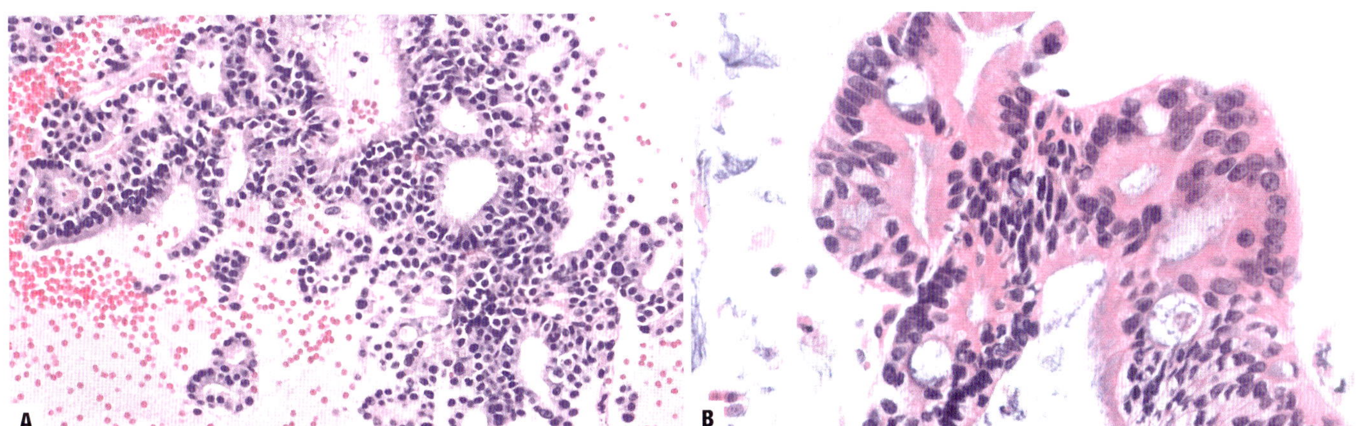

Fig. 9.23 **A** Acinar cell carcinoma. Tissue fragment from a cell block shows a tissue fragment with a cribriform architecture, with polarized nuclei oriented to the glandular holes, prominent nucleoli, and granular eccentric cytoplasm, rather than the mucinous cytoplasm of adenocarcinoma (H&E). **B** Ductal adenocarcinoma. This cell block shows a tissue fragment of columnar glandular cells with a cribriform architecture similar to that of acinar cell carcinoma, but the eccentric cytoplasm is mucinous rather than granular (H&E).

Neuroendocrine tumour

Weynand B
Reid MD
Sigel C

Definition

Pancreatic neuroendocrine tumours (PanNETs) are well-differentiated epithelial tumours with neuroendocrine differentiation.

Clinical features and imaging

PanNETs are indolent, malignant, slow-growing tumours measuring > 5 mm, whereas tumours < 5 mm are known as neuroendocrine microtumours. The biological behaviour of an individual PanNET is unpredictable. Non-functioning PanNETs are often discovered incidentally or present with nonspecific symptoms from local or metastatic spread. Functioning tumours are defined by the specific syndrome associated with hormone production, for example, insulinoma with hypoglycaemic syndrome. PanNETs present as round, well-demarcated, highly vascularized, solid or cystic (10–15%) tumours. In contrast, ductal adenocarcinoma presents as an irregularly shaped hypoechoic mass. PanNETs are usually observed in patients aged 40–60 years and are mostly sporadic lesions, but 10% occur in cancer predisposition syndromes such as multiple endocrine neoplasia type 1, von Hippel–Lindau syndrome, or neurofibromatosis 1 {346}.

Histopathology

PanNETs have a characteristic organoid architecture composed of cell nests and/or trabeculae separated by numerous capillaries. Stroma can be either very scant or abundant and fibrotic, sometimes with calcifications or amyloid {237}. The tumour is composed of a monotonous, polygonal cell population, with round to oval nuclei featuring salt-and-pepper granular chromatin and eccentric plasmacytoid cytoplasm.

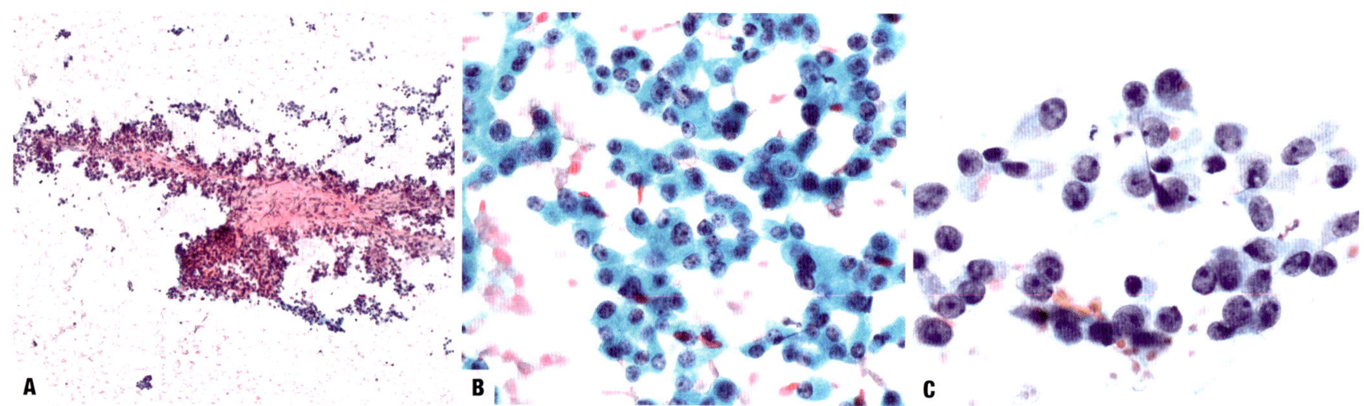

Fig. 9.24 Well-differentiated neuroendocrine tumour (NET). **A** This well-differentiated NET is composed of tissue fragments with fibrovascular cores resembling branching papillae covered in tumour cells, mimicking a solid pseudopapillary neoplasm (Pap). **B** The classic plasmacytoid cells of NETs have salt-and-pepper (intermingled coarse and fine) chromatin and eccentric granular cytoplasm (Pap). **C** Nucleoli can be seen and should not be used as a criterion to separate pancreatic NET (PanNET) from acinar cell carcinoma (Pap).

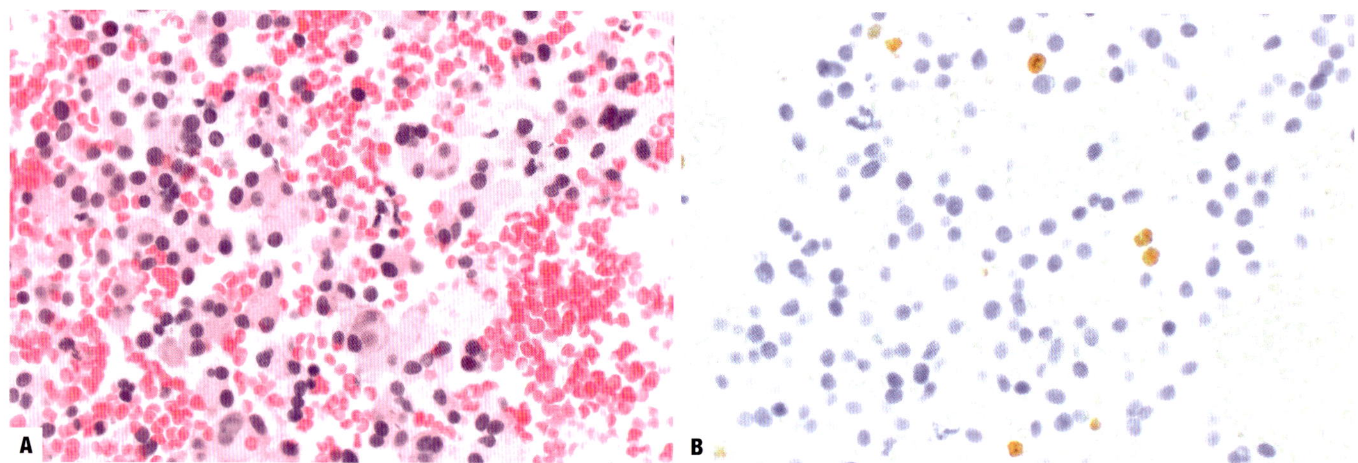

Fig. 9.25 Well-differentiated neuroendocrine tumour (NET), grade 1. **A** In this cell block, the tumour cells are uniform and monotonous without necrosis or mitotic activity (H&E). See Ki-67 (**B**) for grading. **B** Ki-67 ICC shows < 3% nuclear positivity.

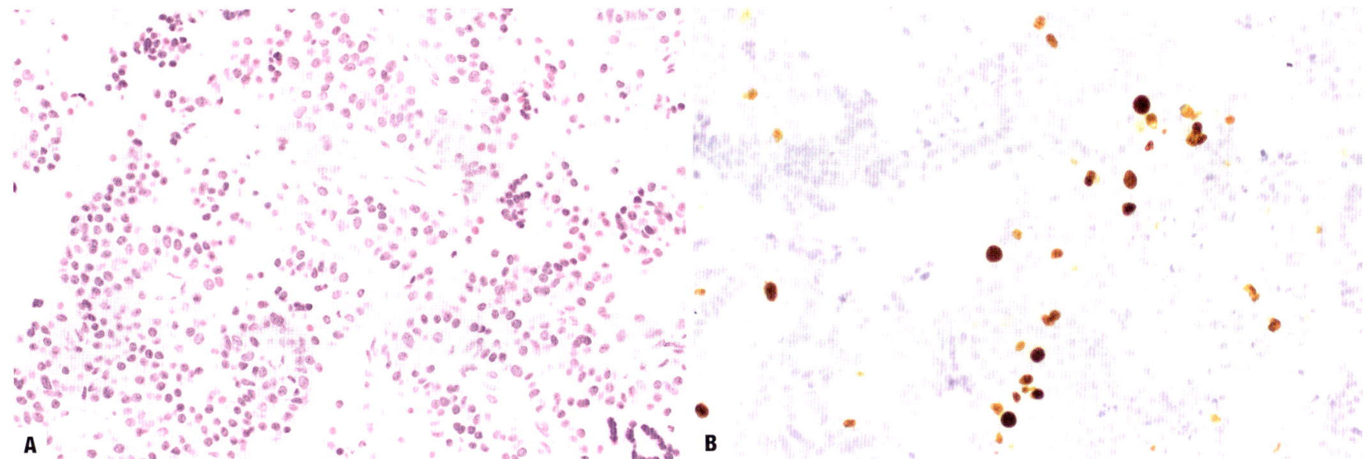

Fig. 9.26 Well-differentiated neuroendocrine tumour (NET), grade 2. **A** This cell block shows uniform and monotonous tumour cells without necrosis or mitotic activity (H&E). See Ki-67 (**B**) for grading. **B** Cell block preparation: Ki-67 ICC shows 3–20% nuclear positivity.

PanNETs are subdivided into three grades, G1, G2, and G3, depending on their proliferative index, as determined by Ki-67 ICC and/or mitotic activity (see Table 9.06).

Key diagnostic cytopathological features

- Usually highly cellular smears
- Loosely cohesive and occasionally 3D tissue fragments and dispersed individual cells
- Epithelioid or plasmacytoid cells, occasionally with minimal cytoplasm
- Round to ovoid nuclei, occasionally angulated
- Smooth, dense nuclear membranes, coarsely stippled salt-and-pepper chromatin
- Nucleoli may be present and even prominent
- Cytoplasm is dense, with fine granularity occasionally noted
- Background is clean, without necrosis

Reference(s): {931,96,219,775}

Discussion and differential diagnosis

PanNET can be non-functioning, i.e. non-syndromic, or functioning, with specific hormone production responsible for a clinical syndrome.

The classic morphology of PanNET is characterized by singly dispersed and loosely cohesive tissue fragments of plasmacytoid cells with oval, eccentric nuclei and coarsely stippled salt-and-pepper chromatin. With increasing grade, PanNET may develop more abundant cytoplasm, mitotic activity, apoptosis, and necrosis but pleomorphism is not associated with a higher-grade neoplasm.

Table 9.06 Classification and grading of pancreatic neuroendocrine neoplasms (PanNENs)

Tumour type	Differentiation	Mitotic count	Ki-67
G1 NET	Well differentiated	< 2/mm^2	< 3%
G2 NET	Well differentiated	2–20/mm^2	3–20%
G3 NET	Well differentiated	> 20/mm^2	> 20%
NEC, small cell type	Poorly differentiated	> 20/mm^2	> 20% (usually > 50%)
NEC, large cell type	Poorly differentiated	> 20/mm^2	> 20% (usually > 50%)

NEC, neuroendocrine carcinoma; NET, neuroendocrine tumour.

The differential diagnosis of PanNET varies according to tumour grade and the presence of variant morphology, but it generally includes other cellular neoplasms with poorly cohesive cytoarchitecture and epithelioid morphology, such as solid pseudopapillary neoplasm (SPN), acinar cell carcinoma, the large cell type of poorly differentiated pancreatic neuroendocrine carcinoma (PanNEC), adenocarcinoma, and metastatic epithelioid neoplasms. PanNET variations include the oncocytic variant with abundant granular cytoplasm; the lipid-rich PanNET with cytoplasmic lipid droplets; pleomorphic PanNET, which shows a degenerative type of endocrine atypia that has no clinical significance; and rhabdoid PanNET {931,96,219}. Oncocytic PanNETs are more pleomorphic, mitotically active, and have prominent nucleoli. They are more clinically aggressive than classic PanNET and resemble acinar cell carcinoma {129,931}. Lipid-rich PanNETs, which may be associated with von Hippel–Lindau syndrome {780}, contain variably sized cytoplasmic lipid droplets, which may rupture tumour cells, making plasmacytoid features difficult to appreciate. The differential diagnosis of lipid-rich PanNET is with metastatic clear cell renal cell carcinoma or primary renal cell carcinoma and adrenocortical neoplasms when the PanNET is located in the pancreatic tail. Pleomorphic PanNET shows threefold anisonucleosis or greater, and if bizarre nuclei are noted it may mimic ductal adenocarcinoma or lymphoma. Rhabdoid PanNETs have striking eosinophilic cytoplasmic protein inclusions that may be mistaken for amyloid, rhabdomyosarcoma, or the Russell bodies of plasma cells.

PanNET may also show prominent papillary growth, thus resembling SPN. In contrast to SPN cells, the cells of PanNET have coarser chromatin, lack nuclear grooves, include cercariform cells (cells with long, slender cytoplasmic tails), and have matrix {718}.

Acinar cell carcinoma has prominent nucleoli and more consistently clumped chromatin than PanNET. A specific diagnosis of PanNET and distinction from the other parenchymal-rich, stromal-poor tumours of acinar cell carcinoma and SPN often requires ICC evaluation.

High-grade (G3) PanNET and large cell–type poorly differentiated PanNEC can be a difficult differential diagnosis, sometimes only distinguished by genotyping. Notably, compared

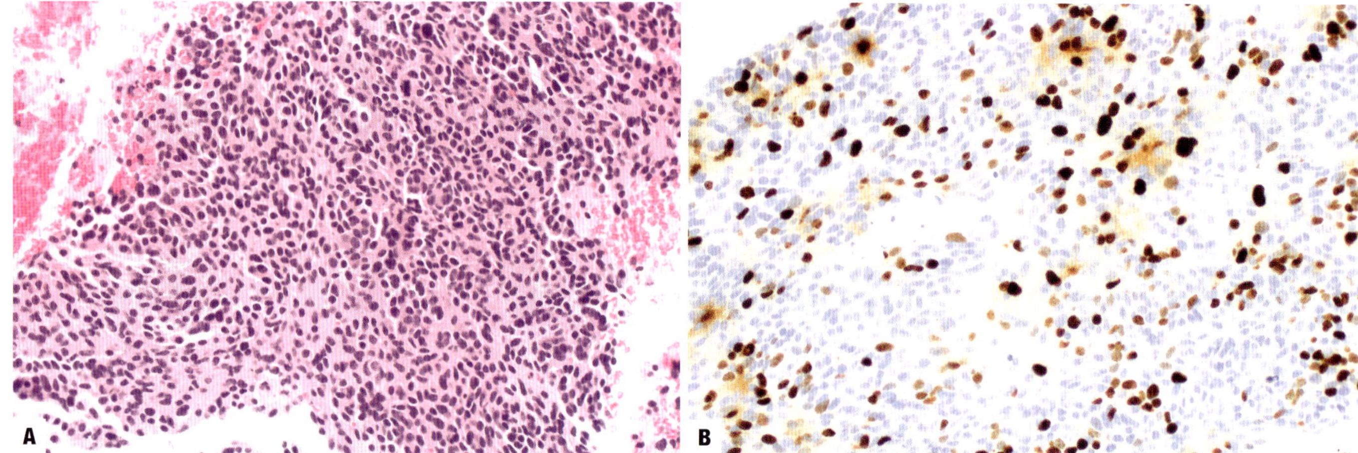

Fig. 9.27 Well-differentiated neuroendocrine tumour (NET), grade 3. **A** Cell block showing the cytomorphology of the tumour cells as well differentiated, i.e. not small cell or large cell poorly differentiated neuroendocrine carcinoma, although they do show more nuclear atypia and mitotic activity than low-grade pancreatic NETs (PanNETs) (H&E). **B** Cell block Ki-67 ICC shows nuclear expression in > 20% of the tumour cells.

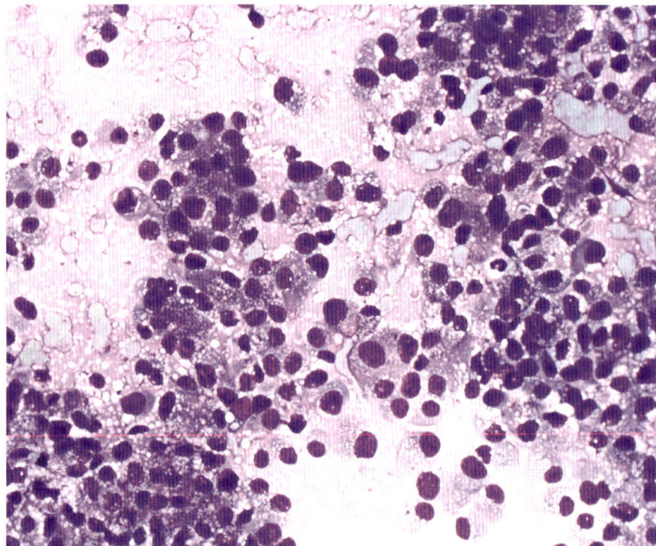

Fig. 9.28 Well-differentiated neuroendocrine tumour (NET), lipid-rich type. Lipid-rich well-differentiated NET cells have abundant small lipid droplets in the abundant eccentric cytoplasm (Giemsa).

with PanNET, PanNEC has more extensive necrosis and markedly elevated mitotic activity and Ki-67 labelling; it may be associated with adenocarcinoma, and it occurs in patients with no history of prior PanNET. Pleomorphic, oncocytic, clear cell, and lipid-rich variants of PanNET can be distinguished from adenocarcinoma and metastatic neoplasms such as melanoma or renal cell carcinoma by ICC demonstration of neuroendocrine differentiation and a low proliferative index.

Ancillary testing

By definition, PanNETs express neuroendocrine markers by ICC, such as chromogranin A and synaptophysin {678}. In resection specimens, their grade is determined by evaluating the Ki-67 proliferation index in ≥ 500 tumour cells in areas of the highest labelling. Grading is subdivided into G1 (Ki-67 < 3%), G2 (Ki-67 3–20%) and G3 (Ki-67 > 20%). Grading on cytopathological material is still a matter of debate. PanNETs are characterized by a heterogeneous distribution of proliferating cells, especially in G2 lesions {287}. Nevertheless, when taken in a linear manner using absolute numbers, the Ki-67 index correlates with

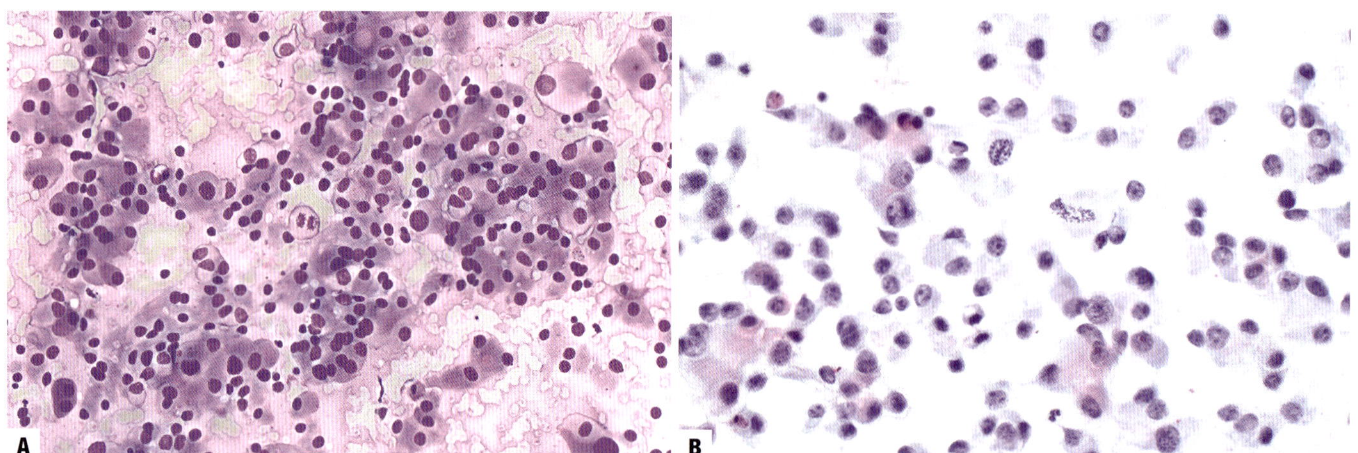

Fig. 9.29 Well-differentiated neuroendocrine tumour (NET), oncocytic type. **A** Oncocytic well-differentiated NET is composed of single dispersed cells with abundant eccentric granular cytoplasm and round to oval nuclei with increased mitotic activity (Giemsa). **B** Oncocytic well-differentiated NET cells are large cells with eccentric eosinophilic granular cytoplasm, coarse chromatin, prominent nucleoli, and relatively plentiful mitoses (Pap).

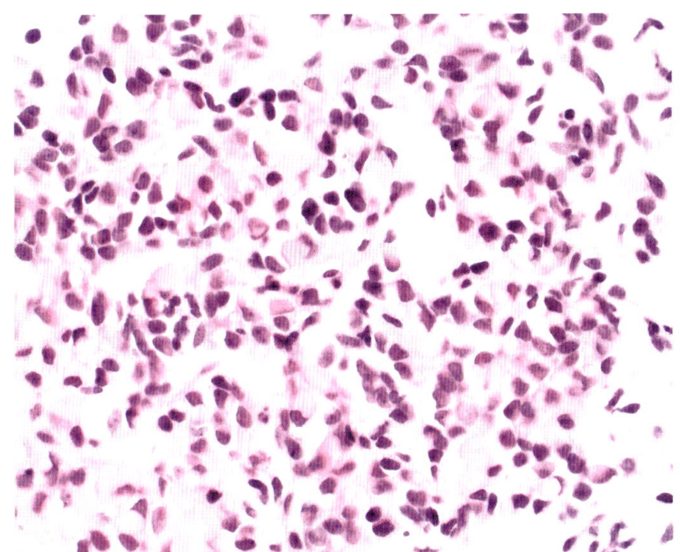

Fig. 9.30 Well-differentiated neuroendocrine tumour (NET), rhabdoid type. This rhabdoid well-differentiated NET is composed of cells with abundant eccentric cytoplasm containing prominent eosinophilic inclusions, which may indent or distort the nuclei (cell block, H&E).

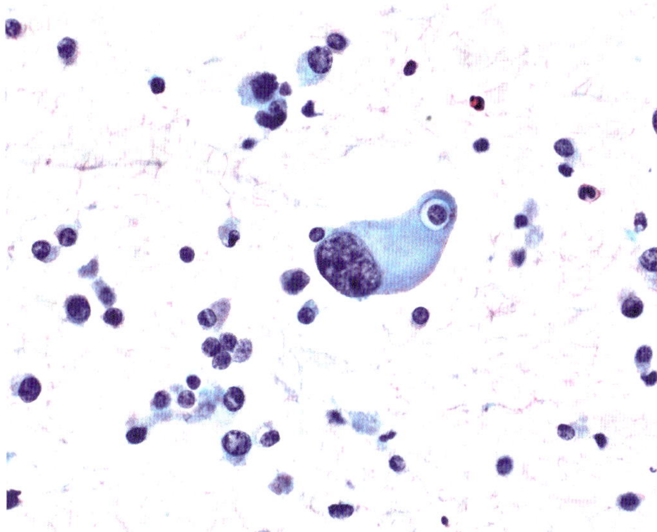

Fig. 9.31 Well-differentiated neuroendocrine tumour (NET), pleomorphic type. Pleomorphic well-differentiated NET shows striking fivefold anisonucleosis with scattered bizarre tumour giant cells surrounded by more classic plasmacytoid cells (Pap).

progression-free and overall survival {773,82,209}. Furthermore, cytohistopathological correlation for grade improves with smaller (< 20 mm) tumours and with counting ≥ 2000 cells, and it depends on the counting method {865,287,677}. Eyeballing (less precise counting) should be avoided, because it gives inaccurate results; a manual count via a microscope and/or on digitized slides is the most appropriate {677,361}.

Molecular analysis is not currently standard in therapeutic management or prognostication, but it may be useful for distinguishing high-grade PanNET from PanNEC (see Table 9.07). The most common genetic alterations of PanNET are *MEN1*, *ATRX*, and *DAXX*, which are not seen in PanNEC {525}. *RB1*, *TP53*, *SMAD4*, and *KRAS* mutations are more compatible with PanNEC {432,841}.

Table 9.07 Immunocytochemical and genetic alterations in G3 pancreatic neuroendocrine tumour (PanNET) compared with pancreatic neuroendocrine carcinoma (PanNEC)

Diagnosis	ICC for diagnosis	ICC for molecular markers	Genetic mutations
PanNET, G3	Strong expression of chromogranin A, synaptophysin, and INSM1	ATRX, DAXX: loss of nuclear expression SSTR2: retained expression	*MEN1*, *ATRX*, and *DAXX* {525}
PanNEC	Usually strong expression of synaptophysin, focal or absent chromogranin A, variable intensity of INSM1 {533}	p53: mutated pattern SMAD4: loss of nuclear expression RB1: loss of nuclear staining	*RB1*, *TP53*, *SMAD4*, and *KRAS* {432}

Neuroendocrine carcinoma

Weynand B
Reid MD
Sigel C

Definition

Pancreatic neuroendocrine carcinoma (PanNEC) is a high-grade malignant epithelial neoplasm with neuroendocrine differentiation.

Clinical features and imaging

PanNEC has a similar clinical presentation to pancreatic adenocarcinoma, with pain, jaundice, and nonspecific abdominal symptoms. Most PanNECs are metastatic at diagnosis. On CT and MRI, PanNECs appear as large pancreatic masses with heterogeneous enhancement due to necrotic and haemorrhagic changes. They can also be cystic. They tend to have a lower rate of vascular encasement than pancreatic adenocarcinoma. The double-duct sign is also less frequently seen than with pancreatic ductal adenocarcinoma. SSTR imaging is usually negative, but PET-CT is positive, indicating a bad prognosis {191}.

Histopathology

PanNECs show either a small cell morphology analogous to pulmonary small cell carcinoma or an intermediate-sized to large cell morphology characterized by abundant cytoplasm, a large nucleus with vesicular chromatin, and a prominent nucleolus. Architecturally, they are characterized by poorly formed, large trabeculae, solid organoid nests, or diffuse sheets of neoplastic cells {775,784}. Extensive necrosis is often present, and mitotic figures are easily spotted.

Key diagnostic cytopathological features

Small cell type

- Highly cellular smears
- Loose crowded tissue fragments, which occasionally are 3D, and/or dispersed single cells
- Necrosis and crushed cells with chromatinic smearing are common
- Angulated pleomorphic nuclei with moulding
- Hyperchromatic and coarsely stippled chromatin
- Scant nucleoli
- Minimal to imperceptible cytoplasm
- Scattered mitotic figures and apoptotic bodies

Large cell type

- Highly cellular smears
- Loose crowded tissue fragments, which occasionally are 3D, and/or dispersed single cells
- Anisonucleosis is marked
- Thickened, relatively smooth nuclear membrane
- Markedly enlarged nuclei with coarsely stippled chromatin and prominent nucleoli; the nuclei are vesicular in Pap-stained smears
- Moderate to abundant eosinophilic cytoplasm
- Necrosis is common

Discussion and differential diagnosis

PanNECs are poorly differentiated high-grade neoplasms composed of small or intermediate to large cells with high-grade nuclear features and neuroendocrine differentiation by ICC. By definition, the proliferation index determined by Ki-67 is > 20%.

PanNEC must be distinguished from pure or mixed forms of acinar cell carcinoma and high-grade (G3) well-differentiated pancreatic neuroendocrine tumour (PanNET). PanNEC with significant (> 30%) acinar differentiation is regarded as a mixed acinar–neuroendocrine carcinoma. These mixed carcinomas have genetic alterations more similar to pure acinar cell carcinoma than PanNEC despite identical cytopathological features,

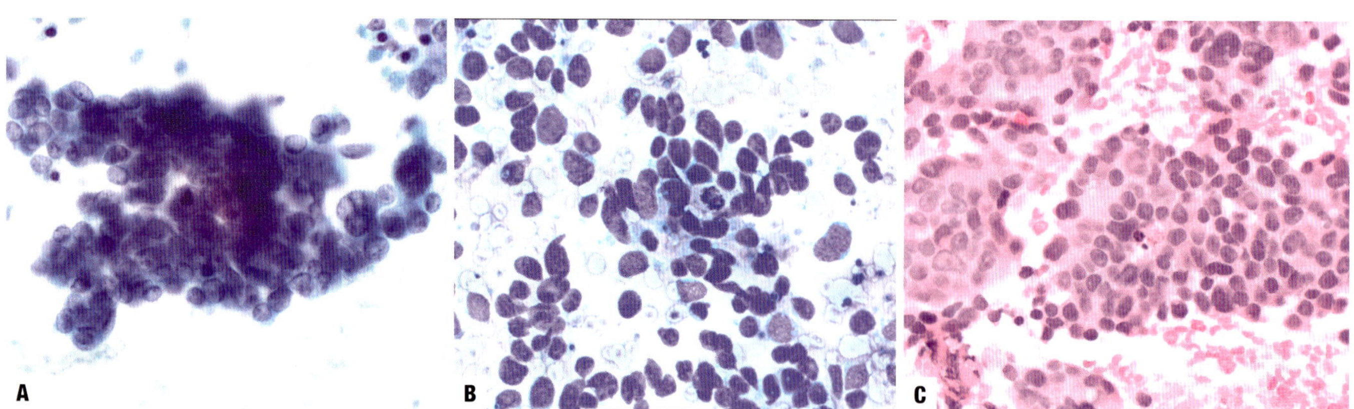

Fig. 9.32 Neuroendocrine carcinoma (NEC), small cell type. **A** Tumour cytomorphology is similar to that of small cell carcinoma of the lung, with nuclear moulding of small cells with hyperchromasia; a mix of fine and coarse, relatively uniformly distributed chromatin; scant cytoplasm; and apoptosis (Pap). **B** Pancreatic NEC (PanNEC), small cell type. Pattern of poorly cohesive small tissue fragments, few intact dispersed single cells, stripped nuclei, and apoptosis, with tumour cells showing a high N:C ratio, nuclear moulding, and abnormal mitoses (Giemsa). **C** Cell block showing tumour cells, which are small with a high N:C ratio and show nuclear moulding and moderate nuclear pleomorphism with some apoptosis (H&E).

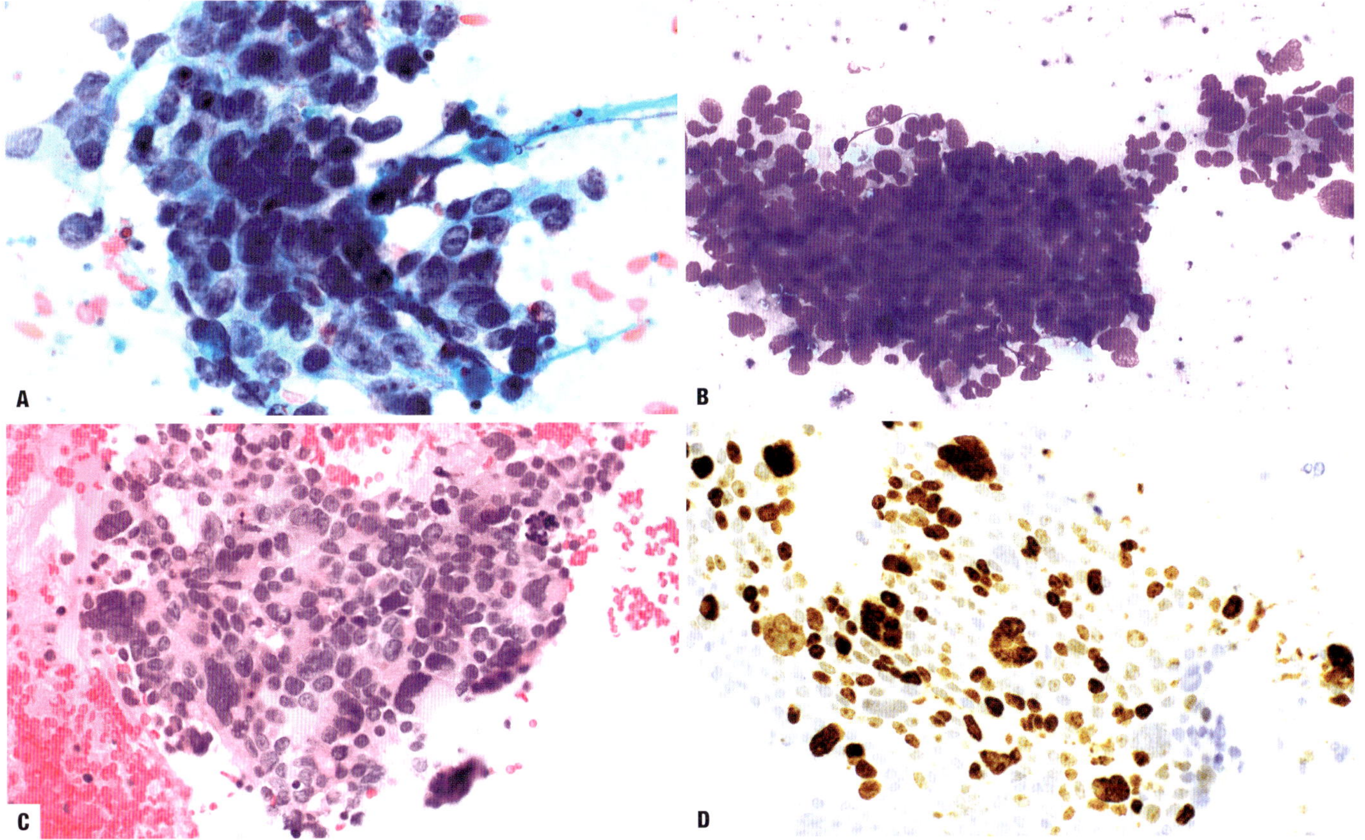

Fig. 9.33 Neuroendocrine carcinoma (NEC), large cell type. **A** Pancreatic NEC (PanNEC), large cell type. The crowded large cells with pleomorphic nuclei show coarse chromatin, prominent nucleoli, and single cell necrosis with apoptotic debris (Pap). **B** Very crowded tissue fragments of large, overtly malignant cells with a high N:C ratio, large nuclei with granular hyperchromatic chromatin, and scant cytoplasm (Giemsa). **C** PanNEC, large cell type. Cell block showing a tissue fragment composed of large cells with eosinophilic cytoplasm and bizarre pleomorphic nuclei, a suggestion of a pseudorosette pattern, and apoptosis (H&E). **D** PanNEC, large cell type. NECs have a high Ki-67 index; here, it is approximately 50% (ICC).

making immunophenotyping essential for accurate diagnosis {72,132,909}.

The most challenging differential diagnosis is with G3 PanNET. PanNEC is not preceded by a history of PanNET and has less plasmacytoid morphology, more irregular nuclei, more pleomorphism, and necrosis {775}. Recognition of a distinct adenocarcinoma component also supports PanNEC. Commonly, genotyping either by ICC surrogate markers or by molecular assays is needed to help distinguish these two morphologically similar but biologically distinct entities (G3 PanNET and PanNEC) {775}. Rarely, adenocarcinomas can have eosinophilic cytoplasm, but they lack the organoid arrangements and coarse chromatin of large cell PanNEC.

Ancillary testing

The neuroendocrine nature of these tumours has to be confirmed by ICC, and expression for synaptophysin is the most frequently retained. Chromogranin A may be less diffusely expressed and a search at high-power magnification for focal cytoplasmic positivity may be necessary. INSM1 may be a valuable adjunct in determining the neuroendocrine nature of these tumours, because it is very specific {533}. Significant acinar differentiation (> 30%) must be excluded with ICC by at least two of the following markers: trypsin, chymotrypsin, or BCL10. The Ki-67 proliferation index is by definition > 20%, but it usually exceeds 50%. Genotyping may be helpful for distinguishing PanNEC from G3 PanNET because *RB1*, *TP53*, *SMAD4*, and *KRAS* mutations are associated with PanNEC {432,841}. Surrogate ICC markers can also be utilized (see Table 9.07, p. 145).

Pancreatoblastoma

Reid MD
Štoos-Veić T

Definition

Pancreatoblastoma is a rare malignant epithelial neoplasm that shows trilineage (i.e. acinar, neuroendocrine, or ductal) differentiation and squamoid nests.

Clinical features and imaging

Pancreatoblastoma is most frequently seen in children, but 30% of cases occur in adults {103,421,613,679}. Although most cases occur sporadically, there is an association with Beckwith–Wiedemann syndrome, familial adenomatous polyposis, and Gardner syndrome {679,417,212,7,392}, which highlights the need for genetic testing and counselling in these patients. Tumours are typically large (mean: 100 mm), and patients present with nonspecific symptoms including abdominal pain, nausea, vomiting, diarrhoea, weight loss, and (rarely) jaundice. Serum AFP elevation may be seen in as many as 60% of children. Serum CEA levels may also be elevated. Approximately 40% present with locally advanced or metastatic disease {421,679}.

On imaging, tumours are usually large, heterogeneous, circumscribed solid masses, but they may show cystic degeneration. The findings can be nonspecific, with benign and malignant tumours in the differential diagnosis {127,335,558, 948}.

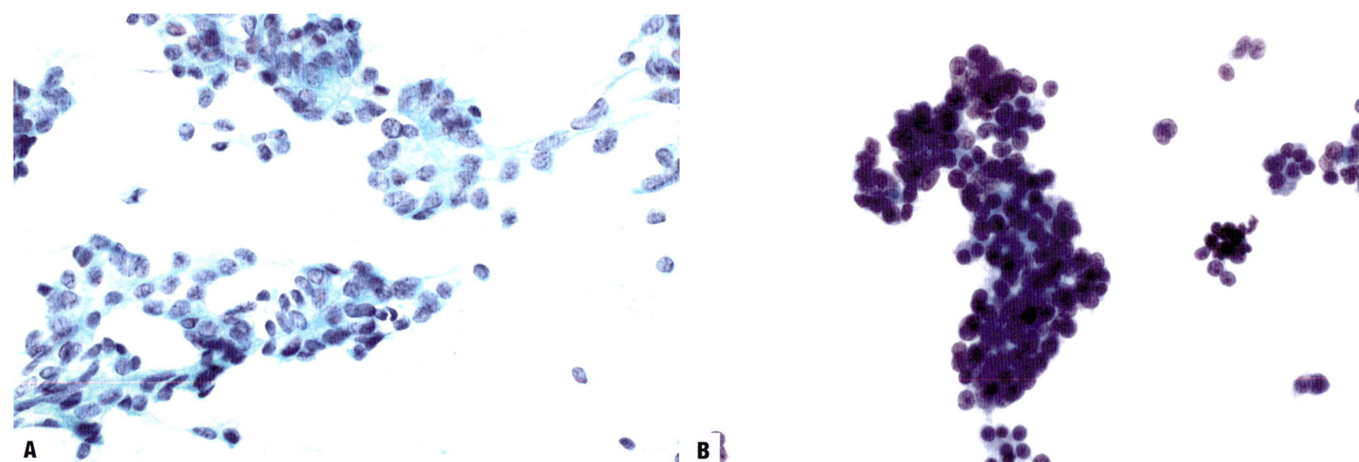

Fig. 9.34 Pancreatoblastoma. **A** Tissue fragments showing vague acinar architecture in some, and composed of blastic cells with a high N:C ratio, round nuclei, powdery immature chromatin, and indistinct nucleoli (Pap). **B** Crowded tissue fragment composed of oval blastic tumour cells with rounded nuclei, immature fine chromatin, and small nucleoli (liquid-based cytopathology, Pap).

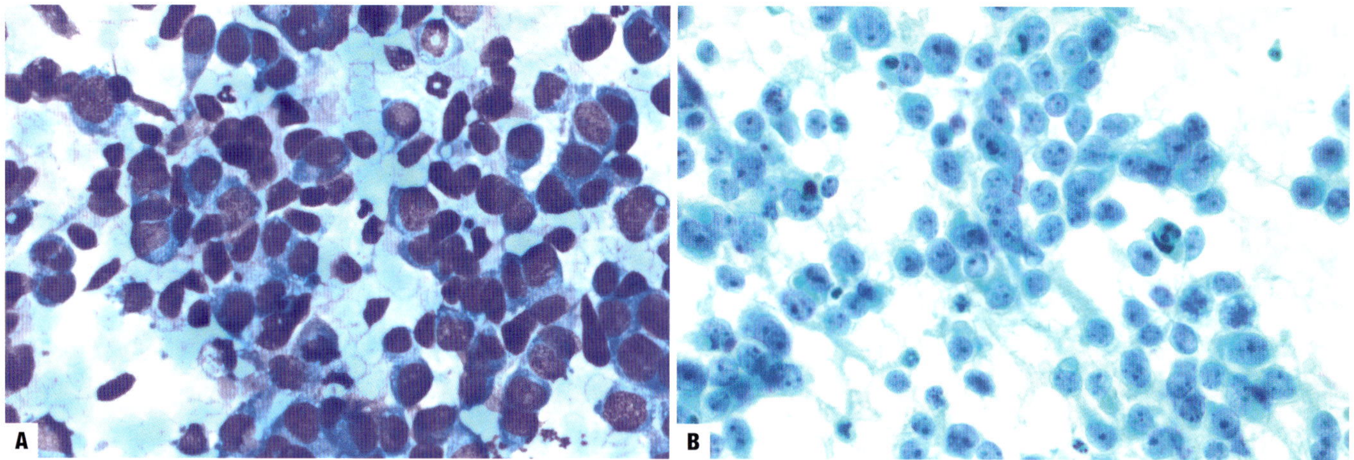

Fig. 9.35 Pancreatoblastoma. **A** These blastic tumour cells are seen in poorly cohesive tissue fragments and as single cells, and they have a high N:C ratio and oval, mildly pleomorphic nuclei showing fine blastic immature chromatin, nucleoli in some cells, and moulding. Single cells resemble lymphoid cells (Giemsa). **B** Small tissue fragments and dispersed single cells are present, and the tumour cells show mildly pleomorphic nuclei varying in size, with fine blastic chromatin and, in this example, prominent nucleoli and single cell necrosis (Pap).

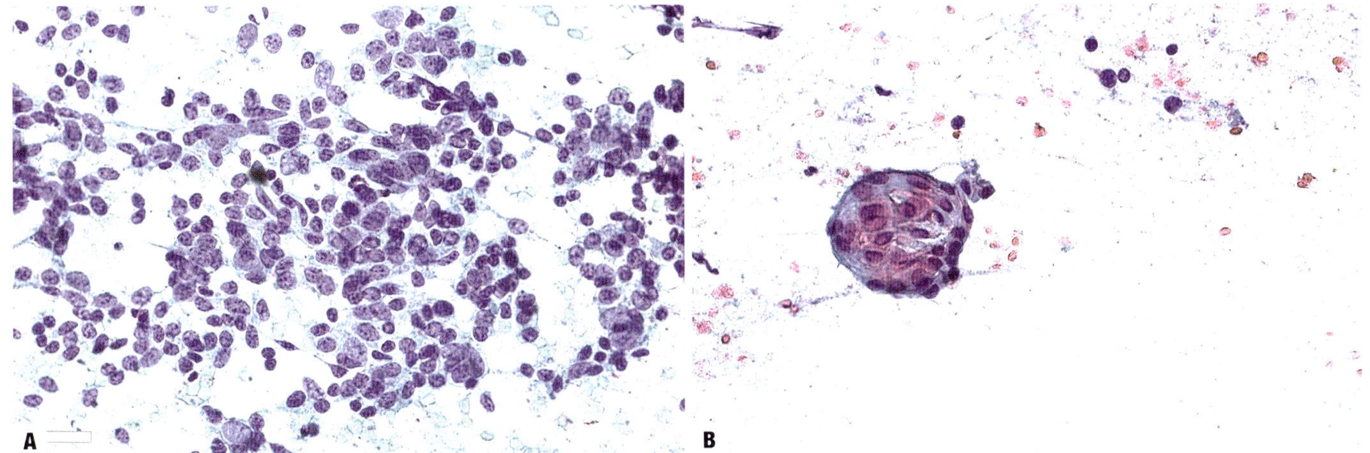

Fig. 9.36 Pancreatoblastoma. **A** Blastic tumour cells show pale, poorly defined cytoplasm; moderate nuclear pleomorphism in size and shape; and focal spindling (Pap). **B** Squamoid nest composed of a tightly whorled group of epithelioid cells with pale cytoplasm, syncytial arrangement, and pale nuclear chromatin (Pap).

Histopathology

Pancreatoblastoma shows solid, trabecular, or acinar growth punctuated with squamoid nests of uniform, polygonal cells containing central nuclei and prominent nucleoli. Acinar growth often predominates, but neuroendocrine differentiation with organoid nests and trabeculae is also commonly seen. Tumours rarely show ductal differentiation. The squamoid nests or morules are the defining hallmark of pancreatoblastoma and are required for the diagnosis.

Key diagnostic cytopathological features

- Hypercellular smears with tissue fragments and singly dispersed cells
- Branching papillae resembling solid pseudopapillary neoplasm may be seen
- Two distinctive cell types: blast-like tumour cells and squamoid nests or morules

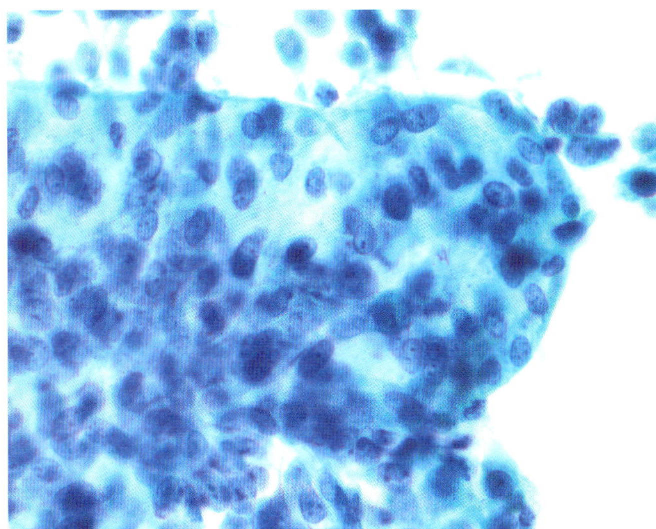

Fig. 9.37 Pancreatoblastoma. This tissue fragment shows a squamoid nest composed of streaming epithelioid cells with pale cytoplasm, syncytial arrangement, and blunt nuclei without nucleoli (Pap).

- Blast-like cells are small (1.5–2 times the diameter of an erythrocyte), with high N:C ratios, scant deep-blue cytoplasm (Giemsa), and round to oval monomorphic nuclei resembling lymphocytes, with delicate, finely granular, immature chromatin and one or two distinct nucleoli (Pap); nuclear moulding may be present
- Squamoid nests consist of swirling squamous cells with increasing cytoplasm centrally
- Spindle cells, immature mesenchyme, and stromal fragments in some tumours

Reference(s): {679,163,296,709,777,988,288,647,674}

Discussion and differential diagnosis

The cytopathology of pancreatoblastoma has only rarely been described in small series {679,182} and case reports {163,296, 709,777,988}.

Because of the trilineage differentiation and the subtlety of the squamoid nests or morules, the cytopathological diagnosis of pancreatoblastoma is challenging. Identifying the two-cell-type population of blast-like cells and squamoid morules assists in the differential diagnosis. Squamoid nests or morules are syncytial tissue fragments of 10–15 streaming, bland, low–N:C ratio epithelioid cells with elongated, blunted nuclei and vesicular chromatin (Pap), and they contain cells with dense light-blue cytoplasm (Giemsa). The morules are much easier to identify in the cell block.

The differential diagnosis includes acinar cell carcinoma, pancreatic neuroendocrine tumours (PanNETs), pancreatic neuroendocrine carcinoma (PanNEC), and solid pseudopapillary neoplasm. Pancreatoblastoma with acinar or neuroendocrine differentiation may morphologically resemble acinar cell carcinoma, PanNET, or PanNEC and require ICC markers. Papillae and nuclear grooves may be seen in pancreatoblastoma, causing misdiagnosis as solid pseudopapillary neoplasm {674}.

Ancillary testing

Pancreatoblastoma is positive for pancytokeratin and, depending on differentiation, may express acinar markers including trypsin, chymotrypsin, BCL10, and/or neuroendocrine markers (most commonly synaptophysin, chromogranin A, CD56, and INSM1).

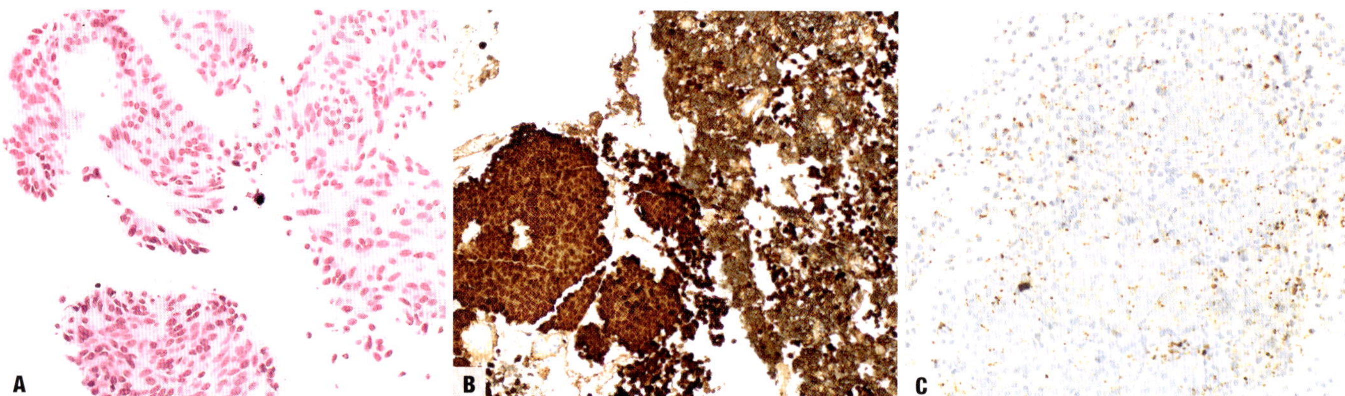

Fig. 9.38 Pancreatoblastoma. **A** Cell block from a pancreatoblastoma showing a two-cell population of smaller blastic cells with a high N:C ratio (left) and a subtle pale pink squamoid morule (right) composed of streaming epithelioid cells with abundant eosinophilic cytoplasm (H&E). **B** Cell block showing a tissue fragment (left) with a subtle squamoid nest that is highlighted by strong nuclear expression for β-catenin (ICC). **C** Cell block tissue fragment shows tumour cells with focal cytoplasmic positivity for chromogranin (ICC).

Squamoid morules are difficult to see on smear and/or cell block and are highlighted by β-catenin immunostain, which shows nuclear labelling in circumscribed or poorly defined morules.

Common molecular alterations include loss of heterozygosity at the short arm of 11p and mutations in *CTNNB1* {7,393,840}. Children with Beckwith–Wiedemann syndrome show loss of heterozygosity at 11p, where the maternal allele is typically lost. The loss of 11p also occurs in > 80% of sporadic pancreatoblastomas. Alterations in the APC/β-catenin pathway have been reported in 50–80% of pancreatoblastomas {7,840}, most often due to mutation of *CTNNB1*, which encodes β-catenin. *APC* gene abnormalities are reported in pancreatoblastomas arising in patients with and without familial adenomatous polyposis {7,937}. Rarely, upregulation of the R-spondin/LGR5/RNF43 module is identified {7,345,937}. *KRAS* mutations and the accumulation of p53, typically found in ductal adenocarcinoma of the pancreas, are not identified. Loss of SMAD4 expression is infrequent.

Solid pseudopapillary neoplasm

Granados R
Stelow EB

Definition

Solid pseudopapillary neoplasm (SPN) is a low-grade malignant pancreatic tumour composed of poorly cohesive epithelial cells forming solid and pseudopapillary structures that lack a specific line of pancreatic epithelial differentiation.

Clinical features and imaging

SPNs occur predominantly in adolescent and young female patients, with a mean age of 28 years, but they may present at any age (range: 7–87 years). They rarely occur in male patients {426,845,276}. They are the second most common pancreatic malignancy in patients aged < 35 years {674}. Patients are often asymptomatic or present with abdominal pain, nausea, vomiting, or a palpable mass. Weight loss, jaundice, and pancreatitis occur rarely {522,458}. Tumours may occur anywhere in the pancreas, being most common in the body and tail {458}. The most common imaging presentation is a well-defined, heterogeneous solid and cystic mass with peripheral calcifications {276}.

Histopathology

SPNs have a heterogeneous architecture with solid and pseudopapillary structures and marked vascularity. Acellular stroma frequently forms cuffs around delicate capillaries. Neoplastic cells typically cling to the vessels as they lose cohesion. The cells are monomorphic and bland with occasional nuclear grooves and cytoplasmic perinuclear vacuoles {455}. Atypical nuclei may be present. Hyaline globules are found within or outside neoplastic cells. Mitoses are rare. Background degeneration can include macrophages and cholesterol granulomas.

Key diagnostic cytopathological features

- Highly cellular smears with branching papillary fronds and single cells
- Three layers in papillary fronds: central vascular cores surrounded by myxoid stroma with an outer layer of neoplastic cells

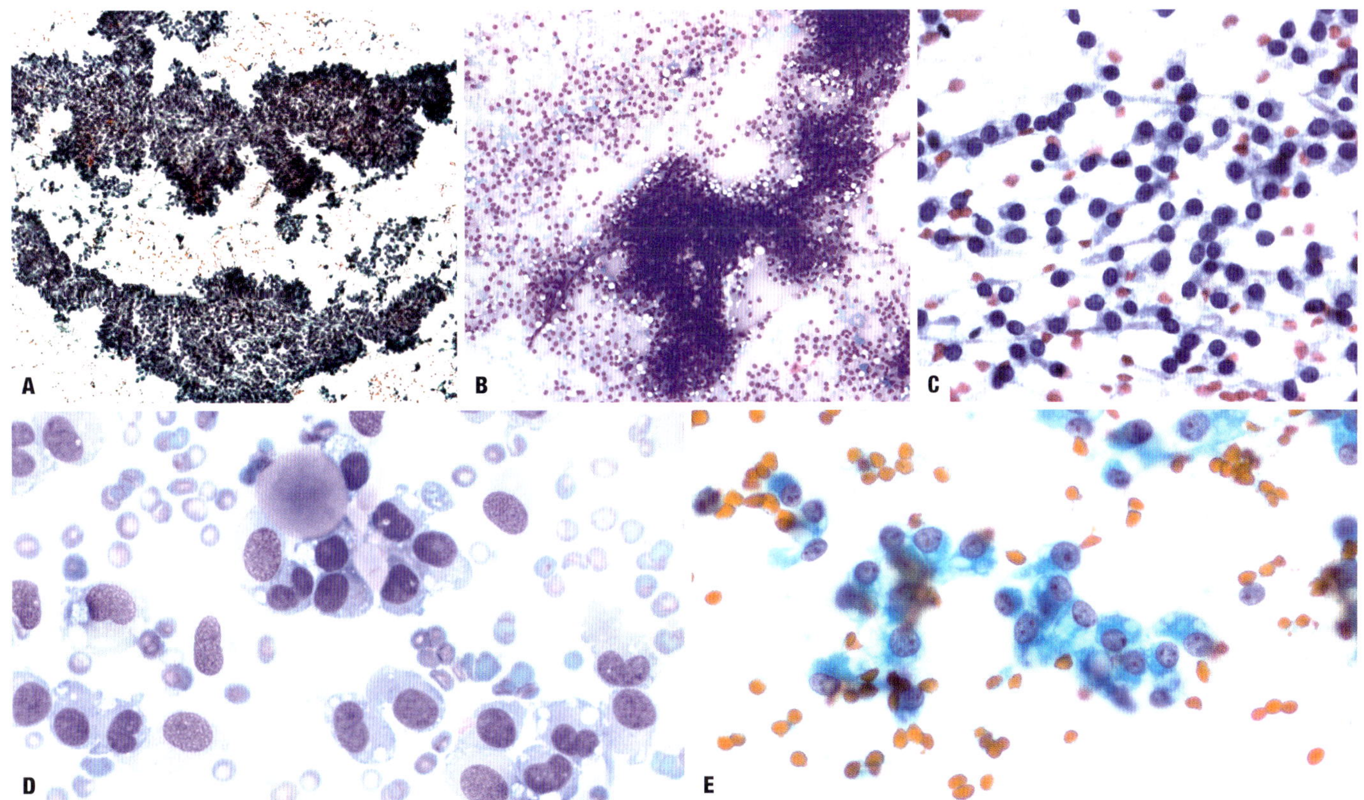

Fig. 9.39 Solid pseudopapillary neoplasm. **A** Highly cellular smears showing tissue fragments with thin vascular strands covered in crowded monotonous polygonal cells resembling papillary tissue fragments (Pap). **B** Smears are highly cellular, with tissue fragments consisting of central thin vascular strands surrounded by crowded tumour cells and with numerous single cells in the background. These tissue fragments resemble papillae (Giemsa). **C** Single cells show round to oval nuclei with indentations in the nuclear envelope and grooves imparting a coffee-bean shape, while the chromatin is evenly distributed, and wispy tags of poorly defined cytoplasm can be seen (Pap). **D** Tumour cells are polygonal, with variable, often scant eccentric cytoplasm; perinuclear cytoplasmic vacuoles; and hyaline globules, which can be intracellular or extracellular (Giemsa). **E** Neoplastic cells with perinuclear cytoplasmic vacuoles; note the cell in the centre at 12 o'clock with a cytoplasmic tail (cercariform cell) (Pap).

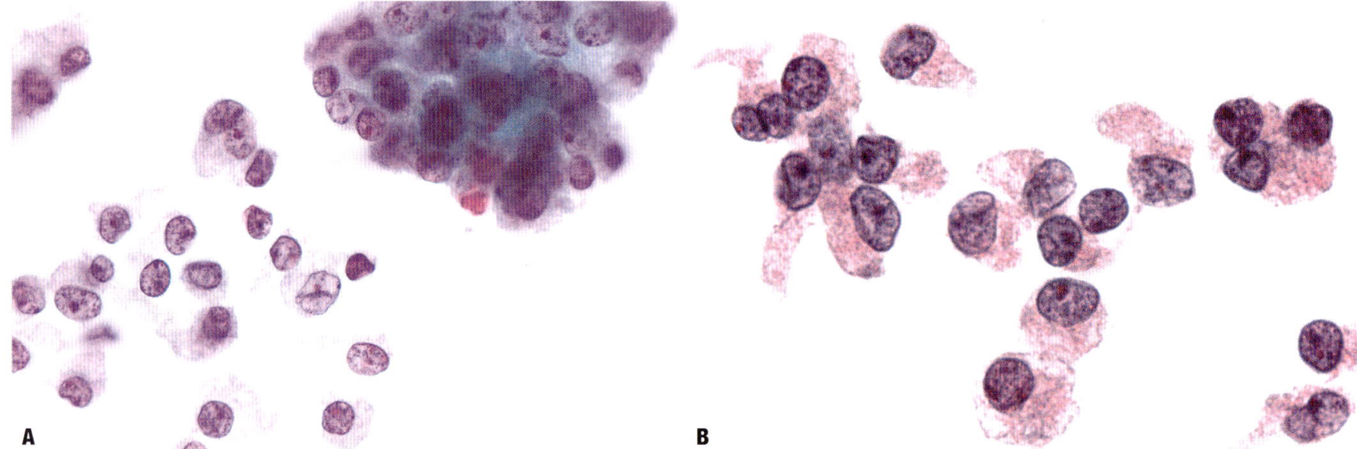

Fig. 9.40 Solid pseudopapillary neoplasm. **A** 3D crowded tissue fragment and dispersed single cells with variable anisonucleosis and nuclear grooves (Pap). **B** Single cells exhibit plasmacytoid shapes with eccentric fragile cytoplasm, with some showing cytoplasmic tails (cercariform cell), binucleation, mildly pleomorphic nuclei, and prominent nucleoli (Pap).

- Myxoid stroma: amphophilic (Pap) or magenta (Giemsa)
- Ball-like structures of myxoid stroma with or without a rim of neoplastic cells
- Monomorphic, medium-sized polygonal or plasmacytoid neoplastic cells with poorly defined cell borders and frequently vacuolated cytoplasm
- Dispersed cells with long, slender cytoplasmic tails (cercariform cells)
- Round to oval nuclei with smooth nuclear membranes, or convoluted or reniform nuclei with nuclear grooves (coffee-bean nuclei)
- Finely granular chromatin
- Prominent nucleoli
- Scant, poorly defined cytoplasm in most cells with perinuclear vacuoles
- Metachromatic (Giemsa), pale pink (H&E and Pap), PAS-positive, diastase-resistant, and Congo red–negative cytoplasmic hyaline globules
- Scarce mitoses
- Background cyst debris with necrosis, multinucleated giant cells, calcifications, cholesterol clefts, and psammoma bodies

Reference(s): {634,539,259,718,779,50,656,630}

Discussion and differential diagnosis

SPNs are typically monomorphic epithelioid neoplasms and show significant cytomorphological overlap with pancreatic neuroendocrine tumours (PanNETs), acinar cell carcinomas, pancreatoblastomas, and some metastatic malignancies such as clear cell renal cell or ovarian carcinoma. FNAB of acinar cell carcinoma contains monomorphic cells in 3D tissue fragments with prominent nucleoli and granular cytoplasm, as well as occasional acinar and papillary structures {774,718}, and it lacks the hyaline globules, nuclear grooves, cercariform cells, and myxoid stroma typical of SPN. SPNs have distinctive feature of small neoplastic cells clinging to the periphery of the perivascular myxoid stroma that clearly highlights the central vessel.

Misclassification of SPN as PanNET is common {314}. Both exhibit plasmacytoid cells, and hyaline globules can occur in

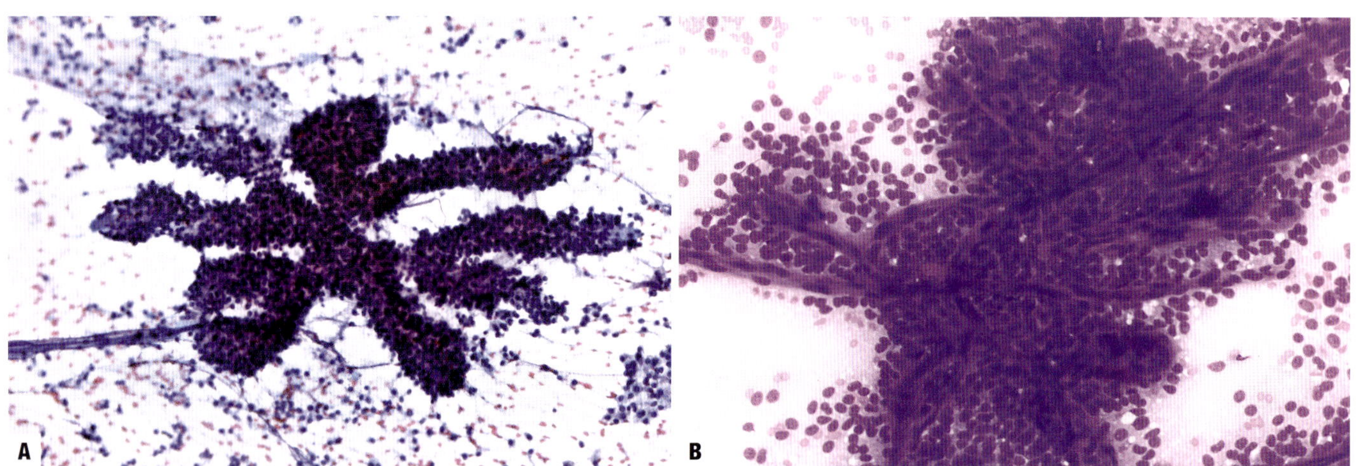

Fig. 9.41 Solid pseudopapillary neoplasm. **A** Tissue fragment showing the papillary architecture that is a characteristic feature of this neoplasm. The centre of the papilla is cleared out, representing the blood vessel and perivascular myxoid stroma (Pap). **B** This tissue fragment shows a central vascular highway of thin, branching and anastomosing capillaries with a small amount of myxoid stroma, surrounded by clinging crowded tumour cells (Giemsa).

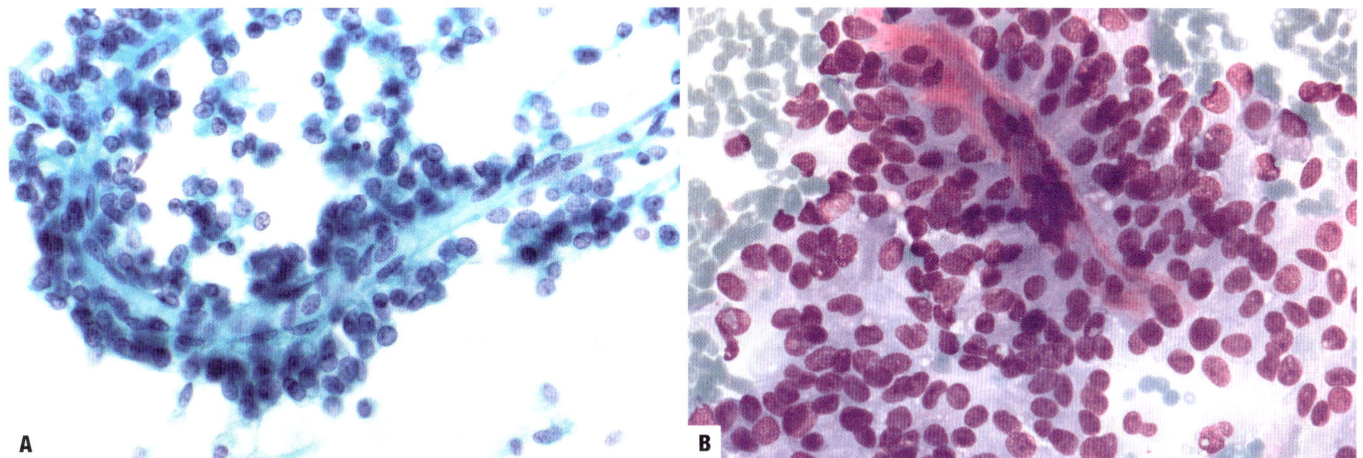

Fig. 9.42 Solid pseudopapillary neoplasm. **A** Tissue fragment resembling a papillary frond with central capillary and clinging neoplastic cells. The second layer of myxoid stroma is thin and difficult to see. Note the scant, poorly defined cytoplasm and bland nuclei (Pap). **B** This tissue fragment shows the second layer of myxoid stroma in the papillary-like fronds as a magenta matrix around the central thin vessel (Giemsa).

PanNET {541}. Distinguishing features for SPN include fine chromatin, nuclear grooves, cercariform cells, and myxoid stroma that is magenta (Giemsa) {550}. Pancreatoblastomas may have papillary groups, but true fibrovascular cores and myxoid matrix are absent {674}. Their primitive cells show moulded nuclei, and squamoid nests or morules are distinctive. Metastatic renal and ovarian carcinomas may have papillary structures, vacuolated cells, and metachromatic hyaline material {509}, but their cytopathological pleomorphism and immunophenotype are distinguishing features {76}.

SPNs with high-grade carcinomas are a subtype of SPN with aggressive behaviour. Their cytopathological features have not been described.

Ancillary testing

The peculiar phenotype of SPN is not specific for any pancreatic cell type, favouring a pluripotential embryonic stem cell origin. SPNs almost universally show nuclear expression of β-catenin by ICC, reflecting point mutations in exon 3 of *CTNNB1* {694}. A pitfall is that some acinar cell carcinomas and PanNETs also harbour mutations in *CTNNB1*, and those tumours will also show nuclear expression of β-catenin, but the nuclear staining in these tumours tends to be patchy rather than diffusely and strongly positive as in SPN. Other commonly expressed markers include CD10, vimentin, synaptophysin, CD56, NSE, and PR. Staining for chromogranin A is usually negative, but a cytoplasmic dot-like staining pattern has been reported {607}. SPN may express cytokeratins AE1/AE3 (expression may range from weak to strong) and CAM5.2, depending on the method of antigen retrieval used. CK7 and CK19 are usually negative {496, 594,356}. α1-Antitrypsin is positive in SPN hyaline globules and in the cytoplasm of pancreatoblastoma cells {606}.

CD99 shows a dot-like paranuclear staining pattern, unique to SPN {718,243}. SPN is also characterized by abnormalities in E-cadherin, either with loss of expression or with aberrant nuclear and cytoplasmic expression, depending on the antibody used {455}. SPN may also stain for melanocytic markers, such as S100, HMB45, and melan-A (MART1) {125,496}.

SOX11, TFE3, LEF1, AR, and claudin-5 staining have also been reported in SPN {400}.

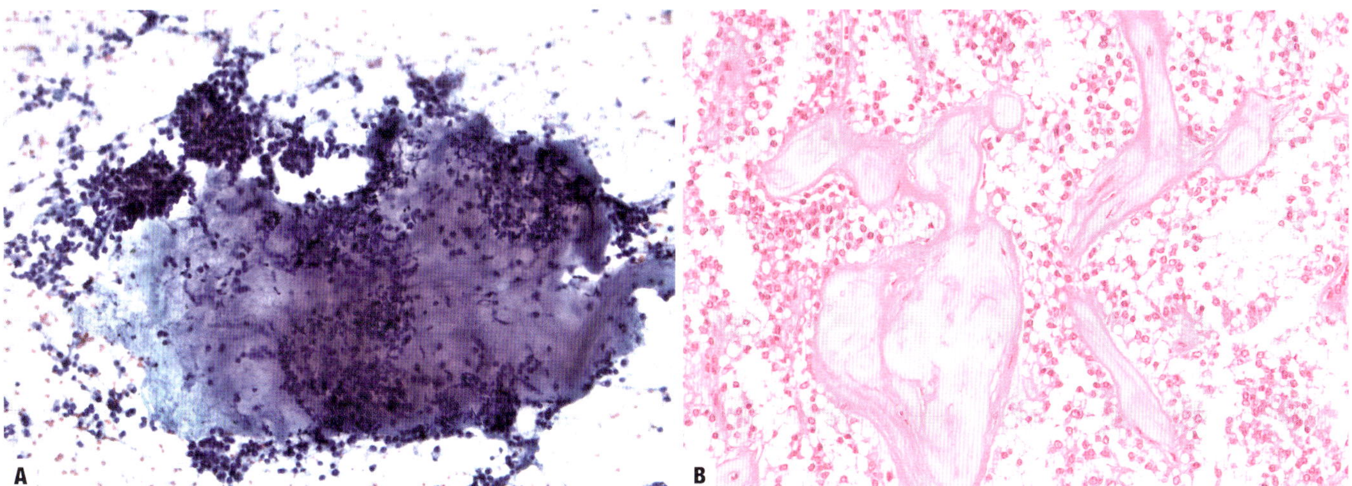

Fig. 9.43 Solid pseudopapillary neoplasm. **A** A large tissue fragment of myxoid stroma is surrounded by small tissue fragments and single dispersed cells (Pap). **B** Fine core needle biopsy shows vacuolated and discohesive tumour cells surrounding the fibrovascular cores, with prominent myxoid stroma (H&E).

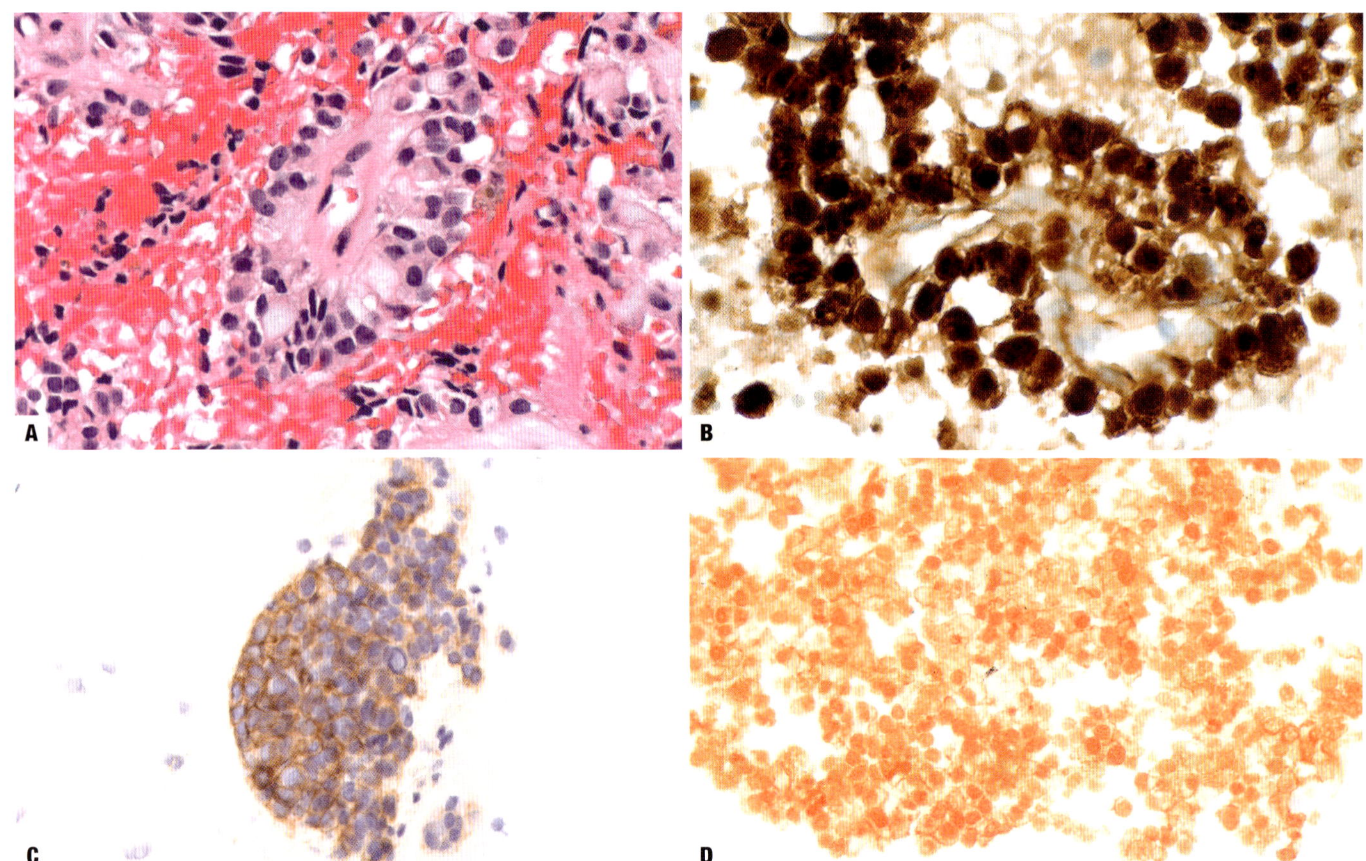

Fig. 9.44 A Solid pseudopapillary neoplasm. Cell block showing tissue fragments with a fibrovascular core with an eosinophilic myxoid rim covered by clinging tumour cells with round to oval nuclei containing occasional nuclear grooves, and scant wispy cytoplasm (H&E). **B** Solid pseudopapillary neoplasm. Cell block tissue fragment showing diffuse, strong nuclear β-catenin staining (ICC, β-catenin). **C** Well-differentiated neuroendocrine tumour (NET). In contrast to solid pseudopapillary tumour, this well-differentiated NET shows β-catenin staining in the cytoplasm but not the nuclei (ICC, β-catenin). **D** Solid pseudopapillary neoplasm. Cell block tissue fragment showing marked diffuse nuclear and cytoplasmic expression of β-catenin (ICC, β-catenin).

Table 9.08 Summary of immunocytochemical stains most useful for the differential diagnosis of solid pseudopapillary neoplasm (SPN), neuroendocrine tumour (NET), acinar cell carcinoma (ACC), and pancreatoblastoma (PB)

Antibody	Pattern	SPN	NET	ACC	PB
AE1/AE3	Cytoplasmic	+ (focal)	+	+	+
α1-Antitrypsin	Hyaline globules or cytoplasm	+	−/+	−	+
AR	Nuclear	+	−/+	−	−
BCL10	Cytoplasmic	−	−	+	+
CAM5.2	Focal	+ (focal)	+	+	+
CD99	Dot-like paranuclear	+	−	−	−
Chymotrypsin	Cytoplasmic	−	−	+	+
Cyclin D1	Nuclear (100%)	−	−	+	+ (squamoid corpuscles)
E-cadherin	Nuclear/cytoplasmic or absent	+	−/+	−	−
LEF1	Nuclear (95%)	+	−	−	−
PR	Nuclear	+	−/+	−/+	+ in stromal components
SOX11	Nuclear	+	−/+	−	−
Synaptophysin	Cytoplasmic	+ (focal)	+	−	−/+
TFE3	Nuclear (75%)	+	−/+	−/+	−
Trypsin	Cytoplasmic	−/+	−/+	+	+

The expression of these markers and the lack of expression of trypsin and BCL10 distinguishes SPN from pancreatoblastoma and acinar cell carcinoma {462}. The pattern of staining for claudins proves helpful in the differential diagnosis as well. SPNs express claudin-5 in a membranous pattern and claudin-7 only in a cytoplasmic pattern. PanNET, acinar cell carcinoma, and pancreatoblastoma show strong membranous expression for claudin-7 and are negative for claudin-5 {149}. The combination of β-catenin, LEF1, and TFE3 in biopsy material was found to have a sensitivity of 100% and a specificity of 91.9% for the diagnosis of SPN {400}. Table 9.08 summarizes a short list of the antibodies that are most relevant in practice for differentiating SPN from other non-ductal neoplasms.

Ki-67 indexes of < 3% are typical, and a high proliferation index is associated with aggressive behaviour {990,400,944}. Gene mutations common in other pancreatic tumours, such as *KRAS*, *TP53*, *SMAD4*, *GNAS*, *RNF43*, and *VHL*, are unusual in SPN {76}.

Chapter 9

Pancreatic lymphomas

Davey DD
Zhang ML

Definition

Pancreatic lymphoma is an extranodal lymphoma with the bulk of disease confined to the pancreas.

Clinical features and imaging

Extranodal lymphomas of the pancreas present either as primary disease in the pancreas, accounting for < 1% of primary pancreatic neoplasms, or (more frequently) as secondary involvement of the pancreas as a result of direct extension from peripancreatic or retroperitoneal lymph nodes in regional or systemic lymphoid neoplasia. Pancreatic lymphoma most commonly affects middle-aged and elderly individuals (mean age: 55–65 years), with a male predominance {205,591,889,987}. The most common types of lymphomas found in the pancreas are non-Hodgkin B-cell lymphomas, with diffuse large B-cell lymphoma (DLBCL) accounting for at least two thirds of cases, and a lesser number of high-grade B-cell lymphomas, follicular lymphomas, extranodal marginal zone lymphomas, and other types. Sporadic cases of T-cell and Hodgkin lymphoma have also been seen. Imaging studies reveal a solid mass most commonly located in the pancreatic head, although multiple masses may be found occasionally. Masses may be detected by a variety of imaging modalities, including CT, MRI, and EUS. Patients most commonly present with gastrointestinal symptoms such as abdominal pain, jaundice, and obstruction. Patients may occasionally present with B symptoms, including fever, night sweats, and weight loss. Serum LDH and CA19-9 may be elevated.

Histopathology

Key histopathological features depend on the type of lymphoma. DLBCL shows effacement of architecture with a diffuse proliferation of medium-sized to large lymphoid cells with variable immunoblastic, centroblastic, or pleomorphic nuclei.

Key diagnostic cytopathological features

- Hypercellularity with dispersed monotonous pattern
- Discohesive cells
- Background lymphoid cytoplasmic fragments (lymphoglandular bodies) with or without necrosis
- DLBCL has medium-sized to large cells with variable concentric, immunoblastic, or scant cytoplasm, and stripped bare nuclei
- Other subtypes may have smaller atypical lymphoid cells or anaplastic features
- Nuclei vary with the subtype of lymphoma
- One or more nucleoli may be prominent, depending on the subtype of lymphoma
- Karyorrhexis and mitoses may be present
- Background may have admixed smaller lymphocytes and other inflammatory cells

Reference(s): {889,987}

Discussion and differential diagnosis

There are two major criteria for the diagnosis of primary pancreatic lymphoma: firstly, the bulk of disease is located within the pancreas, and secondly, the primary clinical presentation must be in the pancreas. Immunodeficiency and EBV infections may play an etiological role in some cases.

The clinical and imaging differential diagnosis of pancreatic lymphoma (see Table 9.09) is pancreatic adenocarcinoma, because this accounts for most of the malignancies in the pancreas. Cytopathological features may be confused with

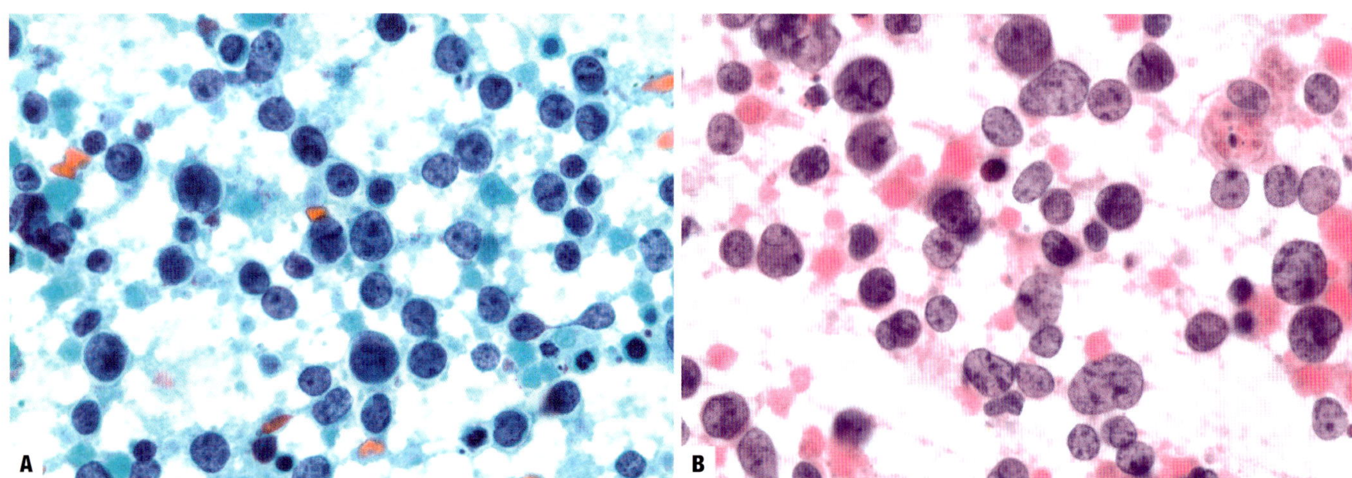

Fig. 9.45 Diffuse large B-cell lymphoma. **A** The malignant cells are present singly and have irregular coarse chromatin distribution and distinct nucleoli. Background cellular necrosis is seen (Pap). **B** The lymphoid cells are dispersed and large, and they have irregular nuclear contours and scant cytoplasm with many stripped nuclei. Nucleoli are prominent. There are no lymphocytes present. There is a tingible-body macrophage at 2 o'clock (Giemsa).

Table 9.09 Differential diagnosis of pancreatic lymphoma

Entity	Key morphology findings	Ancillary tests
DLBCL	Dyscohesive medium-large cells, scant cytoplasm, fine chromatin, nucleoli common	Positive for CD19, CD20, CD79a, and PAX5 B-cell clonality See text for subclassification
Double/triple-hit high-grade B-cell lymphoma	Morphological overlap with DLBCL	Similar to DLBCL Ki-67 index usually high *MYC* and *BCL2* and/or *BCL6* rearrangement
Low-grade B-cell lymphomas	Dyscohesive small to medium-sized cells with scant cytoplasm, condensed chromatin	Positive for CD19, CD20, CD79a, and PAX5 B-cell clonality Other markers vary with type
High-grade and undifferentiated carcinoma	Loosely cohesive cell clusters with crowding, irregular pleomorphic nuclei	Positive for pancytokeratin
Neuroendocrine tumour (NET)	Loose aggregates or dispersed epithelioid or plasmacytoid cells, coarsely stippled chromatin	Positive for chromogranin A, synaptophysin, INSM1 Ki-67 proliferation index varies
Metastatic malignancies	Loose cell aggregates, cells usually pleomorphic	Varies by site: consider kidney, lung, gastrointestinal, melanoma
Chronic or autoimmune pancreatitis	Hypocellular fibrous stroma, fewer small lymphocytes, background reactive epithelial cells	Lymphoid component has mixed T and polyclonal B cells
Splenule, lymphoid tissue	Heterogeneous lymphocytes, histiocytes, capillaries, endothelium	Lymphoid component has mixed T and polyclonal B cells Splenule sinusoids are CD8+

DLBCL, diffuse large B-cell lymphoma.

neuroendocrine tumours (NETs), poorly differentiated carcinomas, acinar cell carcinoma, melanomas, and other metastatic malignancies that may produce a dispersed single cell pattern. Chronic pancreatitis, ectopic splenule, and benign lymph nodes can be challenging to differentiate from low-grade, small-celled lymphomas. Recent consensus guidelines state that cytomorphology alone, without ancillary studies, should not be used to establish a primary diagnosis of lymphoma, and that immunophenotyping by either flow cytometry or ICC is required when these are available {439}. Some series describing the cytopathological evaluation of pancreatic lymphomas report that several passes or repeated biopsies were required to establish a definitive diagnosis {729,889,987}. Histopathological biopsies are suggested if lymphoma is clinically suspected, and sufficient material should be available for ancillary studies {439}.

Ancillary testing

Neoplastic cells in B-cell lymphomas express B-cell antigens including CD19, CD20, CD22, CD79a, and PAX5, but may lack some markers. Subtypes of DLBCL have prognostic and therapeutic relevance: various algorithms including the Hans classifiers and gene signatures can be used to separate the germinal-centre and activated B-cell phenotypes. CD10 expression is present in many germinal-centre cases, and IRF4 (MUM1) is commonly expressed in activated B-cell subtypes; BCL6,

Chapter 9

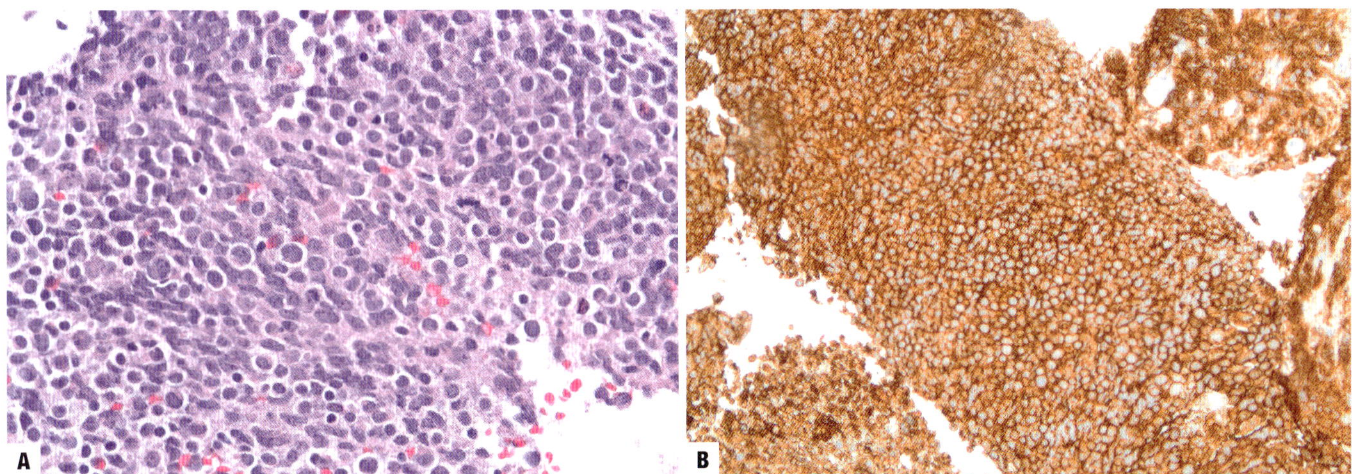

Fig. 9.46 Diffuse large B-cell lymphoma. **A** Cell block showing a tissue fragment of crowded large lymphoid cells showing a variable amount of cytoplasm, with frequent mitoses and focal apoptosis (H&E). **B** Cell block showing diffuse CD20 positivity in the large cells, confirming B-cell monoclonality (ICC). Further ICC and correlation with flow cytometry are required to make a diagnosis of a specific lymphoma.

FOXP1, and other markers can be applied for further classification. Expression of CD5, MYC, and/or BCL2 antigens may confer a worse prognosis, and molecular classifier studies will play an increasing role. It is recommended to evaluate the Ki-67 proliferation index, which generally exceeds 40% in DLBCL. Molecular studies are essential when a high-grade B-cell lymphoma is suspected by cytopathology or a very high Ki-67 index, and one notable type is high-grade B-cell lymphoma with *MYC* and *BCL2* and/or *BCL6* rearrangements (double- or triple-hit lymphoma). Ancillary testing, particularly flow cytometry, is required to establish a definitive diagnosis and further classification of pancreatic lymphoma {439}.

In limited-resource settings, markers including CD45, CD20, CD3, and BCL2 can help establish a general lymphoma diagnosis, and CD5, CD10, CD23, cyclin D1, and Ki-67 can further classify many non-Hodgkin lymphomas {185}.

Metastases to the pancreas

Saieg M
Perez-Machado MA
Tanaka M

Definition

Metastases to the pancreas represent secondary involvement of the pancreas by a malignant neoplasm from another site.

Clinical features and imaging

Metastases to the pancreas represented 43% of all pancreatic masses in an autopsy series of 193 cases {9}. However, they are less frequently encountered in FNAB samples, accounting for 1.8–10.8% of all malignancies diagnosed on FNAB {670,70, 101,227,542,906,464,888,180,245,302,34,41,196,612,793,27, 751,323,73,322,341}. The most common primary site of origin is the kidney (and these are usually renal cell carcinomas), followed by the lung, gastrointestinal tract, skin (which is usually a melanoma), and breast {341,322,546,464,670} (see Table 9.10, p. 160). Any malignancy may metastasize to the pancreas, and the literature is replete with individual case reports or small series describing metastases to the pancreas from various types of neoplasms other than carcinomas {269,456,9,486,695, 341,323,73,322}.

Patients are usually elderly, with a reported age range of 25–89 years, and there is typically a male predominance, similarly to primary carcinomas of the pancreas {101,906,73, 9,464,888,322}. At presentation, most patients have disseminated disease, with rare reports of patients presenting with metastatic disease limited to the pancreas {9,265,510}. The pancreatic metastasis can also be the first sign of cancer in some patients {453}.

Most patients are asymptomatic, because most metastases involve the parenchyma without sclerosis and obstruction of the common bile duct and main pancreatic ducts, which is typical of pancreatic ductal adenocarcinoma (PDAC). When symptoms do occur, patients usually present with weight loss, abdominal pain, steatorrhea, and jaundice {34,546}, which may help in the clinical differential diagnosis with PDAC {234,

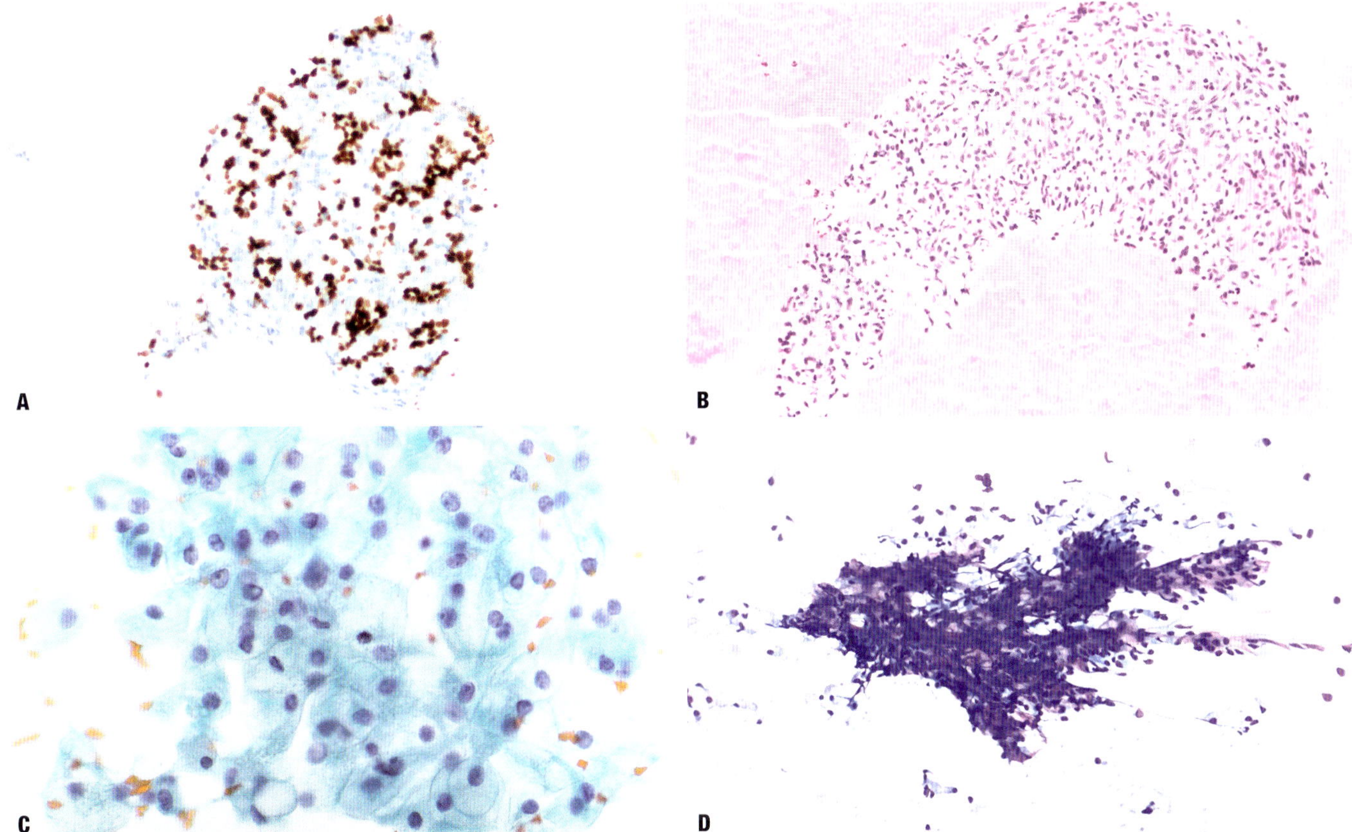

Fig. 9.47 Metastatic renal cell carcinoma. **A** Cell block showing a tissue fragment of carcinoma, showing strongly positive nuclear staining for PAX8. Note that pancreatic neuroendocrine tumours (PanNETs) may also express PAX8, depending on the antibody (ICC). **B** Cell block shows a tissue fragment with a nested pattern, showing nests of neoplastic cells separated by interlacing stroma with some inflammatory cells (H&E). **C** Clear cell renal cell carcinoma exhibiting large cells with abundant foamy cytoplasm and round, mildly pleomorphic, hyperchromatic nuclei with prominent nucleoli. This pattern can be mistaken for the foamy gland pattern of pancreatic ductal adenocarcinoma (Pap). **D** Tissue fragment showing prominent anastomosing vasculature, and large cells with abundant clear to pale eosinophilic cytoplasm and mildly atypical hyperchromatic nuclei (Giemsa).

302,437}. Other features that help identify metastases include multiple lesions, a lack of a retention cyst, main pancreatic duct dilation, and atrophy {793}.

Metastases may present as solitary round or ovoid lesions with variably defined borders usually of the pancreatic head, or as multiple hypervascularized lesions involving the whole gland

Table 9.10 Summary of FNAB series of metastases to the pancreas

Series	Study length (years)	Total cases (FNAB or CNB)	Total cancers	Metastases					
				Total metastases	% of total cases	% of total malignancies	Most common site of origin	Average age, range (years)	M:F ratio
Benning et al., 1992 {70}	n/a	304	176	19	6.3	10.8	Lung	66, 47–79	9:10
Carson et al., 1995 {101}	8	117	n/a	13	11.1	n/a	GI	65, 38–81	10:3
Fritscher-Ravens et al., 2001 {227}	2	112	n/a	12	10.7	n/a	GI/kidney	61, 34–78	4:8
Mesa et al., 2004 {542}	3	468	191	11	2.4	5.8	Lung	n/a	n/a
Volmar et al., 2004 {888}	5	1050	503	20	1.9	4.0	Kidney	61, 40–83	11:9
DeWitt et al., 2005 {180}	6	n/a	n/a	24	2.1	n/a	Kidney	60, 33–83	15:9
Gilbert et al., 2011 {245}	5	1172	n/a	25	2.1	n/a	Kidney	61, 40–80	11:14
Hijioka et al., 2011 {302}	14	n/a	n/a	28	n/a	n/a	Kidney	60, 32–78	13:15
Layfield et al., 2012 {464}	8	2318	222	17	0.7	7.7	Kidney	61, 15–80	14:3
Ardengh et al., 2013 {34}	14	n/a	n/a	32	n/a	n/a	GI	60, 26–84	n/a
Atiq et al., 2013 {41}	5	674	n/a	23	3.4	n/a	Lung	64	10:13
El Hajj et al., 2013 {196}	12	n/a	n/a	49	n/a	n/a	Kidney	63, 30–83	23:26
Olson et al., 2013 {612}	26	5495	2389	42	0.8	1.8	Kidney	Median: 59	23:19
Waters et al., 2014 {906}	10	n/a	1406	66	n/a	4.7	Kidney	63, 40–89	38:28
Smith et al., 2015 {793}	14	2327	n/a	22	0.9	n/a	Kidney	71, 59–83	13:9
Alomari et al., 2016 {27}	7	1346	n/a	31	2.3	n/a	Kidney	66, 49–86	19:12
Raymond et al., 2017 {670}	15	636	221	16	2.5	7.2	Lung	62, 43–82	11:5
Sekulic et al., 2017 {751}	10	1137	594	25	2.1	n/a	Kidney	64, 53–71	13:12
Hou et al., 2018 {323}	8	n/a	n/a	30	n/a	n/a	Kidney	65.5, 25–82	18:12
Betés et al., 2019 {73}	12	1128	n/a	44	3.9	n/a	Kidney	Median: 58.6	28:16
Iaokim et al., 2020 {341}	5	n/a	n/a	7	n/a	n/a	Kidney	67, 61–76	5:2
Hou et al., 2020 {323}	14	3930	n/a	107	2.7	n/a	Kidney	62.4, 34–84	63:44
Median, range	8, 2–26	1132.5, 112–5495	503, 176–2389	25, 7–107	2.3, 0.7–11.1	5.25, 1.8–10.8	n/a	n/a, 15–84	n/a

CNB, core needle biopsy; n/a, not applicable; GI, gastrointestinal tract.

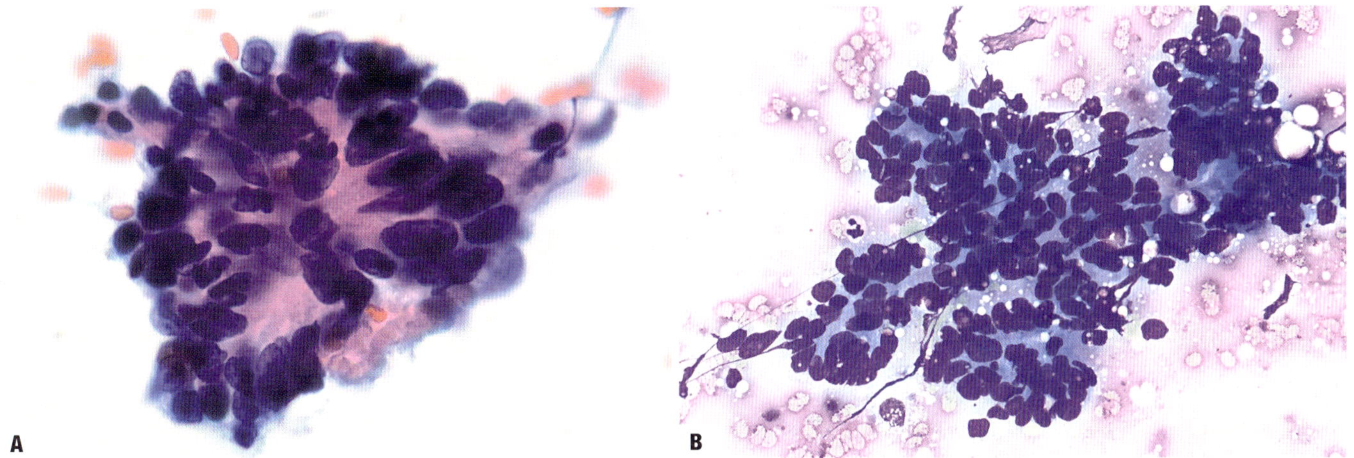

Fig. 9.48 Metastatic colonic adenocarcinoma. **A** Tissue fragment of colonic adenocarcinoma showing columnar cells forming a palisading glandular architecture (Pap). **B** Tissue fragment showing a glandular architecture with columnar cells in a palisading arrangement, along with few small vacuoles in the eccentric cytoplasm and large hyperchromatic, often elongated nuclei (Giemsa).

{546}. This contrasts with the typical irregular, hypoechoic pancreatic head mass presentation of PDAC. Some metastases present as diffusely infiltrating lesions {322,17,751,906,51}. The reported median dimensions of these lesions range from 15 to 40 mm {751,41,302}. Breast carcinoma and small cell neuroendocrine carcinoma (SCNEC) are the two cancers most commonly presenting with diffuse involvement {17}.

The latency period from primary tumour to metastasis is highly variable. Some metastases are detected synchronously with the primary, others not until years later. A long latency period is especially true of renal cell carcinoma, with a reported mean interval of 9.2 years but ranging up to 28 years {51,793,546,888, 751,457}.

The treatment of choice is surgery, which is associated with a better survival, especially for renal cell carcinoma metastases {546,9,623}.

Histopathology

The histopathology of the lesions, as well as cytopathology, varies according to the type of tumour metastatic to the pancreaticobiliary tract. Care is especially warranted for metastatic well-differentiated renal cell carcinoma, which can be confused with the clear cell pattern of PDAC and the clear cell variant of pancreatic neuroendocrine tumour (PanNET) {464}, and for metastatic gastric adenocarcinoma, which tends to be associated with a dense desmoplastic stroma, similarly to PDAC {9}. Melanomas and sarcomas can be difficult to distinguish from undifferentiated carcinomas {9}.

Key diagnostic cytopathological features

- Cytopathology varies according to the type of neoplasm involving the pancreas
- Any cytopathology that is unusual for pancreatic ductal adenocarcinoma should raise suspicion of a metastasis, including a single cell pattern; dirty background; large, prominent nucleoli; and a lack of mucinous cytoplasmic differentiation

Discussion and differential diagnosis

The cytopathological features of the metastatic neoplasm vary according to the primary malignancy. Accordingly, recognition

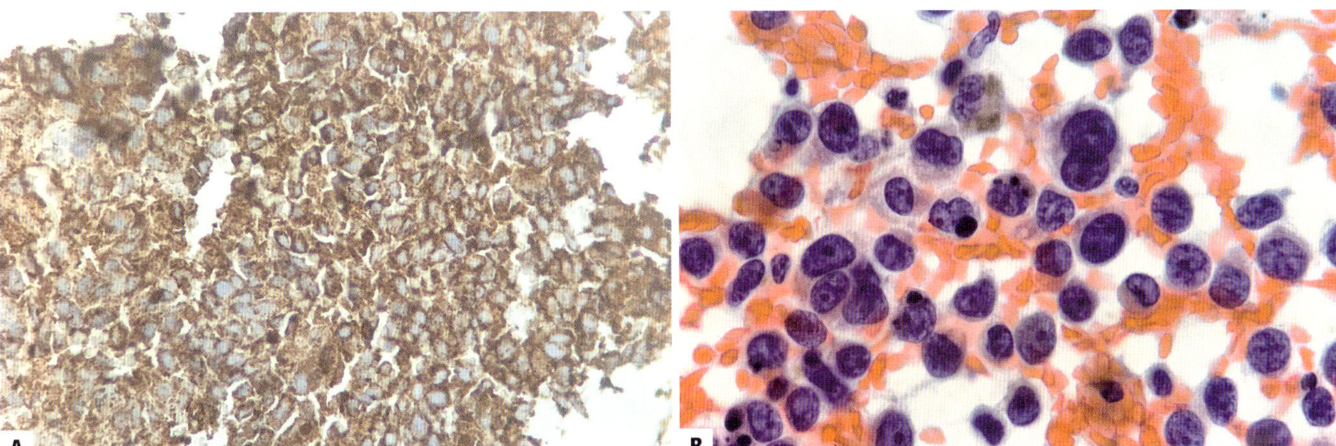

Fig. 9.49 Metastatic melanoma. **A** Cell block shows a large tissue fragment of tumour, which shows positive HMB45 cytoplasmic expression (ICC). **B** Scattered, discohesive large cells with marked anisonucleosis, large prominent nucleoli, and scant non-vacuolated cytoplasm. Some cells show melanin pigment in the cytoplasm, which must be differentiated from haemosiderin in macrophages (Pap).

of malignant elements that are unusual for PDAC should always raise the possibility of a metastasis, especially in cases with a clinical history of a previous malignancy, which is the most important element in making the diagnosis of a metastasis. Identifying such lesions as metastatic is of extreme clinical importance, because they may have a better prognosis than primary PDAC {464}.

FNAB of metastatic renal cell carcinomas can be especially challenging. Well-differentiated renal cell carcinomas exhibit vascularized tissue fragments of polygonal cells with low N:C ratios, abundant foamy or pale cytoplasm in the classic clear cell type, and a prominent single owl-eye nucleolus. The differential diagnosis is with the clear cell variant of PanNET or the foamy gland pattern of PDAC {464,814}. Poorly differentiated metastatic renal carcinoma may also impose challenges and can be confused with PDAC. In addition, FNAB of metastatic renal cell carcinomas can be bloody and hypocellular, owing to their extensive vascularity {623}. In this setting, rapid onsite evaluation (ROSE) is always advisable to guarantee that adequate material is preserved for cell block and ancillary testing {888,670}.

Another common metastatic neoplasm to the pancreas is lung adenocarcinoma, which is difficult to distinguish from PDAC. The characteristic immunoprofile of lung adenocarcinoma, positive for thyroid transcription factor 1 (TTF1) and napsin A, should be helpful. Colonic adenocarcinomas may present with more distinguishing features, such as tall columnar cells in distinctly glandular tissue fragments and a dirty background of necrosis and mucin. Breast carcinomas may show a small tissue fragment and dispersed cell pattern of small to medium-sized cells with eccentric, often non-mucinous cytoplasm and intracytoplasmic lumina. Metastatic squamous cell carcinomas may also be difficult or even impossible to distinguish from primary pancreatic adenosquamous and the rare squamous cell carcinoma. Close correlation to clinical history and identification of areas with adenocarcinomatous elements is therefore mandatory {464}.

Ancillary testing

ICC plays a pivotal role in confirming the nature of the neoplasm involving the pancreas (see Table 9.05, p. 136). Therefore, rinsings of every FNAB needle pass, and if possible a dedicated pass, should be used for a cell block.

ICC markers used will vary according to the clinical history and cytopathology. Clear cell renal cell carcinomas are commonly positive for antibodies against RCCm, PAX8, and CAIX. Other types of renal cell carcinoma express RCCm and PAX8 but do not express CAIX {505}. A word of caution is that primary PanNET is positive for PAX8 {618,721}, depending on the antibody used {488}, and more than half of PDACs may express CAIX {505}. Lung primary adenocarcinomas are positive for TTF1 and napsin A, which are negative in PDAC {77}. Other useful markers include mammaglobin and GATA3 for primary breast carcinomas, and S100, melan-A (MART1), HMB45, and SOX10 for melanomas {155}. SATB2 has been proposed as a specific marker for colorectal carcinoma {120} but is rarely expressed in PDAC, which can also be positive for CDX2. Therefore, when the differential diagnosis includes metastatic colorectal carcinoma, it is best to use a panel including CK7 and CK20 in addition to SATB2 and CDX2. PDAC is typically CK7+/CK20−/+, whereas colorectal carcinoma is CK7−/CK20+. MUC antigens may also be helpful in this scenario, because PDAC is typically EMA (MUC1)+ / MUC2− and colorectal carcinoma is EMA (MUC1)− / MUC2+.

Other lesions (including spindle cell tumours)

Notohara K
Perez-Machado MA

Other malignant haematological and soft tissue neoplasms of the pancreas are extremely rare and easily confused with common pancreatic epithelial neoplasms. Therefore, specific diagnosis is necessary. These neoplasms should be considered in the differential diagnosis when the imaging, cytopathological, or histopathological features are unusual for common pancreatic epithelial neoplasms. Details of these neoplasms are available in relevant volumes of the WHO Classification of Tumours series {910,912,911}.

Leiomyosarcoma

Leiomyosarcoma is the most common pancreatic primary sarcoma {980,964,207}, presenting as a huge mass with a central necrotic cavity {519,207}. The clinical history assists in distinguishing primary leiomyosarcoma from metastatic leiomyosarcoma from the soft tissue or uterus {592}.

Tissue fragments and dispersed cells consisting of spindle atypical cells with elongated, blunt-ended fusiform nuclei are obtained by FNAB with more pleomorphic atypical cells in some cases {187,686}.

ICC for smooth muscle markers including SMA, desmin, and h-caldesmon are necessary for the diagnosis, although none of these markers is specific for smooth muscle differentiation, and cytomorphological features have to be consistent with the diagnosis {592}. Smooth muscle differentiation in dedifferentiated liposarcoma is a differential diagnosis, and overall morphological assessment with ICC or FISH for MDM2 is helpful to make this distinction {446}. Undifferentiated carcinoma and other types of soft tissue tumour are also included in the differential diagnosis.

Gastrointestinal stromal tumour

Gastrointestinal stromal tumours (GISTs) are the most common mesenchymal neoplasm of the gastrointestinal tract and rarely involve the pancreaticobiliary tract {665,942,282,879}.

The majority of GISTs have a spindle cell cytomorphology, and the rest are epithelioid or show a mixed morphology. FNAB smears are typically highly cellular. The spindle cell variant shows closely packed cohesive or sometimes less cohesive tissue fragments, and numerous single, elongated cells. The tumour cells often form fascicles with parallel, side-by-side arrangements of nuclei, with scant cytoplasm. Nuclear palisading is occasionally observed. The neoplastic cells exhibit elongated to wavy nuclei with blunt to tapered ends. The epithelioid variant cells display round nuclei with nucleoli and mimic an epithelial neoplasm {866,449,379}.

GIST is positive for ANO1/DOG1, KIT (CD117), and CD34. Expression of these antigens is dependent on the morphological subtype and mutation status, and additional studies for SDHB, SDHA, and neurofibromin (NF1) may identify GIST with mutations in these genes. The differential diagnosis includes smooth muscle tumours, which are positive for desmin and SMA, and nerve sheath tumours, which are positive for SOX10 and S100. Epithelioid GIST can be mistaken for adenocarcinoma, and a cytokeratin panel positive in the carcinoma can clarify this differential {521,154,379}.

The majority harbour gain-of-function mutations of the *KIT* or *PDGFRA* oncogenes located on chromosome 4 (4q12) {304, 408,295,363,910}. Some 5–10% of GISTs that are wildtype for *KIT* and *PDGFRA* harbour alterations in SDH subunit genes {350,78}, and rarely, mutations occur in *NF1*, *BRAF*, or *KRAS* {548,66,240,910}.

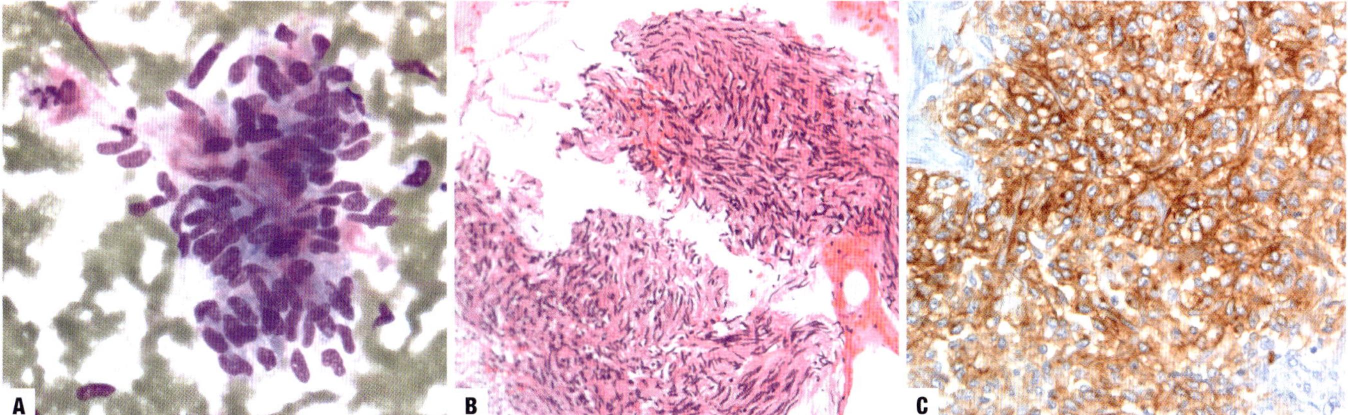

Fig. 9.50 Gastrointestinal stromal tumour. **A** Cohesive tissue fragment showing magenta myxoid stromal strands separating the thin light-blue cytoplasm and elongated hyperchromatic nuclei of the spindle cells. Occasional single detached spindle cells and stripped nuclei are present in the bloody background (Giemsa). **B** Cell block showing tissue fragments consisting of fibrillary stromal collagen strands separating thin spindle cells with hyperchromatic, blunt to fusiform nuclei (H&E). **C** Cell block showing a tissue fragment with diffuse cytoplasmic and membranous staining for KIT (CD117) (ICC).

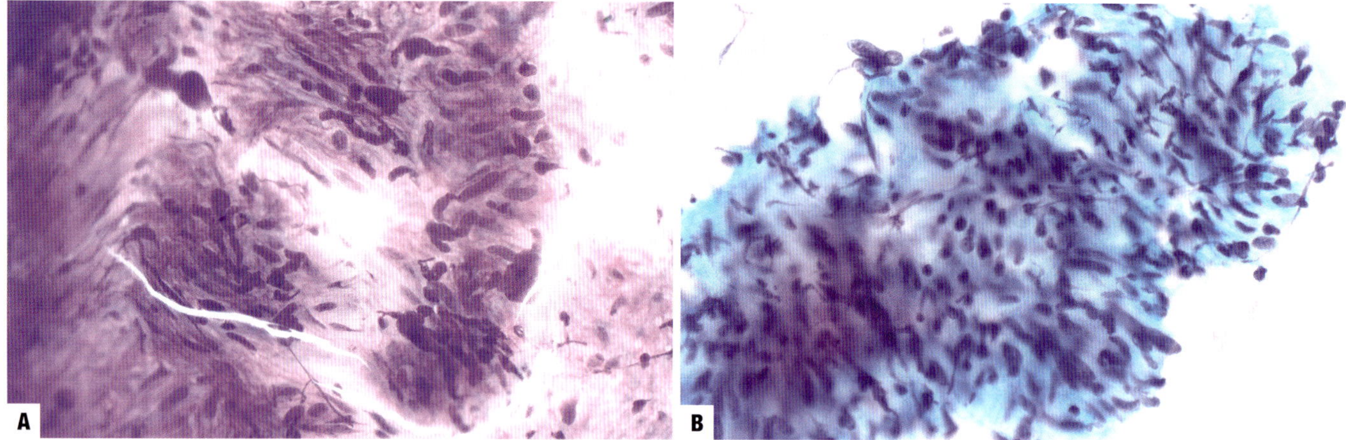

Fig. 9.51 Leiomyosarcoma. **A** Tissue fragment of leiomyosarcoma showing irregular spindle cells arranged in poorly formed fascicles, with large, elongated, pleomorphic nuclei with blunted ends (Giemsa). **B** Tissue fragment of leiomyosarcoma showing spindle cells with elongated large nuclei with blunted ends, which can also be seen as stripped nuclei at the periphery of the tissue fragment (Pap).

Myeloid sarcoma

Myeloid sarcoma is an extramedullary mass-forming myeloblast infiltration with or without mature myeloid lineage cells, which occurs most commonly in adults and occurs with or without acute myeloid leukaemia and myeloproliferative neoplasms {637, 719,342,851}. Subtypes can be distinguished: the blastic type consists of myeloblasts with a scant to moderate rim of basophilic cytoplasm, fine nuclear chromatin, and two to four nucleoli; the immature type consists of myeloblasts, promyelocytes, and eosinophilic myelocytes; and the differentiated type has promyelocytes, eosinophilic myelocytes, and more mature forms and rare crystalline inclusions similar to Charcot–Leyden crystals.

FNAB smears reveal scattered myeloblasts with round or oval nuclei, fine chromatin, and indistinct nucleoli {822,782}. Azurophil granules are seen in the Giemsa. Granulocytic or monocytic maturation may be noted.

Myeloid sarcoma may be confused with malignant lymphoma and undifferentiated carcinoma. Immature myeloid cell markers, i.e. CD33, CD34, CD68/KP1, and KIT, and the mature myeloid cell markers myeloperoxidase and lysozyme, are used for the diagnosis {637}. Molecular cytogenetics studies can be useful. In 55% of cases, myeloid sarcomas are associated with chromosomal abnormalities seen in acute myeloid leukaemia, including monosomy 7, trisomy 8, *KMT2A* (*MLL*) rearrangement, inversion 16, trisomy 4, monosomy 16, 16q−, 5q−, 20q−, and trisomy 11. In a subset of cases, *NPM1* mutations are identified and are frequently associated with myelomonocytic, monocytic, or monoblastic differentiation. The t(8;21)(q22;q22) abnormality is more frequently seen in paediatric cases.

Plasma cell myeloma / plasmacytoma

Pancreatic involvement by plasma cell myeloma has been reported {719,916,697}. Solitary pancreatic plasmacytoma rarely occurs {504}. The imaging features are those of a focal mass or diffuse pancreatic infiltration {719,519,278}.

FNAB smears exhibit monotonous mature plasma cells with variable degrees of atypia, often with plentiful multinucleated tumour cells {723,275}. Immature plasma cells with a large nucleus and prominent nucleolus or pleomorphic plasma cells may be predominant.

Plasma cell myeloma and plasmacytoma are distinguished from reactive conditions and low-grade B-cell lymphomas with plasmacytic differentiation, and they can mimic neuroendocrine tumours (NETs). Undifferentiated carcinoma is a differential diagnosis to immature or pleomorphic plasma cells. CD38 or CD138 immunoreactivity and CD20 negativity should be confirmed to establish the diagnosis. ICC, flow cytometry, or in situ hybridization can be used to demonstrate immunoglobulin light chain monoclonality and is helpful to differentiate between reactive and neoplastic plasma cells.

Follicular dendritic cell sarcoma

Follicular dendritic cell sarcoma and EBV+ inflammatory follicular dendritic cell sarcoma have been rarely reported {487,554}.

Ewing sarcoma

Ewing sarcoma is more common in children and young adults but can also be seen in older age groups, showing a typically huge, poorly defined, and heterogeneously enhancing lesion on imaging {519,596,428}.

FNAB smears are cellular, with tissue fragments and isolated tumour cells {544}. Also, rosette-like structures resembling glands may be seen. The neoplastic cells are monotonous and contain round nuclei with fine chromatin.

Ewing sarcoma raises a cytopathological differential diagnosis with pancreatoblastoma, solid pseudopapillary neoplasm, NETs, neuroendocrine carcinomas (NECs), and malignant lymphoma {704,920}. Ewing sarcoma must be distinguished from other tumours including *CIC*-rearranged sarcoma {962} and sarcoma with *BCOR* genetic alterations {803} in the undifferentiated small round cell sarcomas of the bone and soft tissue category.

Diffuse and strong CD99 immunostaining and NKX2-2 immunoreactivity help diagnose Ewing sarcoma {704}. Gene fusions of the FET gene family, usually *EWSR1*, and ETS family members such as *FLI1* are preferably confirmed.

Other sarcomas

Various primary sarcomas are rarely reported in the pancreas. Retroperitoneal sarcomas can directly invade the pancreas, and sarcomas can metastasize to the pancreas.

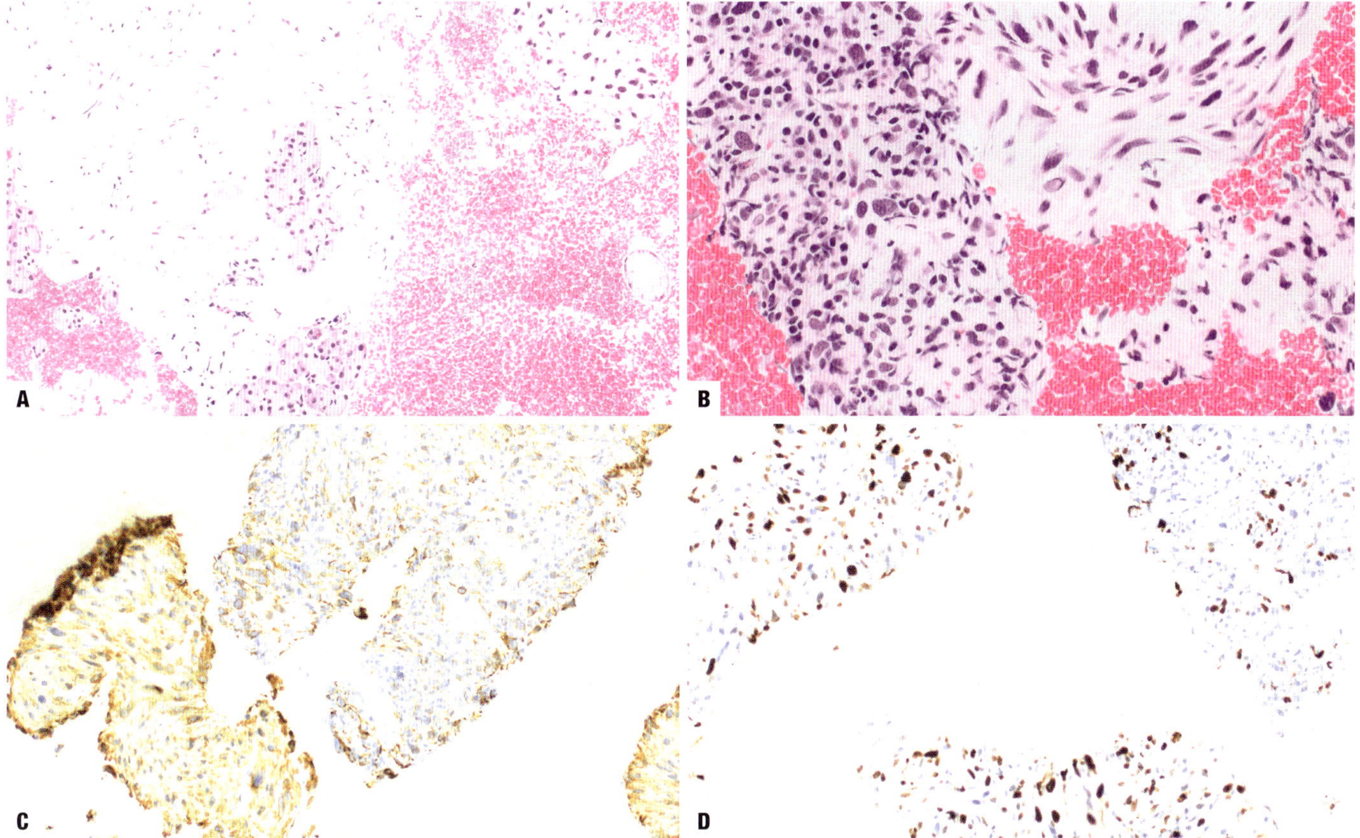

Fig. 9.52 Leiomyosarcoma. **A** Cell block shows hypocellular hyalinized tissue fragment (left) and mildly hypercellular stroma fragment (right) with spindle tumour cells. Note the benign pancreatic acinar tissue fragments (H&E). **B** Cell block shows a hypercellular tissue fragment with variably spindle and polygonal cells showing markedly pleomorphic hyperchromatic nuclei (left), and a mildly cellular tissue fragment with spindle cells and mildly hyperchromatic and enlarged elongated nuclei (right) (H&E). **C** Cell block with tissue fragments of tumour cells showing positive staining for desmin (ICC). **D** Cell block with tissue fragments composed of tumour cells showing positive nuclear staining for Ki-67 (ICC).

Sample reports: Malignant

Layfield LJ
Fukushima N
Kumarasinghe MP
Sigel C

Sample report 1

Clinical and imaging findings: Partly cystic 30 mm mass in head of pancreas.
Specimen adequacy: Satisfactory for evaluation.
Category: Malignant.
Diagnosis: Moderately differentiated ductal adenocarcinoma.

Sample report 2

Clinical and imaging findings: Rounded solid mass in or adjacent to and impinging on the body of the pancreas.
Specimen adequacy: Satisfactory for evaluation.
Category: Malignant.
Diagnosis: Non-Hodgkin lymphoma. See comment.
Comment: Correlation with flow cytometry and concurrent core biopsy (case number) for further classification is required.

Sample report 3

Clinical and imaging findings: Patient with known history of melanoma on upper back.
Specimen adequacy: Satisfactory for evaluation.
Category: Malignant.
Diagnosis: Metastatic melanoma. See comment.
Comment: There is no pigment in the tumour cells, which are dispersed and present in small discohesive tissue fragments of large cells with large pleomorphic nuclei featuring frequent intranuclear pseudoinclusions. The immunoperoxidase for pancytokeratin (CAM5.2) is negative, and stains for melan-A (MART1) and SOX10 are positive, supporting the diagnosis of metastatic amelanotic melanoma.

Sample report 4

Clinical and imaging findings: Irregular mass in body of pancreas.
Specimen adequacy: Satisfactory for evaluation.
Category: Malignant.
Diagnosis: Poorly differentiated neuroendocrine carcinoma (NEC), small cell type. See comment.
Comment: The tumour morphology shows a poorly differentiated carcinoma composed of small cells with nuclear moulding and apoptosis. Immunoperoxidase stains for chromogranin and synaptophysin are positive, supporting neuroendocrine differentiation. Thyroid transcription factor 1 (TTF1) is negative. The proliferation marker Ki-67 shows 80% nuclear positivity.

Sample report 5

Clinical and imaging findings: Irregular mass in head of pancreas.
Specimen adequacy: Satisfactory for evaluation.
Category: Malignant.
Diagnosis: Acinar cell carcinoma. See comment.
Comment: Immunoperoxidase shows the neoplastic cells to be reactive for trypsin and BCL10, and non-reactive for chromogranin and synaptophysin, supporting the diagnosis.

Sample report 6

Clinical and imaging findings: Large mass in head of pancreas.
Specimen adequacy: Satisfactory for evaluation.
Category: Malignant.
Diagnosis: Poorly differentiated neuroendocrine carcinoma (NEC), large cell type. See comment.
Comment: Immunoperoxidase performed on cell block material shows the neoplastic cells to be positive for chromogranin and synaptophysin, supporting neuroendocrine differentiation. There is loss of nuclear staining for RB1 and retention of ATRX and DAXX. Ki-67 proliferation index is 60%. This immunoprofile supports the diagnosis.

Sample report 7

Clinical and imaging findings: Irregular spiculated mass in head of pancreas.
Specimen adequacy: Satisfactory for evaluation.
Category: Malignant.
Diagnosis: Adenocarcinoma of the pancreas, foamy gland pattern.

Sample report 8

Nature of specimen: Mass in tail of pancreas in 21-year-old woman presenting with abdominal discomfort.

Diagnostic summary:
Category: Malignant.
Diagnosis: Solid pseudopapillary neoplasm. See microscopic description.

Microscopic description: These highly cellular smears show branching papillary strands with vascular cores and a focal myxoid stroma, which is magenta in the Giemsa and covered in relatively monotonous polygonal tumour cells with round nuclei with single small nucleoli and occasional grooves. Dispersed single tumour cells, some showing cytoplasmic tails, are present. There is considerable material in the cell block, which is positive for CAM5.2 keratin and β-catenin (diffuse and strong nuclear staining), along with CD10 and CD99 in a perinuclear, dot-like pattern. Trypsin is negative. The Ki-67 proliferation index is 2%.
Comment: The features are those of a solid pseudopapillary neoplasm of the pancreas.

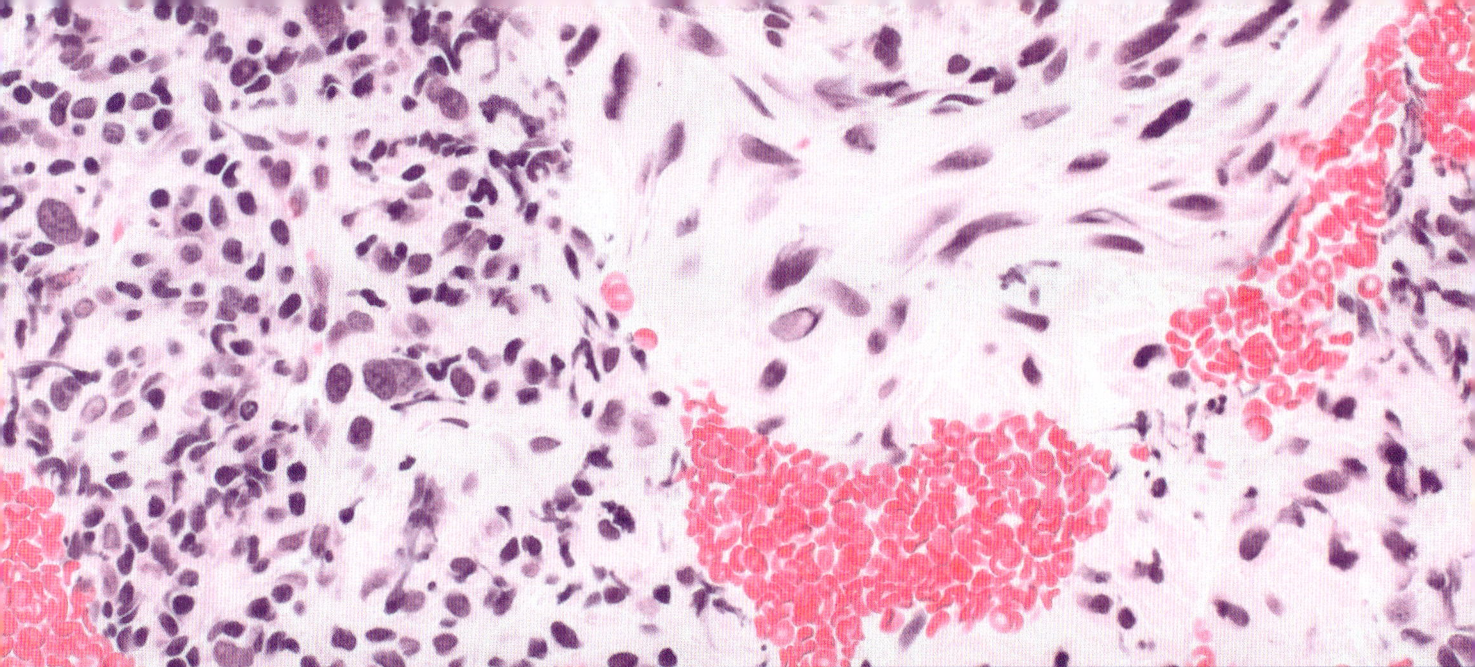

10

Management recommendations for each diagnostic category

Edited by: Centeno BA, Fukushima N, Layfield LJ, Pitman MB, Reid MD, Saieg M, Siddiqui MT, Weynand B

Introduction

Kurtycz D
Klapman J

In bile duct brushing and EUS-FNAB of the pancreas, successful diagnostic outcomes depend on the performance of a dedicated patient care team. The interventionalist must accurately identify and biopsy the target lesion and obtain sufficient cellular material for diagnosis. A good-quality interpretable smear or other satisfactory preparation must be made. Finally, the cytopathologist who analyses the sample must be well-trained and experienced in interpreting the cytopathology and know when to use ancillary techniques. This multidisciplinary approach is often underrecognized in studies published in the literature regarding the sensitivity, specificity, and predictive values of pancreaticobiliary duct brushings and FNAB {197, 199,817,427}.

The patient care team needs to have confidence in the cytopathological diagnosis. To this end, the cytopathology, imaging, and clinical teams should regularly communicate, and when possible, present all case findings at multidisciplinary case conferences. During rapid onsite evaluation (ROSE), a multi-headed microscope or videomicroscopy can quickly acquaint the interventionalist with the cytopathological yield of their procedure. The interventionalist can make this a two-way learning experience by sharing the imaging and ultrasound images of the pancreatic lesion being biopsied. Imaging will inevitably give valuable clues to the diagnosis. This information will narrow the diagnostic possibilities and help optimize the cytopathological interpretation. In cases where small biopsy tissue sampling is necessary, fine core needle biopsy (CNB), using more recently developed sampling devices, can be performed, and ROSE of a cytopathological touch preparation or even smears of these fine cores of tissue can be performed to confirm whether the interventionalist has obtained a diagnostic sample, to provide direction to obtain additional material if needed, and to triage tissue for ancillary tests {807,903,246,598,827}.

The practice of cytopathology continues to evolve. The subspecialty has been experiencing increasing pressure for systematization to minimize variations in reporting. A number of well-accepted standardized systems have been created to standardize diagnostic terminology, improve communication, and generate an environment disposed towards the creation of consistent evidence-based approaches to diagnosis. Based on concepts derived from the latest literature, technology, and biological models, these systems strive to be living entities, with international groups of authors regularly monitoring and revisiting the subject matter to ensure that concepts are current and that the systems are clinically valuable.

Reporting systems all have common aims to improve their clinical utility: firstly, to develop diagnostic categories that are based on dependable cytopathological features and ancillary technologies; secondly, to restrict the use of indeterminate categories such as "Atypical" and "Suspicious for malignancy"; and thirdly, to derive risks of malignancy for each category from the published literature. The following sections will bring together and present summaries from the WHO Reporting System for Pancreaticobiliary Cytopathology of the management options for each category based on the associated risk of malignancy {823,711,306}.

Category: Insufficient/Inadequate/Non-diagnostic

Kumarasinghe MP
Klapman J
Kurtycz D

The risk of malignancy for an "Insufficient/Inadequate/Non-diagnostic" FNAB from the pancreas is relatively high, at 5–25% {792,307,824}, but the risk of malignancy is even higher for an "Insufficient/Inadequate/Non-diagnostic" bile duct brushing, at 28–69% {875,111,192,952,658,468,595}. This is not surprising given the fact that only visible, typically suspicious lesions are sampled. A repeat procedure is generally needed to assess the lesion, whether a mass or a stricture.

Diagnostic yield in pancreatic cytopathology largely depends on the operator's experience, the technique employed, and the use of rapid onsite evaluation (ROSE), which has proved to reduce the number of "Insufficient/Inadequate/Non-diagnostic" samples {299,551,151}. A repeat biopsy might then be needed and may sometimes use a different technique if any of these parameters has led to this categorization. The use of larger-gauge core-like needles has also been associated with a need for fewer needle passes and shorter procedure times {47,206}. In some instances, when repeated cytopathological assessment produces an "Insufficient/Inadequate/Non-diagnostic" result, further clinical management decisions may still be made on the basis of the clinical scenario and imaging.

The nature of the lesion may also be a reason for an "Insufficient/Inadequate/Non-diagnostic" sample, because chronic and autoimmune pancreatitis shows extensive fibrosis and usually produces scant FNAB material. In such situations, an empirical trial of steroids may be appropriate {560}.

For cystic lesions, biochemical analysis is of extreme importance, because high CEA levels (> 192 ng/mL) may be enough to classify the cyst fluid as mucinous {140}, even in the absence of an epithelial component {105}. Molecular analysis of the cyst fluid may also provide significant information for cyst classification and risk of malignancy {787,364}.

Bile duct brushings may be paucicellular or the tissue may be obscured by mechanical crush or preparation artefact, but the criteria for an adequate specimen have not been established, leading to infrequent use of this category for bile duct brushings. An FNAB might be recommended when there is a significant thickening of the wall.

Category: Benign / Negative for malignancy

Saieg M
Klapman J
Pitman MB
Stelow EB

As detailed in Chapter 4: *Diagnostic category: Benign / Negative for malignancy*, most of the lesions categorized as "Benign / Negative for malignancy" have classic cytomorphological features, correlate with the imaging findings, and usually need no further ancillary studies. The risk of malignancy for "Benign" FNAB of the pancreas ranges from 0% to 15% {792,307,824}. Patients with benign lesions can be followed with conservative management; for example, imaging follow-up or medical treatment such as steroids in autoimmune pancreatitis. Surgical intervention can be considered if there are changes such as an increase in size or the development of symptoms.

Cyst fluid analysis with biochemical testing for CEA and amylase is useful for classification of cystic lesions {876,712, 140}: high amylase and low CEA fluid levels are supportive of a pseudocyst, whereas a serous cystadenoma has low CEA and amylase levels. As a pitfall, lymphoepithelial cysts are non-neoplastic cysts but have high CEA levels {668}. Pseudocysts are often drained and not resected, and serous cystadenomas can be followed for subsequent growth and or the development of symptoms.

The risk of malignancy of "Benign" bile duct brushes may be as high as 30% according to retrospective studies {875,111,192, 952,658,468,595}; however, the risk of malignancy of "Benign" lesions is usually calculated by histopathological confirmation and may be overestimated because only clinically suspicious cases are surgically resected after a "Benign" categorization. "Benign" bile duct brushings are generally easier to categorize if normal bile duct epithelium is present, but the definitive diagnosis of malignancy in bile duct brushing samples from inflamed or stented bile ducts is very difficult and has a high false negative rate {699}. False negatives and low sensitivity of cytopathology alone in the evaluation of biliary stricture are a well-known limitation of bile duct brushings {352,44}, and the frequency of cancers that result in a false negative diagnosis may be higher than in samples from pancreatic FNAB. It is important not to misidentify regenerative atypia as malignant, and correlation with imaging findings is highly recommended.

For a lesion to be categorized as "Benign", the sample must be sufficiently cellular and show no cytopathological atypia. If there is a lack of correlation with the clinical and/or imaging diagnoses, the cytopathology report should clearly specify that the cytopathology material may not represent the lesion seen in the imaging owing to sampling error, and recommend to the patient's care team that the imaging should be reviewed and further diagnostic testing should be considered if clinically indicated.

Category: Atypical

Gan Q
Heymann JJ
Klapman J
Roy-Chowdhuri S

The risk of malignancy for the "Atypical" category in EUS-FNAB of a pancreaticobiliary masses ranges from 30% to 40% {792, 307,824}, and for bile duct brushing (BDB) it is much higher, at 25–61% {875,111,192,952,658,468,595}.

For EUS-FNAB of a pancreaticobiliary mass, if an "Atypical" categorization is provided, the procedure may be repeated with the aid of rapid onsite evaluation (ROSE). ROSE allows cytopathologists to request additional material at the time of specimen collection, increasing the possibility that the obtained material is representative and sufficient for diagnostic efficacy, especially in institutions where EUS-FNAB is a new or relatively new procedure {145,169,399,434}. Once sufficient material is obtained, ancillary studies to differentiate benign and malignant lesions include ICC and molecular testing. Loss of expression of SMAD4 (DPC4), a finding in about 55% of pancreatic ductal adenocarcinomas (PDACs), supports a PDAC diagnosis {870}. Several ICC markers, including VHL protein, S100, IMP3, and maspin, among others, have shown promise in distinguishing PDAC from reactive ducts, although further testing and large-scale study are needed to validate their practical use {495}. In order to diagnose non-PDAC malignancy, ICC is extremely useful; for example, synaptophysin, chromogranin, pankeratin, and INSM1 are diagnostic of pancreatic neuroendocrine tumour (PanNET); β-catenin, SOX11, PR, E-cadherin, LEF1, and CD10 confirm solid pseudopapillary neoplasm; trypsin, chymotrypsin, and BCL10 confirm acinar cell carcinoma; trypsin, chymotrypsin, cyclin D1, and β-catenin confirm pancreatoblastoma; primary site-specific markers such as GATA3, TTF1, and PAX8 can confirm a specific metastasis; and IgG and IgG4 can assist in the diagnosis of autoimmune pancreatitis. Flow cytometry is essential in almost all cases of pancreatic lymphoproliferative disorders {106}.

For EUS-FNAB of pancreatic cystic lesions, the number of "Atypical" cases is expected to be low, because a majority will be included in the "Benign" category {711}. Ideally, management will incorporate the correlation of clinical history, imaging findings, and cyst fluid biochemical and/or molecular test results {808}.

For an "Atypical" categorization in BDB, FISH has been recommended in combination with routine cytopathology for the evaluation of pancreaticobiliary strictures {54,585,885}. Recent studies have also shown that molecular testing could significantly increase the sensitivity of detecting malignancy {281,788, 733}. However, there are caveats regarding the use of FISH and molecular testing as ancillary tests in "Atypical" BDB cases. The first is in regard to the findings that some isolated trisomies can be seen in premalignant lesions in patients with primary sclerosing cholangitis and that *KRAS* mutations are seen in cases of low-grade dysplasia {394,326}. The second caveat is that a negative result does not exclude the possibility of malignancy because approximately 20% of malignancies are reported to have no aneusomy by FISH and 25% do not harbour a detectable alteration in genes other than *KRAS* by next-generation sequencing. Therefore, FISH and molecular testing should not be used as standalone tests in "Atypical" BDB specimens at this time. A recommended approach to an "Atypical" BDB is to review the imaging and clinical findings, and if there is concern for a neoplastic process, to consider repeating the procedure or using FNAB to sample any mass lesion.

Other than the above ancillary tests, obtaining a consensus review or second opinion from cytopathologists experienced in pancreaticobiliary cytopathology may be a cost-effective approach. If ancillary testing is not available and the final diagnosis is inconclusive, further workup may include repeat sampling using next-generation biopsy needles with ROSE.

Category: Pancreaticobiliary neoplasm, low-risk/grade

Centeno BA
Klapman J
Pitman MB

The risk of malignancy (ROM) for the "Pancreaticobiliary neoplasm, low-risk/grade (PaN-low)" category is 5–20% {306}, a value calculated from a reclassified study cohort looking at the ROM in the "Neoplastic: other" category in the Papanicolaou Society of Cytopathology (PSC) reporting system, which included both low- and high-risk/grade lesions and had a wide-ranging ROM (14.2–100%) {307}. Cases in the PSC "Neoplastic: other" category with low-grade atypia had a ROM of 4.3%, compared with 90% for those with high-grade atypia {308}. In another study, patients with low-grade atypia had an absolute overall ROM of 14.7% and an absolute ROM of 19.0%, and patients with high-grade atypia had an absolute overall ROM of 83.3% and an absolute ROM of 95.2% {824}.

There are five published guidelines for the management of pancreatic cysts. They include the revised international consensus guidelines {839}, the European evidence-based guidelines

Table 10.01 Indications for surgical resection for intraductal papillary mucinous neoplasm (IPMN) and mucinous cystic neoplasm (MCN) as outlined by current guidelines and the American College of Radiology (ACR) white paper

Guidelines	Cyst type	Absolute indication	Relative indication
ACR (2017) {537}	IPMN or MCN	IPMN or MCN: • Jaundice • Enhancing mural nodule • MPD > 10 mm	Indications for EUS-FNAB: high-risk features: • Mural nodules • Wall thickening • MPD > 7 mm • Peripheral calcifications • Cyst > 25 mm • Interval growth (> 20% in longitudinal axis)
ACG (2018) {201}			Indication for multidisciplinary review: • Jaundice secondary to the cyst • Acute pancreatitis secondary to the cyst • Significantly elevated serum CA19-9 • Any of the following imaging findings: mural nodule, solid component, dilation of MPD > 5 mm, focal dilation of the MPD, mucin-producing cysts ≥ 30 mm • The presence of HGD or pancreatic cancer on cytology
AGA (2015) {878}	MCN	• All MCNs	
	IPMN	• MPD ≥ 5 mm (on MRI and EUS) and solid component • Cytology positive for malignancy	
European evidence-based guidelines (2018) {204}	MCN	• Cyst diameter ≥ 40 mm • Enhancing mural nodule • Symptoms (jaundice, acute pancreatitis, new-onset diabetes mellitus)	
	IPMN	• Positive cytology for malignancy or HGD • Solid mass • Jaundice (tumour-related) • Enhancing mural nodule (≥ 5 mm) • MPD dilatation ≥ 10 mm	• Growth rate ≥ 5 mm per year • Increased levels of serum CA19-9 (> 37 U/mL) • MPD dilatation between 5 and 9.9 mm • Cyst diameter ≥ 40 mm • New-onset diabetes mellitus • Acute pancreatitis (caused by IPMN) • Enhancing mural nodule (< 5 mm)
International consensus guidelines (revised) (2017) {839}	MCN	• All MCNs	
	IPMN	• Cytology suspicious or positive for malignancy, includes cytology with features of HGEA • Jaundice (tumour-related) • Enhancing mural nodule (> 5 mm) • MPD dilatation ≥ 10 mm	• Growth rate ≥ 5 mm over 2 years • Increased levels of serum CA19-9 • MPD dilatation between 5 and 9 mm • Cyst diameter ≥ 30 mm • Acute pancreatitis (caused by IPMN) • Enhancing mural nodule (< 5 mm) • Abrupt change in diameter of MPD with distal atrophy • Lymphadenopathy • Thickened or enhancing cyst walls

ACG, American College of Gastroenterology; AGA, American Gastroenterological Association; HGD, high-grade dysplasia; HGEA, high-grade epithelial atypia; MPD, main pancreatic duct.

on the management of pancreatic cystic neoplasms {204}, the American Gastroenterological Association (AGA) guidelines on the management of asymptomatic pancreatic cystic lesions {878}, the American College of Gastroenterology (ACG) clinical guidelines on the diagnosis and management of pancreatic cystic lesions {201} and the American College of Radiology (ACR) white paper on the management of incidental pancreatic cysts {537}.

All these guidelines use a combination of clinical and imaging findings as absolute or relative indications for surgery, surveillance protocols, and indications for EUS-FNAB for patients with intraductal papillary mucinous neoplasms (see Table 10.01). Four include the cytopathological findings in the decision algorithm, and the presence of a "Malignant" or "Suspicious for malignancy" cytopathology report with high-grade dysplasia will lead to surgical intervention. The white paper published by the ACR is the only one that does not include cytopathology as part of the management algorithm {537}.

Management of low-grade intraductal lesions has been a matter of debate for the past two decades. Management has shifted from resecting all mucinous pancreatic cysts because of their premalignant nature to conservative management and surveillance because most of the lesions are on the very early spectrum of progression to carcinoma, and most patients are elderly with comorbid conditions, making the patient a high-risk surgical candidate. Cytopathology is the best test to accurately distinguish low- from high-grade cysts on the basis of the atypical epithelium in the cyst fluid {140}. Stratifying epithelial atypia into low-grade or high-grade leads to better patient management, because pancreatic cyst fluid FNABs are rarely interpreted as "Suspicious for malignancy" or diagnostic for malignancy owing to their scant cellularity. In the absence of cytopathological high-grade atypia, and in the presence of low-grade atypia, the patient has the option of surveillance depending on the clinical and imaging features {839,648,652}.

Mucinous cystic neoplasms have been considered an absolute indication for surgery in older and some more recent management guidelines, because of the relative ease of the usual distal pancreatectomy versus a lifetime of surveillance for progression to carcinoma {839,878}. More recently, however, there is a move to refer patients for surveillance on the basis of their clinical and imaging findings {204,201,537}. Patients with mucinous cystic neoplasm and low-grade atypia on cytopathology can be referred for surveillance in the absence of other high-risk factors {201,748}.

In the former PSC reporting system, bile duct brushings with low-grade atypia were categorized as "Atypical". This is because clear cytopathological criteria for a definitive diagnosis of biliary intraepithelial neoplasia, low-grade (BilIN-low) were not well defined. In the current WHO Reporting System, features are defined, and these types of samples are placed in the "Pancreaticobiliary neoplasm, low-risk/grade (PaN-low)" category. Similarly, a definitive diagnosis of low-grade pancreatic intraepithelial neoplasia on FNAB is not well defined, but features described in this WHO Reporting System can be used to place these cases in the "PaN-low" category, which is used to encompass low- and intermediate-grade dysplasia. Management options include repeat sampling, preferably with ancillary studies such as FISH {603,979,411,445} or next-generation sequencing {788,281,192,699}.

Category: Pancreaticobiliary neoplasm, high-risk/grade

Pitman MB
Centeno BA
Hoda RS
Klapman J

The estimated risk of malignancy (ROM) of the "Pancreaticobiliary neoplasm, high-risk/grade (PaN-high)" category is 60–95% {306}, a value calculated in part from a reclassified study cohort looking at the ROM in the "Neoplastic: other" category in the Papanicolaou Society of Cytopathology (PSC) reporting system, which included both low- and high-risk/grade lesions and had a wide-ranging ROM (14.2–100%) {307}. Cases in the PSC "Neoplastic: other" category with low-grade atypia had a ROM of 4.3%, compared with 90% for those with high-grade atypia {308}. In another study, patients with low-grade atypia had an absolute overall ROM of 14.7% and an absolute ROM of 19.0%, and patients with high-grade atypia had an absolute overall ROM of 83.3% and an absolute ROM of 95.2% {824}.

The category of "Pancreaticobiliary neoplasm, high-risk/grade (PaN-high)" is used for an intraductal or intracystic lesion at high risk of malignancy and with at least high-grade dysplasia. Lesions within this category are predominantly high-grade intraductal papillary mucinous neoplasms, judging from experience with the "Neoplastic: other" category of the PSC system {307}. The categorization of lesions in this category is based on the cytomorphology of high-grade epithelial atypia {644} and can be supported by the detection of late mutations in the adenoma–carcinoma progression, such as the mutation of *TP53* or loss of SMAD4 or p16 (CDKN2A) {700}.

There are currently five major guidelines on the management of intraductal papillary mucinous neoplasm and mucinous cystic neoplasm: the American College of Radiology (ACR) white paper on the management of incidental pancreatic cysts {537}, the American College of Gastroenterology (ACG) clinical guidelines on the diagnosis and management of incidental pancreatic cysts {201}, the American Gastroenterological Association (AGA) guidelines on the management of asymptomatic pancreatic cystic lesions {878}, the European evidence-based guidelines on the management of pancreatic cystic neoplasms {204}, and the revised international consensus guidelines {839}.

These guidelines and white papers incorporate a combination of clinical findings, imaging features, and cyst fluid analysis with cytopathology to define surveillance strategies and to provide absolute and relative indications for surgical intervention. The surveillance strategies are detailed, and readers are asked to refer to the referenced articles, but the differences between the absolute and relative indications for surgical intervention are summarized in Table 10.01 (p. 174) in *Category: Pancreaticobiliary neoplasm, low-risk/grade*. Most use the terms "positive for malignancy" or "high-grade dysplasia" when addressing the role of cytopathology, and these terms correlate to the "Malignant" category in the WHO Reporting System for Pancreaticobiliary Cytopathology.

Based on the terminology of the WHO Reporting System and the related risk of malignancy (ROM) of a "PaN-high" cytopathology interpretation, a cytopathology report with a "PaN-high" interpretation should also be considered a high-risk test result, warranting surgical resection {201,839,204, 878,537}.

All guidelines emphasize that the decision to intervene with surgical resection should be a shared one between the patient and physician, and the risk of surgical intervention should be weighed against the patient's risk of mortality or morbidity from the surgery and the lifetime risk of developing cancer.

For bile duct brushing (BDB), a definitive classification of "Atypical" as neoplastic is challenging, and few data are available for the accurate cytopathological classification of intraductal bile duct neoplasms {699}. Because established criteria are lacking for the diagnosis of specific premalignant intraductal bile duct neoplasms, most cytopathological interpretations fall into the "Benign", "Malignant", or conventional indeterminate categories ("Atypical" and "Suspicious for malignancy") and not into the "Pancreaticobiliary neoplasm, low-risk/grade (PaN-low)" or "PaN-high" categories. The ROM for BDB is higher per diagnostic category than for FNAB of pancreatic masses, because of a high threshold for a "Malignant" categorization as a result of a significant overlap in reactive or reparative changes and carcinoma, which can be caused by indwelling stents, instrumentation, and underlying inflammatory processes such as in primary sclerosing cholangitis. Using conventional cytopathological categories, an estimated ROM is as high as 25% in the "Negative" category, 50% in the "Atypical" category, and 90% in the "Suspicious for malignancy" categories for this reason. A definitive diagnosis of malignancy is rarely incorrect, with a ROM of 96–100% {875, 111,192,952}. This correlates with the high specificity and low sensitivity of BDB cytopathology.

The management of patients with a bile duct stricture is continued surveillance regardless of a "Benign" interpretation, with increasing consideration of surgical intervention with each diagnostic category. In patients with primary sclerosing cholangitis, there is a 5–10% lifetime risk of developing cholangiocarcinoma, which is a contraindication for liver transplant for most patients, so the detection of bile duct dysplasia is the goal of surveillance {877,85}. To further improve the diagnostic yield of BDB, ancillary techniques have been developed over the past 10–15 years, initially with FISH and more recently with next-generation sequencing. Both tests have shown that when positive and used in combination with BDB cytopathology, the sensitivity for a high-risk stricture with at least high-grade dysplasia increases without decreasing the high specificity of the results {386,483,192,788,733}.

The clinical management for each category for BDB is shown in Table 10.01 (p. 174) in *Category: Pancreaticobiliary neoplasm, low-risk/grade*. Patients with a "Benign" interpretation are generally managed with follow-up dependent on the clinical concern for malignancy. Repeat endoscopic retrograde cholangiopancreatography with cholangioscopy, BDB, and biopsies are warranted when malignancy is suspected, whether the interpretation is "Benign" or higher. The addition of ancillary testing with FISH and/or next-generation sequencing can be considered to increase the support of a "Malignant" categorization if available. The detection of a *KRAS* mutation supports neoplasia rather than reactive changes, and the detection of high-risk mutations, including *TP53* mutation, or *SMAD4* or *CDKN2A* (*P16*) deletion, support a high-risk stricture warranting consideration of surgical intervention {788,192, 699}.

Category: Suspicious for malignancy

Goyal A
Klapman J
Siddiqui MT

The risk of malignancy (ROM) of a "Suspicious for malignancy" categorization is associated with a high ROM of 80–100% for FNAB of the pancreas {792,307,824} and 74–100% for bile duct brushing {875,111,192,952,658,468,595}. On its own, this categorization should not be considered as an indication for surgical resection or initiation of adjuvant therapy {111,752,890,134, 461,307,924,792}. The management of a "Suspicious for malignancy" categorization in the pancreaticobiliary tract depends on various factors, including the clinical presentation, imaging findings, ancillary test results, and patient comorbidities and preferences. The rationale behind such an integrated approach is to further define the patient's ROM in the context of this indeterminate cytopathology interpretation.

Different clinical features or imaging and endoscopic findings or ancillary test results have been emphasized to enable the risk stratification of indeterminate cytopathology interpretations. In a retrospective review of pancreatic lesions, Spier et al. {807} concluded that the EUS findings of lymphadenopathy and vascular involvement were associated with a higher ROM. Other findings were emphasized by Alston et al. {29} in a study of 116 pancreatic EUS-FNAB with suspicious cytopathology: the significant associations of the presence of a mass with a neoplasm and of the clinical finding of weight loss with pancreatic ductal adenocarcinoma. For pancreatobiliary brushings, Volmar et al. {890} also highlighted certain clinical and imaging findings as more likely to be associated with malignancy, i.e. older age, male sex, jaundice, and the presence of a well-defined stricture. Some authors have incorporated different variables to devise predictive models for estimating the probability of malignancy. Fritcher and colleagues {226} generated a multivariable model for pancreaticobiliary strictures based on the patient's age, history of primary sclerosing cholangitis, cytopathology findings, and FISH results. Similarly, Witt et al. {918} proposed a scoring system, termed the "atypical biliary brushing score", for indeterminate bile duct brushing cytopathology that included the patient's age, endoscopic impression, procedure indication, location of stricture, history of primary sclerosing cholangitis, and serum CA19-9 levels.

Ancillary tests such as FISH and next-generation sequencing can be employed to augment the sensitivity of pancreaticobiliary cytopathology and for further risk stratification of indeterminate results. FISH testing and next-generation sequencing have been reported to have a sensitivity of 43–90% and 85%, respectively, for detecting malignancy in bile duct brushings {226,251,192,796,79}. Also, next-generation sequencing has exhibited promising results for the detection of pathogenic alterations in FNAB specimens of solid masses and cystic lesions of the pancreas {247,370,700,364,733}. *KRAS* and/or *GNAS* mutations accompanied with *TP53*, *PIK3CA*, and/or *PTEN* alterations have been shown to have 79% sensitivity and 96% specificity for a mucinous pancreatic cyst with advanced neoplasia {787}.

It is clear that the management of a "Suspicious for malignancy" categorization requires a comprehensive multidisciplinary approach involving the correlation of all the clinical, imaging, and ancillary test data. After evaluating all the information available, the management options may include surgery, repeat sampling, additional imaging, or clinical follow-up. For instance, in a 65-year-old patient with jaundice and a pancreatic mass on imaging, a malignancy is very likely and may prompt surgical intervention. However, in a 40-year-old patient with a history of pancreatitis and a poorly defined lesion on imaging, conservative management with follow-up and repeat sampling may be preferred after a "Suspicious for malignancy" report. Multidisciplinary conferences are the appropriate platforms for discussing and evaluating these different parameters and planning the management of "Suspicious for malignancy" cases.

Category: Malignant

Chhieng DC
Klapman J
Pitman MB

The risk of malignancy of an FNAB of the pancreas interpreted as "Malignant" is 99–100% {792,307,824,306}, and for a bile duct brushing it is 96–100% {875,111,192,952,658,468,595}. False positive interpretations are generally associated with pancreatitis, especially autoimmune pancreatitis {175}. Patients with a "Malignant" cytopathology report that has been correlated with clinical and imaging findings can proceed to definitive treatment, especially if a specific tumour diagnosis has been made. For bile duct lesions, the risk of malignancy is even higher, 99–100%, because of the very high threshold for a definitive "Malignant" interpretation. Improvement in the sensitivity of detecting malignancy on bile duct brushings has been achieved with FISH {226,796} and next-generation sequencing {192,788,733}.

Surgical resection is currently the only means of achieving long-term survival in patients with biopsy-proven pancreatic ductal adenocarcinoma. Unfortunately, only 15–20% of patients present with disease that is amenable to surgery. With the increasing use of neoadjuvant therapies and advances in surgical techniques, the pool of patients for potential surgical resection has been increasing, especially those with borderline resectable disease {397}. For those with locally advanced and/or metastatic disease, systemic therapy with or without radiotherapy is indicated. Eligible candidates can also enrol in clinical trials. Recent gains in the molecular understanding of pancreatic ductal adenocarcinoma have led to the increased use of personalized therapy. One such example would be microsatellite instability; although it is only detected in approximately 1% of patients with the disease, 40% of patients who have microsatellite instability respond to immune checkpoint inhibition and derive improved survival from this therapy {328,469,470}. Microsatellite instability and other genetic mutations can be readily analysed on FNAB cell blocks and residual needle rinses.

Surgical resection is recommended for all functioning pancreatic neuroendocrine tumours (PanNETs) and localized non-functioning PanNETs that do not have widespread metastases. The surgical options include simple enucleation, central pancreatectomy, distal pancreatectomy with or without splenectomy, and the Whipple operation, depending on tumour location {756}. Although some authors recommend conservative observation, (watch and wait) for patients with non-functioning PanNETs measuring < 20 mm, this management option remains controversial {208,527,714,215,759}. Somatostatin analogues are the treatment of choice for the hormone-excess state in PanNET before surgery or if resection cannot be performed.

Complete surgical resection is the only treatment to afford a chance of cure for cholangiocarcinoma {186}. Unfortunately, most tumours are inoperable at the time of presentation. Additional treatment modalities may include stenting, targeted radiotherapy, and systemic chemotherapy {186}.

Surgical management is usually the first line of treatment for less common primary malignancies in the pancreas. If the disease is not resectable, the patients are treated with adjuvant chemotherapy with or without radiotherapy. Lymphomas and metastases are treated according to the stage and disease-specific therapies.

Contributors

AVADHANI, Vaidehi
Emory University
80 Jesse Hill Jr Dr
Atlanta GA 30303

BASTURK, Olca
Memorial Sloan Kettering Cancer Center
1275 York Ave
New York NY 10065

CAI, Guoping
Yale School of Medicine
310 Cedar St, CB506B
New Haven CT 06510

CENTENO, Barbara Ann
Moffitt Cancer Center
12902 USF Magnolia Dr
Tampa FL 33612

CHHIENG, David C.
COLA
9881 Broken Land Pkwy, Suite 200
Columbia MD 21046

CHUTE, Deborah J.
Cleveland Clinic
9500 Euclid Ave, L25
Cleveland OH 44195

CLAYTON, Amy
Mayo Clinic
200 1st St SW
Rochester MN 55905

COCKER, Rubina
Northwell Health
2200 Northern Blvd
Greenvale NY 11548

CREE, Ian A.
International Agency for Research on Cancer
25 Av. Tony Garnier, CS 90627
69366 Lyon, CEDEX 07

DAVEY, Diane D.
University of Central Florida
9885 Leland Dr
Orlando FL 32827

de ANDREA, Carlos E.
Clínica Universidad de Navarra
Av. de Pío XII, 36
31008 Pamplona

DHILLON, Jasreman
H. Lee Moffitt Cancer Center
12902 USF Magnolia Dr
Tampa FL 33612

ELTOUM, Isam A.
University of Alabama at Birmingham
122 HSB, 619 19th St S
Birmingham AL 35249-6823

FIELD, Andrew S.
University of NSW Sydney and
University of Notre Dame Medical Schools
Department of Anatomical Pathology
St Vincent's Hospital Sydney
Victoria St
2010 Darlinghurst NSW

FONSECA, Anil Felix Angelo
Gandhi Medical College/TIMS
Hyderabad, Telangana

FONSECA, Ricardo
Instituto Português de Oncologia de Lisboa
Francisco Gentil
Rua Prof. Lima Basto
1099-023 Lisbon

FUKUSHIMA, Noriyoshi
Jichi Medical University
3311-1 Yakushiji, Shimotsuke
Tochigi 329-0498

GAN, Qiong
University of Texas
MD Anderson Cancer Center
1515 Holcombe Blvd
Houston TX 77030

GOLDMAN-LÉVY, Gabrielle
International Agency for Research on Cancer
25 Av. Tony Garnier, CS 90627
69366 Lyon, CEDEX 07

GÓMEZ-ROMÁN, J. Javier
Hospital Universitario Marqués de Valdecilla,
Universidad de Cantabria, IDIVAL
Av. de Valdecilla, s/n
39008 Santander

GOYAL, Abha
NewYork-Presbyterian/Weill Cornell Medical
Center
525 E 68th St, F-766C
New York NY 10065

GRANADOS, Rosario
Hospital Universitario de Getafe
Carretera de Toledo, Km 12,5, Getafe
28905 Madrid

HEYMANN, Jonas J.
NewYork-Presbyterian/Weill Cornell Medical
Center
525 E 68th St, F-766D
New York NY 10024

HODA, Raza S.
Cleveland Clinic Lerner College of Medicine
Case Western Reserve University
9500 Euclid Ave, L2-125G
Cleveland OH 44195

HooKim, Kim
Cooper University Health Care
1 Cooper Plaza
Camden NJ 08103

ITOI, Takao
Tokyo Medical University
6-7-1 Nishishinjuku, Shinjuku-ku
Tokyo 160-0023

JHALA, Darshana N.
University of Pennsylvania and CMC VAMC
3900 Woodland Ave
Philadelphia PA 19104

JHALA, Nirag
Temple University Hospital
3401 N Broad St, OPB249
Philadelphia PA 19140

KALRA, Naveen
Postgraduate Institute of Medical Education
and Research
Sector 12
Chandigarh 160012

KLAPMAN, Jason
102 Baltic Cir
Tampa FL 33606

KRISHNAN, Kumar*
Massachusetts General Hospital
55 Fruit St
Boston MA 02114

* Indicates disclosure of interests (see p. 183).

KUMARASINGHE, M. Priyanthi
PathWest and University of Western Australia
J Block, QEII Medical Centre
Nedlands WA 6009

KURTYCZ, Daniel
University of Wisconsin
School of Medicine and Public Health
Wisconsin State Laboratory of Hygiene
465 Henry Mall
Madison WI 53706

LAYFIELD, Lester J.
University of Missouri
1 Hospital Dr
Columbia MO 65212

LOZANO, María D.
University of Navarra
Av. de Pío XII, 36
31008 Pamplona

MEHROTRA, Ravi
Centre for Health Innovation and Policy
361, Sector 15A
Noida 20301

NAITO, Yoshiki
Kurume University Hospital
67 Asahimachi
Kurume 830-0011

NOTOHARA, Kenji
Kurashiki Central Hospital
1-1-1 Miwa
Kurashiki 710-8602

OZRETIĆ, Luka
Royal Free Hospital
Pond St
London NW3 2QG

PEREIRA, Stephen P.
University College London
Upper 3rd, Royal Free Hospital, Pond St
London NW3 2QG

PEREZ-MACHADO, Miguel Angel
Royal Free Hospital
Pond St
London NW3 2QG

PITMAN, Martha Bishop*
Harvard Medical School,
Massachusetts General Hospital
55 Fruit St
Boston MA 02114

POLICARPIO NICOLAS, Maria Luisa
Cleveland Clinic
9500 Euclid Ave
Cleveland OH 44195

REID, Michelle D.
Emory University Hospital
1364 Clifton Rd NE, Room G180A
Atlanta GA 30322

ROSENBAUM, Matthew W.
Beth Israel Deaconess Medical Center
330 Brookline Ave, ES-112
Boston MA 02215

ROY-CHOWDHURI, Sinchita
University of Texas
MD Anderson Cancer Center
1515 Holcombe Blvd, Unit 85
Houston TX 77030

SAIEG, Mauro
Santa Casa Medical School
R. Jaguaribe, 155 - Vila Buarque
São Paulo SP 01224-001

SAVIC PRINCE, Spasenija*
University Hospital Basel
Schönbeinstrasse 40
4031 Basel

SCHMITT, Fernando
CINTESIS@RISE (Health Research Network);
Medical Faculty of the University of Porto;
Molecular Pathology Unit, Ipatimup
Rua Júlio Amaral de Carvalho 45
4200-135 Porto

SIDDIQUI, Momin Tipu
NewYork-Presbyterian/Weill Cornell Medical Center
525 E 68th St, F-766A
New York NY 10065

SIGEL, Carlie
Memorial Sloan Kettering Cancer Center
1275 York Ave
New York NY 10065

SINGHI, Aatur D.
University of Pittsburgh Medical Center
200 Lothrop St, Scaife Hall A616.2
Pittsburgh PA 15213

STELOW, Edward B.
University of Virginia School of Medicine
Box 800214
Charlottesville VA 22908-0214

ŠTOOS-VEIĆ, Tajana
University Hospital Dubrava
Avenija Gojka Šuška 6
10000 Zagreb

TANAKA, Mariko
University of Tokyo Hospital
7-3-1 Hongo, Bunkyo-ku
Tokyo 113-8655

TRONCONE, Giancarlo
University of Naples Federico II
Via Sergio Pansini, 5
80128 Naples

VAN DER POL, Christian B.
Juravinski Hospital and Cancer Centre
Hamilton Health Sciences
711 Concession St
Hamilton ON L8V 1C3

VANDENBUSSCHE, Christopher J.
Johns Hopkins Hospital
600 N Wolfe St, Pathology 406
Baltimore MD 21287

WEYNAND, Birgit
UZ Leuven
Herestraat 49
3000 Leuven

YANG, Jack
Medical University of South Carolina
171 Ashley Ave, MSC908
Charleston SC 29425

YOON, Won Jae
Ewha Womans University College of Medicine
25 Magokdong-ro 2-gil, Gangseo-gu
Seoul 07804

ZEN, Yoh
King's College Hospital
Denmark Hill
London SE5 9RS

ZHANG, M. Lisa
Massachusetts General Hospital
55 Fruit St
Boston MA 02114

* Indicates disclosure of interests (see p. 183).

Declaration of interests

Dr Krishnan reports having received personal consultancy fees from Olympus Medical.

Dr Pitman reports having received consultancy fees from Adenocyte LLC.

Dr Savic Prince reports having received personal consultancy fees from MSD Merck Sharp & Dohme for medical, scientific, and usability-related assistance with an open-source PDL1 online platform, and receiving honoraria from Diaceutics Ireland Limited, MSD, AstraZeneca, Boehringer Ingelheim, Roche, Pfizer, Bristol Myers Squibb, Abbott, and Thermo Fisher Scientific.

Sources

Note: For any figure, table, or box not listed below, the original source is this volume; the suggested source citation is

International Academy of Cytology – International Agency for Research on Cancer – World Health Organization Joint Editorial Board. WHO Reporting System for Pancreaticobiliary Cytopathology. Lyon (France): International Agency for Research on Cancer; 2022. (IAC-IARC-WHO cytopathology reporting systems series, 1st ed.; vol. 2). https://publications.iarc.fr/621.

Figures

1.01	Centeno BA
2.01	Brenna W. Casey, Interventional Gastroenterology, Interventional Endoscopy, Massachusetts General Hospital, Harvard Medical School, Boston MA
2.02	Reprinted, with permission from Elsevier, from: Gkolfakis P, Crinò SF, Tziatzios G, et al. Comparative diagnostic performance of end-cutting fine-needle biopsy needles for EUS tissue sampling of solid pancreatic masses: a network meta-analysis. Gastrointest Endosc. 2022 Jun;95(6):1067–77.e15. PMID:35124072
2.03	Reprinted from: Zhang ML, Pitman MB. Practical applications of molecular testing in the cytologic diagnosis of pancreatic cysts. J Mol Pathol. 2021;2(1):11–22. doi:10.3390/jmp2010002.
2.04	Kalra N
2.05	Savic Prince S
2.06	Savic Prince S
2.07A–C	Clayton A
2.08	Lozano MD
2.09	de Andrea CE
2.10	Reprinted, with permission, from: Khan I, Baig M, Bandepalle T, et al. Utility of cyst fluid carcinoembryonic antigen in differentiating mucinous and non-mucinous pancreatic cysts: an updated meta-analysis. Dig Dis Sci. 2022 Sep;67(9):4541–8. PMID:34783970
3.01A,B	Donna Russell, University of Rochester Medical Center, Rochester NY
3.02	Donna Russell, University of Rochester Medical Center, Rochester NY
3.03A	Pitman MB
3.03B	Charles Sturgis, Department of Pathology, Mayo Clinic, Rochester MN
4.01A–C	Pitman MB
4.02A,B	Pitman MB
4.03	Pitman MB
4.04A,B	Pitman MB
4.05	Pitman MB
4.06	Pitman MB
4.07	Pitman MB
4.08A,B	Naito Y
4.09	Naito Y
4.10	Naito Y
4.11	Zen Y
4.12A,B	Zen Y
4.13A,C	Yang J
4.13B	Pitman MB
4.14	Chute DJ
4.15A,B	Reid MD
4.16	Chute DJ
4.17	Reid MD
4.18	Reid MD
4.19	Notohara K
4.20A,B	Notohara K
4.21A,B	Pitman MB
4.22	Pitman MB
4.23A,B	VandenBussche CJ
4.24A,B	VandenBussche CJ
4.25	VandenBussche CJ
4.26A	Naito Y
4.26B	Sigel C
4.26C	Pitman MB
4.27	Perez-Machado MA
4.28A,B	Perez-Machado MA
4.29A,B	Reid MD
4.30	Pitman MB
4.31A–C	Pitman MB
4.32A,B	Reid MD
4.33A–D	Pitman MB
4.34	Pitman MB
4.35A,B	Pitman MB
4.35C	Fonseca R
4.36	Pitman MB
5.01A,D,E	Pitman MB
5.01B	Yang J
5.01C	Heymann JJ
6.01A,B	Tanaka M
6.02A,B	Tanaka M
6.03	Pitman MB
6.04A,B	Sigel C
6.05A–C	Pitman MB
6.06	Pitman MB
6.07A,B	Zen Y
6.08A,B	Cai G
6.09	Pitman MB
7.01A	Fukushima N
7.01B,C	HooKim K
7.02A,B	Zen Y
7.03	Zen Y
7.04	Pitman MB
7.05A–C	Pitman MB
7.06A,B	Pitman MB
7.07A,B	Pitman MB
7.08	Pitman MB
7.09	Pitman MB
7.10	Pitman MB
7.11A–C	Zen Y
7.12A–C	Zen Y
7.13A,C	Pitman MB
7.13B,D	Cai G
7.14A,B	Reid MD
7.15A–C	Reid MD
7.16	Reid MD
7.17	Reid MD
7.18A,B	Basturk O
7.19A,B	Reid MD
7.20	Basturk O
8.01A–D	Goyal A
8.02	Goyal A
9.01A,B	Sigel C
9.01C	Layfield LJ
9.02A	Sigel C
9.02B–D	Pitman MB
9.03A,B	Pitman MB

9.04A,B	Pitman MB
9.05A,B	Sigel C
9.06A,B	Weynand B
9.07	Pitman MB
9.08A,C,D	Weynand B
9.08B	Pitman MB
9.08E	Jhala N
9.09A–D	Pitman MB
9.10	Weynand B
9.11A–C	Pitman MB
9.12A,B	Cocker R
9.12C,D	Weynand B
9.13A,B	Pitman MB
9.13C	Kumarasinghe MP
9.14A	Weynand B
9.14B	Dhillon J
9.15A,B	Weynand B
9.16A	Pitman MB
9.16B–D	Reid MD
9.17	Sigel C
9.18	Sigel C
9.19A	Sigel C
9.19B	Pitman MB
9.20A	Sigel C
9.20B	Pitman MB
9.21A	Sigel C
9.21B	Pitman MB
9.22A	Sigel C
9.22B	Pitman MB
9.23A	Sigel C
9.23B	Pitman MB
9.24A,B	Reid MD
9.24C	Pitman MB
9.25A,B	Reid MD
9.26A,B	Reid MD
9.27A,B	Reid MD
9.28	Reid MD
9.29A,B	Reid MD
9.30	Reid MD
9.31	Reid MD
9.32A–C	Reid MD
9.33A–D	Reid MD
9.34A,B	Reid MD
9.35A,B	Reid MD
9.36A	Reid MD
9.36B	Adapted, with permission, from: Reid MD, Bhattarai S, Graham RP, et al. Pancreatoblastoma: cytologic and histologic analysis of 12 adult cases reveals helpful criteria in their diagnosis and distinction from common mimics. Cancer Cytopathol. 2019 Nov;127(11):708–19. PMID:31581358
9.37	Reid MD
9.38A–C	Reid MD
9.39A,D	Pitman MB
9.39B,E	Centeno BA
9.39C	Lozano MD
9.40A,B	Granados R
9.41A	Lozano MD
9.41B	Pitman MB
9.42A	Pitman MB
9.42B	Centeno BA
9.43A	Lozano MD
9.43B	Granados R
9.44A–C	Pitman MB
9.44D	Granados R
9.45A,B	Zhang ML
9.46A,B	Zhang ML
9.47A,B	Centeno BA
9.47C	Pitman MB
9.47D	Saieg M
9.48A,B	Saieg M
9.49A,B	Saieg M
9.50A–C	Centeno BA
9.51A,B	Reid MD
9.52A–D	Reid MD

Tables

1.01	Hoda RS
1.02	Hoda RS
2.01	Eltoum IA
2.02	Centeno BA
2.03	Centeno BA
2.04	Lozano MD
2.05	Lozano MD
2.06	Singhi AD
4.01	Zen Y
4.02	Notohara K
9.01	Centeno BA
9.02	Centeno BA
9.03	Jhala N
9.04	Weynand B
9.05	Jhala N
9.06	Centeno BA
9.07	Centeno BA
9.08	Centeno BA
9.09	Davey DD
9.10	Saieg M
10.01	Centeno BA

Boxes

2.01	Eltoum IA
2.02	Lozano MD

Images on the cover

Top left	Fig. 4.23A: VandenBussche CJ
Bottom left	Fig. 9.18: Sigel C
Top centre	Fig. 2.06: Savic Prince S
Bottom centre	Fig. 9.16C: Reid MD
Top right	Fig. 2.05: Savic Prince S
Bottom right	Fig. 9.42B: Centeno BA

Images on the chapter title pages

Chapter 1	Fig. 9.08C: Weynand B
Chapter 2	Fig. 2.05: Savic Prince S
Chapter 3	Fig. 3.02: Donna Russell, University of Rochester Medical Center, Rochester NY
Chapter 4	Fig. 4.02A: Pitman MB
Chapter 5	Fig. 5.01B: Yang J
Chapter 6	Fig. 6.07A: Zen Y
Chapter 7	Fig. 7.05C: Pitman MB
Chapter 8	Fig. 8.02: Goyal A
Chapter 9	Fig. 9.16A: Pitman MB
Chapter 10	Fig. 9.52B: Reid MD

References

1. Abdelgawwad MS, Alston E, Eltoum IA. The frequency and cancer risk associated with the atypical cytologic diagnostic category in endoscopic ultrasound-guided fine-needle aspiration specimens of solid pancreatic lesions: a meta-analysis and argument for a Bethesda system for reporting cytopathology of the pancreas. Cancer Cytopathol. 2013 Nov;121(11):620–8. PMID:23881871

2. Abdelkader A, Hunt B, Hartley CP, et al. Cystic lesions of the pancreas: differential diagnosis and cytologic-histologic correlation. Arch Pathol Lab Med. 2020 Jan;144(1):47–61. PMID:31538798

3. Abe K, Suda K, Arakawa A, et al. Different patterns of p16INK4A and p53 protein expressions in intraductal papillary-mucinous neoplasms and pancreatic intraepithelial neoplasia. Pancreas. 2007 Jan;34(1):85–91. PMID:17198188

4. Abendroth CS, Dabbs DJ. Immunocytochemical staining of unstained versus previously stained cytologic preparations. Acta Cytol. 1995 May-Jun;39(3):379–86. PMID:7539200

5. Abou-Alfa GK, Sahai V, Hollebecque A, et al. Pemigatinib for previously treated, locally advanced or metastatic cholangiocarcinoma: a multicentre, open-label, phase 2 study. Lancet Oncol. 2020 May;21(5):671–84. PMID:32203698

6. Abraham SC, Wu TT, Hruban RH, et al. Genetic and immunohistochemical analysis of pancreatic acinar cell carcinoma: frequent allelic loss on chromosome 11p and alterations in the APC/beta-catenin pathway. Am J Pathol. 2002 Mar;160(3):953–62. PMID:11891193

7. Abraham SC, Wu TT, Klimstra DS, et al. Distinctive molecular genetic alterations in sporadic and familial adenomatous polyposis-associated pancreatoblastomas : frequent alterations in the APC/beta-catenin pathway and chromosome 11p. Am J Pathol. 2001 Nov;159(5):1619–27. PMID:11696422

8. Adsay NV, Adair CF, Heffess CS, et al. Intraductal oncocytic papillary neoplasms of the pancreas. Am J Surg Pathol. 1996 Aug;20(8):980–94. PMID:8712298

9. Adsay NV, Andea A, Basturk O, et al. Secondary tumors of the pancreas: an analysis of a surgical and autopsy database and review of the literature. Virchows Arch. 2004 Jun;444(6):527–35. PMID:15057558

10. Adsay NV, Hasteh F, Cheng JD, et al. Lymphoepithelial cysts of the pancreas: a report of 12 cases and a review of the literature. Mod Pathol. 2002 May;15(5):492–501. PMID:12011254

11. Adsay NV, Pierson C, Sarkar F, et al. Colloid (mucinous noncystic) carcinoma of the pancreas. Am J Surg Pathol. 2001 Jan;25(1):26–42. PMID:11145249

12. Adsay NV, Zamboni G. Paraduodenal pancreatitis: a clinico-pathologically distinct entity unifying "cystic dystrophy of heterotopic pancreas", "para-duodenal wall cyst", and "groove pancreatitis". Semin Diagn Pathol. 2004 Nov;21(4):247–54. PMID:16273943

13. Adsay V, Logani S, Sarkar F, et al. Foamy gland pattern of pancreatic ductal adenocarcinoma: a deceptively benign-appearing variant. Am J Surg Pathol. 2000 Apr;24(4):493–504. PMID:10757396

14. Adsay V, Mino-Kenudson M, Furukawa T, et al. Pathologic evaluation and reporting of intraductal papillary mucinous neoplasms of the pancreas and other tumoral intraepithelial neoplasms of pancreatobiliary tract: recommendations of Verona consensus meeting. Ann Surg. 2016 Jan;263(1):162–77. PMID:25775066

15. Ahls MG, Niedergethmann M, Dinter D, et al. Case report: intraductal tubulopapillary neoplasm of the pancreas with unique clear cell phenotype. Diagn Pathol. 2014 Jan 20;9:11. PMID:24443801

16. Ahmad-Nielsen SA, Bruun Nielsen MF, Mortensen MB, et al. Frequency of mismatch repair deficiency in pancreatic ductal adenocarcinoma. Pathol Res Pract. 2020 Jun;216(6):152985. PMID:32360245

17. Ahmed S, Johnson PT, Hruban R, et al. Metastatic disease to the pancreas: pathologic spectrum and CT patterns. Abdom Imaging. 2013 Feb;38(1):144–53. PMID:22349804

18. Ainechi S, Lee H. Updates on precancerous lesions of the biliary tract: biliary precancerous lesion. Arch Pathol Lab Med. 2016 Nov;140(11):1285–9. PMID:27788047

19. Aishima S, Fujita N, Mano Y, et al. Different roles of S100P overexpression in intrahepatic cholangiocarcinoma: carcinogenesis of perihilar type and aggressive behavior of peripheral type. Am J Surg Pathol. 2011 Apr;35(4):590–8. PMID:21412073

20. Aishima S, Oda Y. Pathogenesis and classification of intrahepatic cholangiocarcinoma: different characters of perihilar large duct type versus peripheral small duct type. J Hepatobiliary Pancreat Sci. 2015 Feb;22(2):94–100. PMID:25181580

21. Ajaj Saieg M, Munson V, Colletti S, et al. Impact of pancreatic cyst fluid CEA levels on the classification of pancreatic cysts using the Papanicolaou Society of Cytology terminology system for pancreaticobiliary cytology. Diagn Cytopathol. 2017 Feb;45(2):101–6. PMID:28110503

22. Akita M, Fujikura K, Ajiki T, et al. Intracholecystic papillary neoplasms are distinct from papillary gallbladder cancers: a clinicopathologic and exome-sequencing study. Am J Surg Pathol. 2019 Jun;43(6):783–91. PMID:30807303

23. Aksoy-Altinboga A, Baglan T, Umudum H, et al. Diagnostic value of S100p, IMP3, maspin, and pVHL in the differantial diagnosis of pancreatic ductal adenocarcinoma and normal/chronic pancreatitis in fine needle aspiration biopsy. J Cytol. 2018 Oct-Dec;35(4):247–51. PMID:30498299

24. Albers K, Fuchs E. The molecular biology of intermediate filament proteins. Int Rev Cytol. 1992;134:243–79. PMID:1374743

26. Ali A, Brown V, Denley S, et al. Expression of KOC, S100P, mesothelin and MUC1 in pancreatico-biliary adenocarcinomas: development and utility of a potential diagnostic immunohistochemistry panel. BMC Clin Pathol. 2014 Jul 23;14:35. PMID:25071419

27. Alomari AK, Ustun B, Aslanian HR, et al. Endoscopic ultrasound-guided fine-needle aspiration diagnosis of secondary tumors involving the pancreas: an institution's experience. Cytojournal. 2016 Jan 28;13:1. PMID:26955395

28. Alston E, Bae S, Eltoum IA. Atypical cytologic diagnostic category in EUS-FNA of the pancreas: follow-up, outcomes, and predictive models. Cancer Cytopathol. 2014 Jun;122(6):428–34. PMID:24436110

29. Alston EA, Bae S, Eltoum IA. Suspicious cytologic diagnostic category in endoscopic ultrasound-guided FNA of the pancreas: follow-up and outcomes. Cancer Cytopathol. 2016 Jan;124(1):53–7. PMID:26335261

30. Aly FZ, Mostofizadeh S, Jawaid S, et al. Effect of single operator cholangioscopy on accuracy of bile duct cytology. Diagn Cytopathol. 2020 Dec;48(12):1230–6. PMID:32770823

31. Amato E, Molin MD, Mafficini A, et al. Targeted next-generation sequencing of cancer genes dissects the molecular profiles of intraductal papillary neoplasms of the pancreas. J Pathol. 2014 Jul;233(3):217–27. PMID:24604757

32. Andea A, Sarkar F, Adsay VN. Clinicopathological correlates of pancreatic intraepithelial neoplasia: a comparative analysis of 82 cases with and 152 cases without pancreatic ductal adenocarcinoma. Mod Pathol. 2003 Oct;16(10):996–1006. PMID:14559982

33. Aoki Y, Mizuma M, Hata T, et al. Intraductal papillary neoplasms of the bile duct consist of two distinct types specifically associated with clinicopathological features and molecular phenotypes. J Pathol. 2020 May;251(1):38–48. PMID:32100878

34. Ardengh JC, Lopes CV, Kemp R, et al. Accuracy of endoscopic ultrasound-guided fine-needle aspiration in the suspicion of pancreatic metastases. BMC Gastroenterol. 2013 Apr 11;13:63. PMID:23578194

35. Arena M, Eusebi LH, Pellicano R, et al. Endoscopic ultrasound core needle for diagnosing of solid pancreatic lesions: Is rapid on-site evaluation really necessary? Minerva Med. 2017 Dec;108(6):547–53. PMID:28750500

36. Argani P, Shaukat A, Kaushal M, et al. Differing rates of loss of DPC4 expression and of p53 overexpression among carcinomas of the proximal and distal bile ducts. Cancer. 2001 Apr 1;91(7):1332–41. PMID:11283934

37. Arora A, Rajesh S, Mukund A, et al. Clinicoradiological appraisal of 'paraduodenal pancreatitis': pancreatitis outside the pancreas! Indian J Radiol Imaging. 2015 Jul-Sep;25(3):303–14. PMID:26288527

38. Khashab MA, Chithadi KV, Acosta RD, et al. Antibiotic prophylaxis for GI endoscopy. Gastrointest Endosc. 2015 Jan;81(1):81–9. PMID:25442089

39. Aslam A, Wasnik AP, Shi J, et al. Intraductal papillary neoplasm of the bile duct (IPNB): CT and MRI appearance with radiology-pathology correlation. Clin Imaging. 2020 Oct;66:10–7. PMID:32438236

40. Aslan DL, Jessurun J, Gulbahce HE, et al. Endoscopic ultrasound-guided fine needle aspiration features of a pancreatic neoplasm with predominantly intraductal growth and prominent tubular cytomorphology: intraductal tubular carcinoma of the pancreas? Diagn Cytopathol. 2008 Nov;36(11):833–9. PMID:18831024

41. Atiq M, Bhutani MS, Ross WA, et al. Role of endoscopic ultrasonography in evaluation of metastatic lesions to the pancreas: a tertiary cancer center experience. Pancreas. 2013 Apr;42(3):516–23. PMID:23211369

42. Attam R, Arain MA, Bloechl SJ, et al. "Wet suction technique (WEST)": a novel way to enhance the quality of EUS-FNA aspirate. Results of a prospective, single-blind, randomized, controlled trial using a 22-gauge needle for EUS-FNA of solid lesions. Gastrointest Endosc. 2015;81(6):1401–7. PMID:25733127

43. Augustin J, Gabignon C, Scriva A, et al. Testing for ROS1, ALK, MET, and HER2 rearrangements and amplifications in a large series of biliary tract adenocarcinomas. Virchows Arch. 2020 Jul;477(1):33–45. PMID:32447492

44. Avadhani V, Hacihasanoglu E, Memis B, et al. Cytologic predictors of malignancy in bile duct brushings: a multi-reviewer analysis of 60 cases. Mod Pathol. 2017 Sep;30(9):1273–86. PMID:28664934

45. Badiyan SN, Molitoris JK, Chuong MD, et al. The role of radiation therapy for pancreatic cancer in the adjuvant and neoadjuvant settings. Surg Oncol Clin N Am. 2017 Jul;26(3):431–53. PMID:28576181

46. Banales JM, Cardinale V, Carpino G, et al. Expert consensus document: Cholangiocarcinoma: current knowledge and future perspectives consensus statement from the European Network for the Study of Cholangiocarcinoma (ENS-CCA). Nat Rev Gastroenterol Hepatol. 2016 May;13(5):261–80. PMID:27095655

47. Bang JY, Kirtane S, Krall K, et al. In memoriam: Fine-needle aspiration, birth: fine-needle biopsy: the changing trend in endoscopic ultrasound-guided tissue acquisition. Dig Endosc. 2019 Mar;31(2):197–202. PMID:30256458

48. Bang JY, Navaneethan U, Hasan MK, et al. Endoscopic ultrasound-guided specimen collection and evaluation techniques affect diagnostic accuracy. Clin Gastroenterol Hepatol. 2018 Nov;16(11):1820–1828.e4. PMID:29535060

49. Banks PA, Bollen TL, Dervenis C, et al. Classification of acute pancreatitis 2012: revision of the Atlanta classification and definitions by international consensus. Gut. 2013 Jan;62(1):102–11. PMID:23100216

50. Bardales RH, Centeno B, Mallery JS, et al. Endoscopic ultrasound-guided fine-needle aspiration cytology diagnosis of solid-pseudopapillary tumor of the pancreas: a rare neoplasm of elusive origin but characteristic cytomorphologic features. Am J Clin Pathol. 2004 May;121(5):654–62. PMID:15151205

51. Baron TH. Endoscopic US for metastases to the pancreas: chasing the satellites. Gastrointest Endosc. 2005 May;61(6):697–9. PMID:15855974

52. Barr Fritcher EG, Caudill JL, Blue JE, et al. Identification of malignant cytologic criteria in pancreatobiliary brushings with corresponding positive fluorescence in situ hybridization results. Am J Clin Pathol. 2011 Sep;136(3):442–9. PMID:21846921

53. Barr Fritcher EG, Kipp BR, Voss JS, et al. Primary sclerosing cholangitis patients with serial polysomy fluorescence in situ hybridization results are at increased risk of cholangiocarcinoma. Am J Gastroenterol. 2011 Nov;106(11):2023–8. PMID:21844920

54. Barr Fritcher EG, Voss JS, Brankley SM, et al. An optimized set of fluorescence in situ hybridization probes for detection of pancreatobiliary tract cancer in cytology brush samples. Gastroenterology. 2015 Dec;149(7):1813–1824.e1. PMID:26327129

55. Basar O, Brugge WR. My treatment approach: pancreatic cysts. Mayo Clin Proc. 2017 Oct;92(10):1519–31. PMID:28890216
56. Basar O, Yuksel O, Yang DJ, et al. Feasibility and safety of microforceps biopsy in the diagnosis of pancreatic cysts. Gastrointest Endosc. 2018 Jul;88(1):79–86. PMID:29510146
57. Basturk O, Adsay V, Askan G, et al. Intraductal tubulopapillary neoplasm of the pancreas: a clinicopathologic and immunohistochemical analysis of 33 cases. Am J Surg Pathol. 2017 Mar;41(3):313–25. PMID:27984235
58. Basturk O, Berger MF, Yamaguchi H, et al. Pancreatic intraductal tubulopapillary neoplasm is genetically distinct from intraductal papillary mucinous neoplasm and ductal adenocarcinoma. Mod Pathol. 2017 Dec;30(12):1760–72. PMID:28776573
59. Basturk O, Chung SM, Hruban RH, et al. Distinct pathways of pathogenesis of intraductal oncocytic papillary neoplasms and intraductal papillary mucinous neoplasms of the pancreas. Virchows Arch. 2016 Nov;469(5):523–32. PMID:27591765
60. Basturk O, Hong SM, Wood LD, et al. A revised classification system and recommendations from the Baltimore Consensus Meeting for Neoplastic Precursor Lesions in the Pancreas. Am J Surg Pathol. 2015 Dec;39(12):1730–41. PMID:26559377
61. Basturk O, Khayyata S, Klimstra DS, et al. Preferential expression of MUC6 in oncocytic and pancreatobiliary types of intraductal papillary neoplasms highlights a pyloropancreatic pathway, distinct from the intestinal pathway, in pancreatic carcinogenesis. Am J Surg Pathol. 2010 Mar;34(3):364–70. PMID:20139757
62. Basturk O, Weigelt B, Adsay V, et al. Sclerosing epithelioid mesenchymal neoplasm of the pancreas - a proposed new entity. Mod Pathol. 2020 Mar;33(3):456–67. PMID:31383964
63. Basturk O, Zamboni G, Klimstra DS, et al. Intraductal and papillary variants of acinar cell carcinomas: a new addition to the challenging differential diagnosis of intraductal neoplasms. Am J Surg Pathol. 2007 Mar;31(3):363–70. PMID:17325477
64. Bätge B, Bosslet K, Sedlacek HH, et al. Monoclonal antibodies against CEA-related components discriminate between pancreatic duct type carcinomas and nonneoplastic duct lesions as well as nonduct type neoplasias. Virchows Arch A Pathol Anat Histopathol. 1986;408(4):361–74. PMID:3004013
65. Bayne LJ, Beatty GL, Jhala N, et al. Tumor-derived granulocyte-macrophage colony-stimulating factor regulates myeloid inflammation and T cell immunity in pancreatic cancer. Cancer Cell. 2012 Jun 12;21(6):822–35. PMID:22698406
66. Belinsky MG, Rink L, Cai KQ, et al. Somatic loss of function mutations in neurofibromin 1 and MYC associated factor X genes identified by exome-wide sequencing in a wild-type GIST case. BMC Cancer. 2015 Nov 10;15:887. PMID:26555092
67. Bellevicine C, Malapelle U, Vigliar E, et al. How to prepare cytological samples for molecular testing. J Clin Pathol. 2017 Oct;70(10):819–26. PMID:28739858
68. Bellizzi AM, Stelow EB. Pancreatic cytopathology: a practical approach and review. Arch Pathol Lab Med. 2009 Mar;133(3):388–404. PMID:19260745
69. Belsley NA, Pitman MB, Lauwers GY, et al. Serous cystadenoma of the pancreas: limitations and pitfalls of endoscopic ultrasound-guided fine-needle aspiration biopsy. Cancer. 2008 Apr 25;114(2):102–10. PMID:18260088
70. Benning TL, Silverman JF, Berns LA, et al. Fine needle aspiration of metastatic and hematologic malignancies clinically mimicking pancreatic carcinoma. Acta Cytol. 1992 Jul-Aug;36(4):471–6. PMID:1636336
71. Bergeron JP, Perry KD, Houser PM, et al. Endoscopic ultrasound-guided pancreatic fine-needle aspiration: potential pitfalls in one institution's experience of 1212 procedures. Cancer Cytopathol. 2015 Feb;123(2):98–107. PMID:25410732
72. Bergmann F. [Pancreatic acinar neoplasms : comparative molecular characterization]. Pathologe. 2016 Nov;37(Suppl 2):191–5. German. PMID:27807633
73. Betés M, González Vázquez S, Bojórquez A, et al. Metastatic tumors in the pancreas: the role of endoscopic ultrasound-guided fine-needle aspiration. Rev Esp Enferm Dig. 2019 May;111(5):345–50. PMID:30746956
74. Betz BL, Dixon CA, Weigelin HC, et al. The use of stained cytologic direct smears for ALK gene rearrangement analysis of lung adenocarcinoma. Cancer Cytopathol. 2013 Sep;121(9):489–99. PMID:23536384
75. Beyer G, Habtezion A, Werner J, et al. Chronic pancreatitis. Lancet. 2020 Aug 15;396(10249):499–512. PMID:32798493
76. Bhatnagar R, Olson MT, Fishman EK, et al. Solid-pseudopapillary neoplasm of the pancreas: cytomorphologic findings and literature review. Acta Cytol. 2014;58(4):347–55. PMID:24969629
77. Bishop JA, Sharma R, Illei PB. Napsin A and thyroid transcription factor-1 expression in carcinomas of the lung, breast, pancreas, colon, kidney, thyroid, and malignant mesothelioma. Hum Pathol. 2010 Jan;41(1):20–5. PMID:19740516
77A. Blandamura S, Parenti A, Famengo B, et al. Three cases of pancreatic serous cystadenoma and endocrine tumour. J Clin Pathol. 2007 Mar;60(3):278–82. PMID:16644876
78. Boikos SA, Pappo AS, Killian JK, et al. Molecular subtypes of KIT/PDGFRA wild-type gastrointestinal stromal tumors: a report from the National Institutes of Health Gastrointestinal Stromal Tumor Clinic. JAMA Oncol. 2016 Jul 1;2(7):922–8. PMID:27011036
79. Boldorini R, Paganotti A, Sartori M, et al. Fluorescence in situ hybridisation in the cytological diagnosis of pancreatobiliary tumours. Pathology. 2011 Jun;43(4):335–9. PMID:21519286
80. Bollen TL, Wessels FJ. Radiological workup of cystic neoplasms of the pancreas. Visc Med. 2018 Jul;34(3):182–90. PMID:30140683
81. Borhani AA, Fasanella KE, Iranpour N, et al. Lymphoepithelial cyst of pancreas: spectrum of radiological findings with pathologic correlation. Abdom Radiol (NY). 2017 Mar;42(3):877–83. PMID:27738791
82. Boutsen L, Jouret-Mourin A, Borbath I, et al. Accuracy of pancreatic neuroendocrine tumour grading by endoscopic ultrasound-guided fine needle aspiration: analysis of a large cohort and perspectives for improvement. Neuroendocrinology. 2018;106(2):158–66. PMID:28494461
83. Bowlus CL, Olson KA, Gershwin ME. Evaluation of indeterminate biliary strictures. Nat Rev Gastroenterol Hepatol. 2016 Jan;13(1):28–37. PMID:26526122
84. Boxhoorn L, Voermans RP, Bouwense SA, et al. Acute pancreatitis. Lancet. 2020 Sep 5;396(10252):726–34. PMID:32891214
85. Boyd S, Vannas M, Jokelainen K, et al. Suspicious brush cytology is an indication for liver transplantation evaluation in primary sclerosing cholangitis. World J Gastroenterol. 2017 Sep 7;23(33):6147–54. PMID:28970730
86. Brandt KR, Charboneau JW, Stephens DH, et al. CT- and US-guided biopsy of the pancreas. Radiology. 1993 Apr;187(1):99–104. PMID:8451443
87. Brosens LA, Leguit RJ, Vleggaar FP, et al. EUS-guided FNA cytology diagnosis of paraduodenal pancreatitis (groove pancreatitis) with numerous giant cells: conservative management allowed by cytological and radiological correlation. Cytopathology. 2015 Apr;26(2):122–5. PMID:24650015
88. Brugge WR. Cyst fluid: moving beyond the carcinoembryonic antigen. Gastrointest Endosc. 2015 Dec;82(6):1070–1. PMID:26264436
89. Brugge WR. Diagnosis and management of cystic lesions of the pancreas. J Gastrointest Oncol. 2015 Aug;6(4):375–88. PMID:26261724
90. Brugge WR. The role of EUS in the diagnosis of cystic lesions of the pancreas. Gastrointest Endosc. 2000 Dec;52(6 Suppl):S18–22. PMID:11115943
91. Brugge WR, Lewandrowski K, Lee-Lewandrowski E, et al. Diagnosis of pancreatic cystic neoplasms: a report of the cooperative pancreatic cyst study. Gastroenterology. 2004 May;126(5):1330–6. PMID:15131794
92. Buisine MP, Devisme L, Degand P, et al. Developmental mucin gene expression in the gastroduodenal tract and accessory digestive glands. II. Duodenum and liver, gallbladder, and pancreas. J Histochem Cytochem. 2000 Dec;48(12):1667–76. PMID:11101635
93. Burford H, Baloch Z, Liu X, et al. E-cadherin/beta-catenin and CD10: a limited immunohistochemical panel to distinguish pancreatic endocrine neoplasm from solid pseudopapillary neoplasm of the pancreas on endoscopic ultrasound-guided fine-needle aspirates of the pancreas. Am J Clin Pathol. 2009 Dec;132(6):831–9. PMID:19926573
94. Burnett AS, Calvert TJ, Chokshi RJ. Sensitivity of endoscopic retrograde cholangiopancreatography standard cytology: 10-y review of the literature. J Surg Res. 2013 Sep;184(1):304–11. PMID:23866788
95. Cai G, Bernstein J, Aslanian HR, et al. Endoscopic ultrasound-guided fine-needle aspiration biopsy of autoimmune pancreatitis: diagnostic clues and pitfalls. J Am Soc Cytopathol. 2015 Jul-Aug;4(4):211–7. PMID:31051756
96. Canberk S, LiVolsi VA, Baloch Z. Oncocytic lesions of the neuroendocrine system. Adv Anat Pathol. 2014 Mar;21(2):69–82. PMID:24508690
97. Canepa M, Yao R, Nam GH, et al. Cytomorphology of intraductal papillary neoplasm of the biliary tract. Diagn Cytopathol. 2019 Sep;47(9):922–6. PMID:31116517
98. Canto MI, Almario JA, Schulick RD, et al. Risk of neoplastic progression in individuals at high risk for pancreatic cancer undergoing long-term surveillance. Gastroenterology. 2018 Sep;155(3):740–751.e2. PMID:29803839
99. Capurso G, Archibugi L, Petrone MC, et al. Slow-pull compared to suction technique for EUS-guided sampling of pancreatic solid lesions: a meta-analysis of randomized controlled trials. Endosc Int Open. 2020 May;8(5):E636–43. PMID:32355882
100. Carr RA, Yip-Schneider MT, Simpson RE, et al. Pancreatic cyst fluid glucose: rapid, inexpensive, and accurate diagnosis of mucinous pancreatic cysts. Surgery. 2018 Mar;163(3):600–5. PMID:29241991
101. Carson HJ, Green LK, Castelli MJ, et al. Utilization of fine-needle aspiration biopsy in the diagnosis of metastatic tumors to the pancreas. Diagn Cytopathol. 1995 Feb;12(1):8–13. PMID:7789254
102. Carvalho D, Loureiro R, Pavão Borges V, et al. Paraduodenal pancreatitis: three cases with different therapeutic approaches. GE Port J Gastroenterol. 2017 Mar;24(2):89–94. PMID:28848788
103. Cavallini A, Falconi M, Bortesi L, et al. Pancreatoblastoma in adults: a review of the literature. Pancreatology. 2009;9(1-2):73–80. PMID:19077457
104. Centeno BA. Metastases, secondary tumors, and lymphomas of the pancreas. Monogr Clin Cytol. 2020;26:109–21. PMID:32987382
105. Centeno BA, Pitman MB. Fine needle aspiration biopsy of the pancreas. New York (NY): Taylor & Francis; 1999.
106. Centeno BA, Stelow EB, Pitman MB, editors. Pancreatic cytohistology. Cambridge (UK): Cambridge University Press; 2015. (Cytohistology of small tissue samples series)
107. Centeno BA, Stockwell JW, Lewandrowski KB. Cyst fluid cytology and chemical features in a case of lymphoepithelial cyst of the pancreas: a rare and difficult preoperative diagnosis. Diagn Cytopathol. 1999 Nov;21(5):328–30. PMID:10527479
108. Centeno BA, Thomas SC. Non-neoplastic and neoplastic cysts of the pancreas. Monogr Clin Cytol. 2020;26:53–73. PMID:32987387
109. Centeno BA, Thomas SC. Non-neoplastic masses of the pancreas. Monogr Clin Cytol. 2020;26:42–52. PMID:32987396
110. Chadwick BE. Beyond cytomorphology: expanding the diagnostic potential for biliary cytology. Diagn Cytopathol. 2012 Jun;40(6):536–41. PMID:22619128
111. Chadwick BE, Layfield LJ, Witt BL, et al. Significance of atypia in pancreatic and bile duct brushings: follow-up analysis of the categories atypical and suspicious for malignancy. Diagn Cytopathol. 2014 Apr;42(4):285–91. PMID:24167030
112. Chai SM, Herba K, Kumarasinghe MP, et al. Optimizing the multimodal approach to pancreatic cyst fluid diagnosis: developing a volume-based triage protocol. Cancer Cytopathol. 2013 Feb;121(2):86–100. PMID:22961878
113. Chaiteerakij R, Barr Fritcher EG, Angsuwatcharakon P, et al. Fluorescence in situ hybridization compared with conventional cytology for the diagnosis of malignant biliary tract strictures in Asian patients. Gastrointest Endosc. 2016 Jun;83(6):1228–35. PMID:26684604
114. Chan ES, Alexander J, Swanson PE, et al. PDX-1, CDX-2, TTF-1, and CK7: a reliable immunohistochemical panel for pancreatic neuroendocrine neoplasms. Am J Surg Pathol. 2012 May;36(5):737–43. PMID:22498824
115. Chang KJ, Katz KD, Durbin TE, et al. Endoscopic ultrasound-guided fine-needle aspiration. Gastrointest Endosc. 1994 Nov-Dec;40(6):694–9. PMID:7859967
116. Chang YR, Park JK, Jang JY, et al. Incidental pancreatic cystic neoplasms in an asymptomatic healthy population of 21,745 individuals: large-scale, single-center cohort study. Medicine (Baltimore). 2016 Dec;95(51):e5535. PMID:28002329
117. Chantrill LA, Nagrial AM, Watson C, et al. Precision medicine for advanced pancreas cancer: the Individualized Molecular Pancreatic Cancer Therapy (IMPaCT) trial. Clin Cancer Res. 2015 May 1;21(9):2029–37. PMID:25896973
118. Chari ST, Kloeppel G, Zhang L, et al. Histopathologic and clinical subtypes of autoimmune pancreatitis: the Honolulu consensus document. Pancreas. 2010 Jul;39(5):549–54. PMID:20562576
119. Charlesworth M, Verbeke CS, Falk GA, et al. Pancreatic lesions in von Hippel-Lindau disease? A systematic review and meta-synthesis of the literature. J Gastrointest Surg. 2012 Jul;16(7):1422–8. PMID:22370733
120. Chauhan A, Sanchez-Avila M, Manivel J, et al. Optimization of immunophenotypic panel to differentiate upper from lower gastrointestinal adenocarcinomas: analysis of new and traditional markers. Appl Immunohistochem Mol Morphol. 2021 Jan;29(1):13–9. PMID:33295746

121. Chavali P, Prayaga AK, Tandon A, et al. Utility of immunochemistry in cytology. J Cytol. 2016 Apr-Jun;33(2):71–5. PMID:27279681
122. Chebib I, Albanese E, Scourtas A, et al. Inspissated cyst fluid in endoscopic ultrasound-guided fine needle aspiration of pancreatic cysts. Diagn Cytopathol. 2018 May;46(5):395–9. PMID:29476610
123. Chen AL, Misdraji J, Brugge WR, et al. Acinar cell cystadenoma: a challenging cytology diagnosis, facilitated by Moray® micro-forceps biopsy. Diagn Cytopathol. 2017 Jun;45(6):557–60. PMID:28236434
124. Chen B, Zhao Y, Gu J, et al. Papanicolaou Society of Cytopathology new guidelines have a greater ability of risk stratification for pancreatic endoscopic ultrasound-guided fine-needle aspiration specimens. Oncotarget. 2017 Jan 31;8(5):8154–61. PMID:28042957
125. Chen C, Jing W, Gulati P, et al. Melanocytic differentiation in a solid pseudopapillary tumor of the pancreas. J Gastroenterol. 2004 Jun;39(6):579–83. PMID:15235877
126. Chen L, Huang K, Himmelfarb EA, et al. Diagnostic value of maspin in distinguishing adenocarcinoma from benign biliary epithelium on endoscopic bile duct biopsy. Hum Pathol. 2015 Nov;46(11):1647–54. PMID:26362203
127. Chen M, Zhang H, Hu Y, et al. Adult pancreatoblastoma: a case report and clinicopathological review of the literature. Clin Imaging. 2018 Jul-Aug;50:324–9. PMID:29753278
128. Chen S, Lin J, Wang X, et al. EUS-guided FNA cytology of pancreatic neuroendocrine tumour (PanNET): a retrospective study of 132 cases over an 18-year period in a single institution. Cytopathology. 2014 Dec;25(6):396–403. PMID:24635775
129. Chen S, Wang X, Lin J. Fine needle aspiration of oncocytic variants of pancreatic neuroendocrine tumor: a report of three misdiagnosed cases. Acta Cytol. 2014;58(2):131–7. PMID:24335139
130. Chhieng DC, Benson E, Eltoum I, et al. MUC1 and MUC2 expression in pancreatic ductal carcinoma obtained by fine-needle aspiration. Cancer. 2003 Dec 25;99(6):365–71. PMID:14681945
131. Chi Z, Wu HH, Cramer H, et al. Cytomorphological features useful to prevent errors in the diagnosis of pancreatic adenocarcinoma by fine needle aspiration cytology. Acta Cytol. 2017;61(1):7–16. PMID:27889759
132. Chmielecki J, Hutchinson KE, Frampton GM, et al. Comprehensive genomic profiling of pancreatic acinar cell carcinomas identifies recurrent RAF fusions and frequent inactivation of DNA repair genes. Cancer Discov. 2014 Dec;4(12):1398–405. PMID:25266736
133. Choi JY, Kim MJ, Lee JY, et al. Typical and atypical manifestations of serous cystadenoma of the pancreas: imaging findings with pathologic correlation. AJR Am J Roentgenol. 2009 Jul;193(1):136–42. PMID:19542405
134. Choi WT, Swanson PE, Grieco VS, et al. The outcomes of "atypical" and "suspicious" bile duct brushings in the identification of pancreaticobiliary tumors: follow-up analysis of surgical resection specimens. Diagn Cytopathol. 2015 Nov;43(11):885–91. PMID:26221777
135. Chu LC, Singhi AD, Haroun RR, et al. The many faces of pancreatic serous cystadenoma: radiologic and pathologic correlation. Diagn Interv Imaging. 2017 Mar;98(3):191–202. PMID:27614585
136. Chuang SC, Lee KT, Tsai KB, et al. Immunohistochemical study of DPC4 and p53 proteins in gallbladder and bile duct cancers. World J Surg. 2004 Oct;28(10):995–1000. PMID:15573254
137. Chute DJ, Stelow EB. Fine-needle aspiration features of paraduodenal pancreatitis (groove pancreatitis): a report of three cases. Diagn Cytopathol. 2012 Dec;40(12):1116–21. PMID:21548125
138. Cibas ES, Ali SZ. The 2017 Bethesda system for reporting thyroid cytopathology. Thyroid. 2017 Nov;27(11):1341–6. PMID:29091573
139. Cibas ES, Ducatman BS. Cytology: diagnostic principles and clinical correlates. 5th ed. New York (NY): Elsevier; 2019.
140. Cizginer S, Turner BG, Bilge AR, et al. Cyst fluid carcinoembryonic antigen is an accurate diagnostic marker of pancreatic mucinous cysts. Pancreas. 2011 Oct;40(7):1024–8. PMID:21775920
141. Cohen MB, Egerter DP, Holly EA, et al. Pancreatic adenocarcinoma: regression analysis to identify improved cytologic criteria. Diagn Cytopathol. 1991;7(4):341–5. PMID:1935510
142. Cohen MB, Wittchow RJ, Johlin FC, et al. Brush cytology of the extrahepatic biliary tract: comparison of cytologic features of adenocarcinoma and benign biliary strictures. Mod Pathol. 1995 Jun;8(5):498–502. PMID:7675767
143. Colán-Hernández J, Sendino O, Loras C, et al. Antibiotic prophylaxis is not required for endoscopic ultrasonography-guided fine-needle aspiration of pancreatic cystic lesions, based on a randomized trial. Gastroenterology. 2020 May;158(6):1642–1649.e1. PMID:31972236
144. Collins BT. Serous cystadenoma of the pancreas with endoscopic ultrasound fine needle aspiration biopsy and surgical correlation. Acta Cytol. 2013;57(3):241–51. PMID:23635954
145. Collins BT, Murad FM, Wang JF, et al. Rapid on-site evaluation for endoscopic ultrasound-guided fine-needle biopsy of the pancreas decreases the incidence of repeat biopsy procedures. Cancer Cytopathol. 2013 Sep;121(9):518–24. PMID:23983161
146. Collins JA, Ali SZ, VandenBussche CJ. Pancreatic cytopathology. Surg Pathol Clin. 2016 Dec;9(4):661–76. PMID:27926365
147. Colonna J, Plaza JA, Frankel WL, et al. Serous cystadenoma of the pancreas: clinical and pathological features in 33 patients. Pancreatology. 2008;8(2):135–41. PMID:18382099
148. Colovic RB, Grubor NM, Micev MT, et al. Cystic lymphangioma of the pancreas. World J Gastroenterol. 2008 Nov 28;14(44):6873–5. PMID:19058318
149. Comper F, Antonello D, Beghelli S, et al. Expression pattern of claudins 5 and 7 distinguishes solid-pseudopapillary from pancreatoblastoma, acinar cell and endocrine tumors of the pancreas. Am J Surg Pathol. 2009 May;33(5):768–74. PMID:19194274
150. Conrad R, Castelino-Prabhu S, Cobb C, et al. Cytopathology of the pancreatobiliary tract-the agony, and sometimes, the ease of it. J Gastrointest Oncol. 2013 Jun;4(2):210–9. PMID:23730518
151. Conti CB, Cereatti F, Grassia R. Endoscopic ultrasound-guided sampling of solid pancreatic masses: the fine needle aspiration or fine needle biopsy dilemma. Is the best needle yet to come? World J Gastrointest Endosc. 2019 Aug 16;11(8):454–71. PMID:31523377
152. Conway AB, Cook SM, Samad A, et al. Large platelet aggregates in endoscopic ultrasound-guided fine-needle aspiration of the pancreas and peripancreatic region: a clue for the diagnosis of intrapancreatic or accessory spleen. Diagn Cytopathol. 2013 Aug;41(8):661–72. PMID:22045629
153. Conwell DL, Lee LS, Yadav D, et al. American Pancreatic Association Practice Guidelines in Chronic Pancreatitis: evidence-based report on diagnostic guidelines. Pancreas. 2014 Nov;43(8):1143–62. PMID:25333398
154. Costa F, Casaca R, Monteiro C, et al. Oesophageal GIST. BMJ Case Rep. 2020 Oct 31;13(10):e238058. PMID:33130586
155. Cowan ML, VandenBussche CJ. Cancer of unknown primary: ancillary testing of cytologic and small biopsy specimens in the era of targeted therapy. Cancer Cytopathol. 2018 Aug;126 Suppl 8:724–37. PMID:30156769
156. Crippa S, Capurso G, Cammà C, et al. Risk of pancreatic malignancy and mortality in branch-duct IPMNs undergoing surveillance: a systematic review and meta-analysis. Dig Liver Dis. 2016 May;48(5):473–9. PMID:26965783
157. da Cunha Santos G, Saieg MA, Troncone G, et al. Cytological preparations for molecular analysis: a review of technical procedures, advantages and limitations for referring samples for testing. Cytopathology. 2018 Apr;29(2):125–32. PMID:29575423
158. Dabbs DJ, Abendroth CS, Grenko RT, et al. Immunocytochemistry on the ThinPrep processor. Diagn Cytopathol. 1997 Nov;17(5):388–92. PMID:9360054
159. Dabbs DJ, Wang X. Immunocytochemistry on cytologic specimens of limited quantity. Diagn Cytopathol. 1998 Feb;18(2):166–9. PMID:9484646
160. da Cunha Santos G, Saieg MA. Preanalytic specimen triage: smears, cell blocks, cytospin preparations, transport media, and cytobanking. Cancer Cytopathol. 2017 Jun;125 S6:455–64. PMID:28609003
161. Daly MB, Pal T, Berry MP, et al. Genetic/familial high-risk assessment: breast, ovarian, and pancreatic, Version 2.2021, NCCN Clinical Practice Guidelines in Oncology. J Natl Compr Canc Netw. 2021 Jan 6;19(1):77–102. PMID:33406487
162. Das KK, Xiao H, Geng X, et al. mAb Das-1 is specific for high-risk and malignant intraductal papillary mucinous neoplasm (IPMN). Gut. 2014 Oct;63(10):1626–34. PMID:24277729
163. Das S, Ghosh R, Sen A, et al. Fine needle aspiration cytology diagnosis of a pancreatoblastoma in an infant: case report with a summary of prior published cases. Cytopathology. 2016 Dec;27(6):479–82. PMID:27038102
164. Date K, Okabayashi T, Shima Y, et al. Clinicopathological features and surgical outcomes of intraductal tubulopapillary neoplasm of the pancreas: a systematic review. Langenbecks Arch Surg. 2016 Jun;401(4):439–47. PMID:27001682
165. de Bellis M, Sherman S, Fogel EL, et al. Tissue sampling at ERCP in suspected malignant biliary strictures (part 2). Gastrointest Endosc. 2002 Nov;56(5):720–30. PMID:12397282
166. de Biase D, Acquaviva G, Visani M, et al. Molecular diagnostic of solid tumor using a next generation sequencing custom-designed multi-gene panel. Diagnostics (Basel). 2020 Apr 23;10(4):250. PMID:32340363
167. de Biase D, Visani M, Acquaviva G, et al. The role of next-generation sequencing in the cytologic diagnosis of pancreatic lesions. Arch Pathol Lab Med. 2018 Apr;142(4):458–64. PMID:29565213
168. de Moura DTH, McCarty TR, Jirapinyo P, et al. Endoscopic ultrasound fine-needle aspiration versus fine-needle biopsy for lymph node diagnosis: a large multicenter comparative analysis. Clin Endosc. 2020 Sep;53(5):600–10. PMID:31794654
169. de Moura DTH, McCarty TR, Jirapinyo P, et al. Evaluation of endoscopic ultrasound fine-needle aspiration versus fine-needle biopsy and impact of rapid on-site evaluation for pancreatic masses. Endosc Int Open. 2020 Jun;8(6):E738–47. PMID:32490158
170. de Moura DTH, Ryou M, de Moura EGH, et al. Endoscopic ultrasound-guided fine needle aspiration and endoscopic retrograde cholangiopancreatography-based tissue sampling in suspected malignant biliary strictures: a meta-analysis of same-session procedures. Clin Endosc. 2020 Jul;53(4):417–28. PMID:31684700
171. Del Poggio P, Buonocore M. Cystic tumors of the liver: a practical approach. World J Gastroenterol. 2008 Jun 21;14(23):3616–20. PMID:18595127
172. Denda T, Kamoshida S, Kawamura J, et al. Optimal antigen retrieval for ethanol-fixed cytologic smears. Cancer Cytopathol. 2012 Jun 25;120(3):167–76. PMID:22434540
173. Denda T, Kamoshida S, Kawamura J, et al. Rapid immunocytochemistry with simple heat-induced antigen retrieval technique for improvement in the quality of cytological diagnosis. J Histochem Cytochem. 2013 Dec;61(12):920–30. PMID:24004858
174. Deshpande V, Gupta R, Sainani N, et al. Subclassification of autoimmune pancreatitis: a histologic classification with clinical significance. Am J Surg Pathol. 2011 Jan;35(1):26–35. PMID:21164284
175. Deshpande V, Mino-Kenudson M, Brugge WR, et al. Endoscopic ultrasound guided fine needle aspiration biopsy of autoimmune pancreatitis: diagnostic criteria and pitfalls. Am J Surg Pathol. 2005 Nov;29(11):1464–71. PMID:16224213
176. Deshpande V, Zen Y, Chan JK, et al. Consensus statement on the pathology of IgG4-related disease. Mod Pathol. 2012 Sep;25(9):1181–92. PMID:22596100
177. De Souza AL, Saif MW. Platinum-based therapy in adenosquamous pancreatic cancer: experience at two institutions. JOP. 2014 Mar 10;15(2):144–6. PMID:24618440
178. Detlefsen S, Sipos B, Feyerabend B, et al. Pancreatic fibrosis associated with age and ductal papillary hyperplasia. Virchows Arch. 2005 Nov;447(5):800–5. PMID:16021508
179. Detlefsen S, Zamboni G, Frulloni L, et al. Clinical features and relapse rates after surgery in type 1 autoimmune pancreatitis differ from type 2: a study of 114 surgically treated European patients. Pancreatology. 2012 May-Jun;12(3):276–83. PMID:22687385
180. DeWitt J, Jowell P, Leblanc J, et al. EUS-guided FNA of pancreatic metastases: a multicenter experience. Gastrointest Endosc. 2005 May;61(6):689–96. PMID:15855973
181. Dhall D, Klimstra DS. The cellular composition of osteoclastlike giant cell-containing tumors of the pancreatobiliary tree. Am J Surg Pathol. 2008 Feb;32(2):335–7. PMID:18223338
182. Dhillon J. Non-ductal tumors of the pancreas. Monogr Clin Cytol. 2020;26:92–108. PMID:32987393
183. Di Mitri R, Mocciaro F, Antonini F, et al. Stylet slow-pull vs. standard suction technique for endoscopic ultrasound-guided fine needle biopsy in pancreatic solid lesions using 20 gauge Procore™ needle: a multicenter randomized trial. Dig Liver Dis. 2020 Feb;52(2):178–84. PMID:31601535
184. Dim DC, Jiang F, Qiu Q, et al. The usefulness of S100P, mesothelin, fascin, prostate stem cell antigen, and 14-3-3 sigma in diagnosing pancreatic adenocarcinoma in cytological specimens obtained by endoscopic ultrasound guided fine-needle aspiration. Diagn Cytopathol. 2014 Mar;42(3):193–9. PMID:21538952
185. Disanto MG, Ambrosio MR, Rocca BJ, et al. Optimal minimal panels of immunohistochemistry for diagnosis of B-cell lymphoma for application in countries with limited resources and for triaging cases before referral to specialist centers. Am J Clin Pathol. 2016 May;145(5):687–95. PMID:27247372
186. Doherty B, Nambudiri VE, Palmer WC. Update on the diagnosis and treatment of cholangiocarcinoma. Curr Gastroenterol Rep. 2017 Jan;19(1):2. PMID:28110453
187. Domanski HA, Akerman M, Rissler P, et al. Fine-needle aspiration of soft tissue leiomyosarcoma: an analysis of the most

common cytologic findings and the value of ancillary techniques. Diagn Cytopathol. 2006 Sep;34(9):597–604. PMID:16900474
188. D'Onofrio M, De Robertis R, Barbi E, et al. Ultrasound-guided percutaneous fine-needle aspiration of solid pancreatic neoplasms: 10-year experience with more than 2,000 cases and a review of the literature. Eur Radiol. 2016 Jun;26(6):1801–7. PMID:26373764
189. Dowen SE, Crnogorac-Jurcevic T, Gangeswaran R, et al. Expression of S100P and its novel binding partner S100PBPR in early pancreatic cancer. Am J Pathol. 2005 Jan;166(1):81–92. PMID:15632002
190. Doxtader EE, Sturgis CD, Dyhdalo KS. Cystic pancreatic schwannoma diagnosed by endoscopic ultrasound-guided fine needle aspiration. Diagn Cytopathol. 2018 Oct;46(10):883–5. PMID:30146793
191. Dromain C, Déandréis D, Scoazec JY, et al. Imaging of neuroendocrine tumors of the pancreas. Diagn Interv Imaging. 2016 Dec;97(12):1241–57. PMID:27876341
192. Dudley JC, Zheng Z, McDonald T, et al. Next-generation sequencing and fluorescence in situ hybridization have comparable performance characteristics in the analysis of pancreaticobiliary brushings for malignancy. J Mol Diagn. 2016 Jan;18(1):124–30. PMID:26596524
193. Dumonceau JM, Delhaye M, Charette N, et al. Challenging biliary strictures: pathophysiological features, differential diagnosis, diagnostic algorithms, and new clinically relevant biomarkers - part 1. Therap Adv Gastroenterol. 2020 Jun 16;13:1756284820927292. PMID:32595761
194. Duorui N, Shi B, Zhang T, et al. The contemporary trend in worsening prognosis of pancreatic acinar cell carcinoma: a population-based study. PLoS One. 2020 Dec 17;15(12):e0243164. PMID:33332471
195. Eisen GM, Dominitz JA, Faigel DO, et al. Guidelines for credentialing and granting privileges for endoscopic ultrasound. Gastrointest Endosc. 2001 Dec;54(6):811–4. PMID:11726873
196. El Hajj II, LeBlanc JK, Sherman S, et al. Endoscopic ultrasound-guided biopsy of pancreatic metastases: a large single-center experience. Pancreas. 2013 Apr;42(3):524–30. PMID:23146924
197. Elek G, Györkeres T, Schäfer E, et al. Early diagnosis of pancreatobiliary duct malignancies by brush cytology and biopsy. Pathol Oncol Res. 2005;11(3):145–55. PMID:16195768
198. El Hussein S, Khader SN. Cytopathology of anaplastic carcinoma of the pancreas: review of a rare entity and description of a variant with signet ring cell features. Diagn Cytopathol. 2019 Sep;47(9):956–60. PMID:31254330
199. Eloubeidi MA, Jhala D, Chhieng DC, et al. Yield of endoscopic ultrasound-guided fine-needle aspiration biopsy in patients with suspected pancreatic carcinoma. Cancer. 2003 Oct 25;99(5):285–92. PMID:14579295
200. Eloubeidi MA, Tamhane A, Jhala N, et al. Agreement between rapid onsite and final cytologic interpretations of EUS-guided FNA specimens: implications for the endosonographer and patient management. Am J Gastroenterol. 2006 Dec;101(12):2841–7. PMID:17026562
201. Elta GH, Enestvedt BK, Sauer BG, et al. ACG Clinical Guideline: diagnosis and management of pancreatic cysts. Am J Gastroenterol. 2018 Apr;113(4):464–79. PMID:29485131
202. Ercan M, Aziret M, Bal A, et al. Pancreatic schwannoma: a rare case and a brief literature review. Int J Surg Case Rep. 2016;22:101–4. PMID:27084984
203. Esposito I, Hruban RH, Verbeke C, et al. Guidelines on the histopathology of chronic pancreatitis. Recommendations from the working group for the international consensus guidelines for chronic pancreatitis in collaboration with the International Association of Pancreatology, the American Pancreatic Association, the Japan Pancreas Society, and the European Pancreatic Club. Pancreatology. 2020 Jun;20(4):586–93. PMID:32414657
204. European Study Group on Cystic Tumours of the Pancreas. European evidence-based guidelines on pancreatic cystic neoplasms. Gut. 2018 May;67(5):789–804. PMID:29574408
205. Facchinelli D, Sina S, Boninsegna E, et al. Primary pancreatic lymphoma: clinical presentation, diagnosis, treatment, and outcome. Eur J Haematol. 2020 Oct;105(4):468–75. PMID:32542880
206. Facciorusso A, Wani S, Triantafyllou K, et al. Comparative accuracy of needle sizes and designs for EUS tissue sampling of solid pancreatic masses: a network meta-analysis. Gastrointest Endosc. 2019 Dec;90(6):893–903.e7. PMID:31310744
207. Fadaee N, Sefa T, Das A, et al. Pancreatic leiomyosarcoma: a diagnostic challenge and literature review. BMJ Case Rep. 2019 Nov 27;12(11):e231529. PMID:31780603
208. Falconi M, Bartsch DK, Eriksson B, et al. ENETS Consensus Guidelines for the management of patients with digestive neuroendocrine neoplasms of the digestive system: well-differentiated pancreatic non-functioning tumors. Neuroendocrinology. 2012;95(2):120–34. PMID:22261872
209. Farrell JM, Pang JC, Kim GE, et al. Pancreatic neuroendocrine tumors: accurate grading with Ki-67 index on fine-needle aspiration specimens using the WHO 2010/ENETS criteria. Cancer Cytopathol. 2014 Oct;122(10):770–8. PMID:25044931
210. Feldmann G, Beaty R, Hruban RH, et al. Molecular genetics of pancreatic intraepithelial neoplasia. J Hepatobiliary Pancreat Surg. 2007;14(3):224–32. PMID:17520196
211. Fernández-del Castillo C, Adsay NV. Intraductal papillary mucinous neoplasms of the pancreas. Gastroenterology. 2010 Sep;139(3):708–713.e1–2. PMID:20650278
212. Ferrari A, Brecht IB, Gatta G, et al. Defining and listing very rare cancers of paediatric age: consensus of the Joint Action on Rare Cancers in cooperation with the European Cooperative Study Group for Pediatric Rare Tumors. Eur J Cancer. 2019 Mar;110:120–6. PMID:30785015
213. Ferrucci JT Jr, Wittenberg J, Mueller PR, et al. Diagnosis of abdominal malignancy by radiologic fine-needle aspiration biopsy. AJR Am J Roentgenol. 1980 Feb;134(2):323–30. PMID:6766240
214. Fetsch PA, Simsir A, Brosky K, et al. Comparison of three commonly used cytologic preparations in effusion immunocytochemistry. Diagn Cytopathol. 2002 Jan;26(1):61–6. PMID:11782091
215. Finkelstein P, Sharma R, Picado O, et al. Pancreatic neuroendocrine tumors (panNETs): analysis of overall survival of nonsurgical management versus surgical resection. J Gastrointest Surg. 2017 May;21(5):855–66. PMID:28255853
216. Finkelstein SD, Bibbo M, Kowalski TE, et al. Mutational analysis of cytocentrifugation supernatant fluid from pancreatic solid mass lesions. Diagn Cytopathol. 2014 Aug;42(8):719–25. PMID:24265269
217. Finkelstein SD, Bibbo M, Loren DE, et al. Molecular analysis of centrifugation supernatant fluid from pancreaticobiliary duct samples can improve cancer detection. Acta Cytol. 2012;56(4):439–47. PMID:22846349
218. Fischer MA, Donati O, Heinrich S, et al. Intraductal oncocytic papillary neoplasm of the pancreas: a radio-pathological case study. JOP. 2010 Jan 8;11(1):49–54. PMID:20065553
219. Fite JJ, Ali SZ, VandenBussche CJ. Fine-needle aspiration of a pancreatic neuroendocrine tumor with prominent rhabdoid features. Diagn Cytopathol. 2018 Jul;46(7):600–3. PMID:29359517
220. Fitzpatrick MJ, Hernandez-Barco YG, Krishnan K, et al. Diagnostic yield of the SharkCore EUS-guided fine-needle biopsy. J Am Soc Cytopathol. 2019 Jul-Aug;8(4):212–9. PMID:31076375
221. Fitzpatrick MJ, Hernandez-Barco YG, Krishnan K, et al. Evaluating triage protocols for endoscopic ultrasound-guided fine needle biopsies of the pancreas. J Am Soc Cytopathol. 2020 Sep-Oct;9(5):396–404. PMID:32620535
222. Fong ZV, Brownlee SA, Qadan M, et al. The clinical management of cholangiocarcinoma in the United States and Europe: a comprehensive and evidence-based comparison of guidelines. Ann Surg Oncol. 2021 May;28(5):2660–74. PMID:33646431
223. Fonseca R, Pitman MB. Lymphangioma of the pancreas: a multimodal approach to pre-operative diagnosis. Cytopathology. 2013 Jun;24(3):172–6. PMID:21810124
224. Forsmark CE, Vege SS, Wilcox CM. Acute pancreatitis. N Engl J Med. 2016 Nov 17;375(20):1972–81. PMID:27959604
225. Fowler LJ, Lachar WA. Application of immunohistochemistry to cytology. Arch Pathol Lab Med. 2008 Mar;132(3):373–83. PMID:18318580
226. Fritcher EG, Kipp BR, Halling KC, et al. A multivariable model using advanced cytologic methods for the evaluation of indeterminate pancreatobiliary strictures. Gastroenterology. 2009 Jun;136(7):2180–6. PMID:19232347
227. Fritscher-Ravens A, Sriram PV, Krause C, et al. Detection of pancreatic metastases by EUS-guided fine-needle aspiration. Gastrointest Endosc. 2001 Jan;53(1):65–70. PMID:11154491
228. Fujikura K, Akita M, Ajiki T, et al. Recurrent mutations in APC and CTNNB1 and activated Wnt/β-catenin signaling in intraductal papillary neoplasms of the bile duct: a whole exome sequencing study. Am J Surg Pathol. 2018 Dec;42(12):1674–85. PMID:30212390
229. Fujikura K, Fukumoto T, Ajiki T, et al. Comparative clinicopathological study of biliary intraductal papillary neoplasms and papillary cholangiocarcinomas. Histopathology. 2016 Dec;69(6):950–61. PMID:27410028
230. Fujiwara H, Kohno N, Nakaya S, et al. Lymphoepithelial cyst of the pancreas with sebaceous differentiation. J Gastroenterol. 2000;35(5):396–401. PMID:10832677
231. Fukushima N, Zamboni G. Mucinous cystic neoplasms of the pancreas: update on the surgical pathology and molecular genetics. Semin Diagn Pathol. 2014 Nov;31(6):467–74. PMID:25441310
232. Furmanczyk PS, Grieco VS, Agoff SN. Biliary brush cytology and the detection of cholangiocarcinoma in primary sclerosing cholangitis: evaluation of specific cytomorphologic features and CA19-9 levels. Am J Clin Pathol. 2005 Sep;124(3):355–60. PMID:16191503
233. Furuhata A, Minamiguchi S, Mikami Y, et al. Intraductal tubulopapillary neoplasm with expansile invasive carcinoma of the pancreas diagnosed by endoscopic ultrasonography-guided fine needle aspiration: a case report. Diagn Cytopathol. 2014 Apr;42(4):314–20. PMID:24339429
234. Gagovic V, Spier BJ, DeLee RJ, et al. Endoscopic ultrasound fine-needle aspiration characteristics of primary adenocarcinoma versus other malignant neoplasms of the pancreas. Can J Gastroenterol. 2012 Oct;26(10):691–6. PMID:23061060
235. Gailey MP, Stence AA, Jensen CS, et al. Multiplatform comparison of molecular oncology tests performed on cytology specimens and formalin-fixed, paraffin-embedded tissue. Cancer Cytopathol. 2015 Jan;123(1):30–9. PMID:25186473
236. Galanis C, Zamani A, Cameron JL, et al. Resected serous cystic neoplasms of the pancreas: a review of 158 patients with recommendations for treatment. J Gastrointest Surg. 2007 Jul;11(7):820–6. PMID:17440789
237. Gambella A, Falco EC, Metovic J, et al. Amyloid-rich pancreatic neuroendocrine tumors: a potential diagnostic pitfall in endoscopic ultrasound-guided fine needle aspiration cytology (EUS-FNAC). Endocr Pathol. 2021 Jun;32(2):318–25. PMID:32399832
238. Gao L, Li ZS, Jin ZD, et al. Undifferentiated carcinoma with osteoclast-like giant cells of the pancreas diagnosed by endoscopic ultrasonography-guided fine-needle aspiration. Chin Med J (Engl). 2009 Jul 5;122(13):1598–600. PMID:19719957
239. Garcia-Carracedo D, Turk AT, Fine SA, et al. Loss of PTEN expression is associated with poor prognosis in patients with intraductal papillary mucinous neoplasms of the pancreas. Clin Cancer Res. 2013 Dec 15;19(24):6830–41. PMID:24132918
240. Gasparotto D, Rossi S, Polano M, et al. Quadruple-negative GIST is a sentinel for unrecognized neurofibromatosis type 1 syndrome. Clin Cancer Res. 2017 Jan 1;23(1):273–82. PMID:27390349
241. Geramizadeh B, Moughali M, Shahim-Aein A, et al. False negative and false positive rates in common bile duct brushing cytology, a single center experience. Gastroenterol Hepatol Bed Bench. 2018 Fall;11(4):296–300. PMID:30425807
242. Gheonea DI, Ciurea ME, Săftoiu A, et al. Quantitative RT-PCR analysis of MMR genes on EUS-guided FNA samples from focal pancreatic lesions. Hepatogastroenterology. 2012 May;59(115):916–20. PMID:22020914
243. Ghosh R, Mallik SR, Mathur SR, et al. CD 99 immunocytochemistry in solid pseudopapillary tumor of pancreas: a study on fine-needle aspiration cytology smears. J Cytol. 2013 Jul;30(3):151–5. PMID:24130404
244. Gilani SM, Adeniran AJ, Cai G. Endoscopic ultrasound-guided fine needle aspiration cytologic evaluation of intraductal papillary mucinous neoplasm and mucinous cystic neoplasms of pancreas. Am J Clin Pathol. 2020 Sep 8;154(4):559–70. PMID:32589187
245. Gilbert CM, Monaco SE, Cooper ST, et al. Endoscopic ultrasound-guided fine-needle aspiration of metastases to the pancreas: a study of 25 cases. Cytojournal. 2011;8:7. PMID:21713016
246. Gimeno-García AZ, Elwassief A. How to improve the success of endoscopic ultrasound guided fine needle aspiration cytology in the diagnosis of pancreatic lesions. J Interv Gastroenterol. 2012 Jan-Mar;2(1):31–6. PMID:22586548
246A. Gkolfakis P, Crinò SF, Tziatzios G, et al. Comparative diagnostic performance of end-cutting fine-needle biopsy needles for EUS tissue sampling of solid pancreatic masses: a network meta-analysis. Gastrointest Endosc. 2022 Jun;95(6):1067–77.e15. PMID:35124072
247. Gleeson FC, Kerr SE, Kipp BR, et al. Targeted next generation sequencing of endoscopic ultrasound acquired cytology from ampullary and pancreatic adenocarcinoma has the potential to aid patient stratification for optimal therapy selection. Oncotarget. 2016 Aug 23;7(34):54526–36. PMID:27203738
248. Gokozan HN, Michael CW. Nondiagnostic fine-needle aspirates of the pancreas: a root cause analysis. Cancer Cytopathol. 2020 Oct;128(10):704–14. PMID:32525623

249. Goldberg BB, Pollack HM. Ultrasonic aspiration transducer. Radiology. 1972 Jan;102(1):187–9. PMID:5008144

250. Goldman ML, Naib ZM, Galambos JT, et al. Preoperative diagnosis of pancreatic carcinoma by percutaneous aspiration biopsy. Am J Dig Dis. 1977 Dec;22(12):1076–82. PMID:930906

251. Gonda TA, Glick MP, Sethi A, et al. Polysomy and p16 deletion by fluorescence in situ hybridization in the diagnosis of indeterminate biliary strictures. Gastrointest Endosc. 2012 Jan;75(1):74–9. PMID:22100297

252. Gong Y, Sun X, Michael CW, et al. Immunocytochemistry of serous effusion specimens: a comparison of ThinPrep vs cell block. Diagn Cytopathol. 2003 Jan;28(1):1–5. PMID:12508174

253. Gonzalez Obeso E, Murphy E, Brugge W, et al. Pseudocyst of the pancreas: the role of cytology and special stains for mucin. Cancer. 2009 Apr 25;117(2):101–7. PMID:19365837

254. Goodman P, Kumar D, Balachandran S. Lymphoepithelial cyst of the pancreas. Abdom Imaging. 1994 Mar-Apr;19(2):157–9. PMID:8199550

255. Gordon-Weeks AN, Jones K, Harriss E, et al. Systematic review and meta-analysis of current experience in treating IPNB: clinical and pathological correlates. Ann Surg. 2016 Apr;263(4):656–63. PMID:26501712

256. Govil H, Reddy V, Kluskens L, et al. Brush cytology of the biliary tract: retrospective study of 278 cases with histopathologic correlation. Diagn Cytopathol. 2002 May;26(5):273–7. PMID:11992366

257. Goyal A, Abdul-Karim FW, Yang B, et al. Interobserver agreement in the cytologic grading of atypia in neoplastic pancreatic mucinous cysts with the 2-tiered approach. Cancer Cytopathol. 2016 Dec;124(12):909–16. PMID:27525382

258. Goyal A, Sharaiha RZ, Alperstein SA, et al. Cytologic diagnosis of adenocarcinoma on bile duct brushings in the presence of stent associated changes: a retrospective analysis. Diagn Cytopathol. 2018 Oct;46(10):826–32. PMID:30144340

259. Granter SR, DiNisco S, Granados R. Cytologic diagnosis of papillary cystic neoplasm of the pancreas. Diagn Cytopathol. 1995 Jun;12(4):313–9. PMID:7544719

260. Gress F, Gottlieb K, Cummings O, et al. Endoscopic ultrasound characteristics of mucinous cystic neoplasms of the pancreas. Am J Gastroenterol. 2000 Apr;95(4):961–5. PMID:10763945

261. Gress TM, Wallrapp C, Frohme M, et al. Identification of genes with specific expression in pancreatic cancer by cDNA representational difference analysis. Genes Chromosomes Cancer. 1997 Jun;19(2):97–103. PMID:9172000

262. Groot VP, Thakker SS, Gemenetzis G, et al. Lessons learned from 29 lymphoepithelial cysts of the pancreas: institutional experience and review of the literature. HPB (Oxford). 2018 Jul;20(7):612–20. PMID:29530477

263. Guan H, Gurda G, Lennon AM, et al. Intraductal tubulopapillary neoplasm of the pancreas on fine needle aspiration: case report with differential diagnosis. Diagn Cytopathol. 2014 Feb;42(2):156–60. PMID:22807417

264. Guo Y, Yuan F, Deng H, et al. Paranuclear dot-like immunostaining for CD99: a unique staining pattern for diagnosing solid-pseudopapillary neoplasm of the pancreas. Am J Surg Pathol. 2011 Jun;35(6):799–806. PMID:21566515

265. Gutiérrez Zurimendi G, Llarena Ibarguren R, Lecumberri Castaños D, et al. [Pancreatic metastasis of primary kidney cancer: a presentation of a series of clinical cases and revision of the literature.]. Arch Esp Urol. 2020 Mar;73(2):147–54. Spanish. PMID:32124846

266. Haaga JR, Alfidi RJ. Precise biopsy localization by computer tomography. Radiology. 1976 Mar;118(3):603–7. PMID:1251009

267. Habashi S, Draganov PV. Pancreatic pseudocyst. World J Gastroenterol. 2009 Jan 7;15(1):38–47. PMID:19115466

268. Hacihasanoglu E, Memis B, Pehlivanoglu B, et al. Factors impacting the performance characteristics of bile duct brushings: a clinico-cytopathologic analysis of 253 patients. Arch Pathol Lab Med. 2018 Jul;142(7):863–70. PMID:29582676

269. Hadzri MH, Rosemi S. Pancreatic metastases from ovarian carcinoma–diagnosis by endoscopic ultrasound-guided fine needle aspiration. Med J Malaysia. 2012 Apr;67(2):210–1. PMID:22822646

270. Haeberle L, Schramm M, Goering W, et al. Molecular analysis of cyst fluids improves the diagnostic accuracy of pre-operative assessment of pancreatic cystic lesions. Sci Rep. 2021 Feb 3;11(1):2901. PMID:33536452

271. Hall-Craggs MA, Lees WR. Fine-needle aspiration biopsy: pancreatic and biliary tumors. AJR Am J Roentgenol. 1986 Aug;147(2):399–403. PMID:3487961

272. Hammel PR, Vilgrain V, Terris B, et al. Pancreatic involvement in von Hippel-Lindau disease. The Groupe Francophone d'Etude de la Maladie de von Hippel-Lindau. Gastroenterology. 2000 Oct;119(4):1087–95. PMID:11040195

273. Hanaoka T, Okuwaki K, Imaizumi H, et al. Pancreatic schwannoma diagnosed by endoscopic ultrasound-guided fine-needle aspiration. Intern Med. 2021 May 1;60(9):1389–95. PMID:33250465

274. Hancke S, Holm HH, Koch F. Ultrasonically guided percutaneous fine needle biopsy of the pancreas. Surg Gynecol Obstet. 1975 Mar;140(3):361–4. PMID:1114427

275. Handa U, Chhabra S, Mohan H. Plasma cell tumours: cytomorphological features in a series of 12 cases diagnosed on fine needle aspiration cytology. Cytopathology. 2010 Jun;21(3):186–90. PMID:19416310

276. Hansen CP, Kristensen TS, Storkholm JH, et al. Solid pseudopapillary neoplasm of the pancreas: clinical-pathological features and management, a single-center experience. Rare Tumors. 2019 Sep 26;11:2036361319878513. PMID:31598207

277. Hansen T, Pedersen H, Brauner V, et al. Control specimens for immunocytochemistry in liquid-based cytology. Cytopathology. 2011 Aug;22(4):243–6. PMID:20482720

278. Hara A, Minaga K, Watanabe T. Diffuse pancreas swelling in a patient with multiple myeloma. Gastroenterology. 2021 Feb;160(3):e6–9. PMID:32569765

279. Hara H, Suda K. Review of the cytologic features of noninvasive ductal carcinomas of the pancreas: differences from invasive ductal carcinoma. Am J Clin Pathol. 2008 Jan;129(1):115–29. PMID:18089497

280. Hara H, Suda K, Oyama T. Two cytologic patterns in invasive ductal adenocarcinoma of the pancreas. Acta Cytol. 2005 Nov-Dec;49(6):611–20. PMID:16450900

281. Harbhajanka A, Michael CW, Janaki N, et al. Tiny but mighty: use of next generation sequencing on discarded cytocentrifuged bile duct brushing specimens to increase sensitivity of cytological diagnosis. Mod Pathol. 2020 Oct;33(10):2019–25. PMID:32457409

282. Harindhanavudhi T, Tanawuttiwat T, Pyle J, et al. Extra-gastrointestinal stromal tumor presenting as hemorrhagic pancreatic cyst diagnosed by EUS-FNA. JOP. 2009 Mar 9;10(2):189–91. PMID:19287116

283. Hart PA, Kamisawa T, Brugge WR, et al. Long-term outcomes of autoimmune pancreatitis: a multicentre, international analysis. Gut. 2013 Dec;62(12):1771–6. PMID:23232048

284. Hart PA, Levy MJ, Smyrk TC, et al. Clinical profiles and outcomes in idiopathic duct-centric chronic pancreatitis (type 2 autoimmune pancreatitis): the Mayo Clinic experience. Gut. 2016 Oct;65(10):1702–9. PMID:26085439

285. Hart PA, Zen Y, Chari ST. Recent advances in autoimmune pancreatitis. Gastroenterology. 2015 Jul;149(1):39–51. PMID:25770706

286. Hartley CP, Mahajan AM, Selvaggi SM, et al. FNA smears of pancreatic ductal adenocarcinoma are superior to formalin-fixed paraffin-embedded tissue as a source of DNA: comparison of targeted KRAS amplification and genotyping in matched preresection and postresection samples. Cancer Cytopathol. 2017 Nov;125(11):838–47. PMID:29024530

287. Hasegawa T, Yamao K, Hijioka S, et al. Evaluation of Ki-67 index in EUS-FNA specimens for the assessment of malignancy risk in pancreatic neuroendocrine tumors. Endoscopy. 2014 Jan;46(1):32–8. PMID:24218309

288. Hasegawa Y, Ishida Y, Kato K, et al. Pancreatoblastoma. A case report with special emphasis on squamoid corpuscles with optically clear nuclei rich in biotin. Acta Cytol. 2003 Jul-Aug;47(4):679–84. PMID:12920766

289. Hashimoto D, Arima K, Yokoyama N, et al. Heterogeneity of KRAS mutations in pancreatic ductal adenocarcinoma. Pancreas. 2016 Sep;45(8):1111–4. PMID:26967456

290. Heath JE, Goicochea LB, Staats PN. Biliary stent-related alterations can be distinguished from adenocarcinoma on bile duct brushings using a limited number of cytologic features. J Am Soc Cytopathol. 2015 Sep-Oct;4(5):282–9. PMID:31051766

291. Hechtman JF, Klimstra DS, Nanjangud G, et al. Performance of DAXX immunohistochemistry as a screen for DAXX mutations in pancreatic neuroendocrine tumors. Pancreas. 2019 Mar;48(3):396–9. PMID:30747827

292. Hedegaard Jensen G, Mortensen MB, Klöppel G, et al. Utility of pVHL, maspin, IMP3, S100P and Ki67 in the distinction of autoimmune pancreatitis from pancreatic ductal adenocarcinoma. Pathol Res Pract. 2020 May;216(5):152925. PMID:32273198

293. Hegyi P, Párniczky A, Lerch MM, et al. International Consensus Guidelines for Risk Factors in Chronic Pancreatitis. Recommendations from the working group for the international consensus guidelines for chronic pancreatitis in collaboration with the International Association of Pancreatology, the American Pancreatic Association, the Japan Pancreas Society, and European Pancreatic Club. Pancreatology. 2020 Jun;20(4):579–85. PMID:32376198

294. Heimbach JK, Sanchez W, Rosen CB, et al. Trans-peritoneal fine needle aspiration biopsy of hilar cholangiocarcinoma is associated with disease dissemination. HPB (Oxford). 2011 May;13(5):356–60. PMID:21492336

295. Heinrich MC, Corless CL, Duensing A, et al. PDGFRA activating mutations in gastrointestinal stromal tumors. Science. 2003 Jan 31;299(5607):708–10. PMID:12522257

296. Henke AC, Kelley CM, Jensen CS, et al. Fine-needle aspiration cytology of pancreatoblastoma. Diagn Cytopathol. 2001 Aug;25(2):118–21. PMID:11477717

297. Henkes DN, Patel SN, Rosenkranz LA, et al. The utility of UroVysion fluorescence in situ hybridization in pancreatic fine-needle aspiration samples directed and obtained by endoscopic ultrasonography. Arch Pathol Lab Med. 2013 Jan;137(1):64–71. PMID:23276176

298. Henry BM, Skinningsrud B, Saganiak K, et al. Development of the human pancreas and its vasculature - an integrated review covering anatomical, embryological, histological, and molecular aspects. Ann Anat. 2019 Jan;221:115–24. PMID:30300687

299. Hewitt MJ, McPhail MJ, Possamai L, et al. EUS-guided FNA for diagnosis of solid pancreatic neoplasms: a meta-analysis. Gastrointest Endosc. 2012 Feb;75(2):319–31. PMID:22248600

300. Heymann JJ, Siddiqui MT. Ancillary techniques in cytologic specimens obtained from solid lesions of the pancreas: a review. Acta Cytol. 2020;64(1-2):103–23. PMID:30970350

301. Hibi Y, Fukushima N, Tsuchida A, et al. Pancreatic juice cytology and subclassification of intraductal papillary mucinous neoplasms of the pancreas. Pancreas. 2007 Mar;34(2):197–204. PMID:17312458

302. Hijioka S, Matsuo K, Mizuno N, et al. Role of endoscopic ultrasound and endoscopic ultrasound-guided fine-needle aspiration in diagnosing metastasis to the pancreas: a tertiary center experience. Pancreatology. 2011;11(4):390–8. PMID:21894056

303. Hirooka Y, Goto H, Itoh A, et al. Case of intraductal papillary mucinous tumor in which endosonography-guided fine-needle aspiration biopsy caused dissemination. J Gastroenterol Hepatol. 2003 Nov;18(11):1323–4. PMID:14535994

304. Hirota S, Isozaki K, Moriyama Y, et al. Gain-of-function mutations of c-kit in human gastrointestinal stromal tumors. Science. 1998 Jan 23;279(5350):577–80. PMID:9438854

305. Hisa T, Nobukawa B, Suda K, et al. Intraductal carcinoma with complex fusion of tubular glands without macroscopic mucus in main pancreatic duct: dilemma in classification. Pathol Int. 2007 Nov;57(11):741–5. PMID:17922686

306. Hoda RS, Arpin RN 3rd, Rosenbaum MW, et al. Risk of malignancy associated with diagnostic categories of the proposed World Health Organization International System for Reporting Pancreaticobiliary Cytopathology. Cancer Cytopathol. 2022 Mar;130(3):195–201. PMID:34623767

307. Hoda RS, Finer EB, Arpin RN 3rd, et al. Risk of malignancy in the categories of the Papanicolaou Society of Cytopathology system for reporting pancreaticobiliary cytology. J Am Soc Cytopathol. 2019 May-Jun;8(3):120–7. PMID:31097287

308. Hoda RS, Lu R, Arpin RN 3rd, et al. Risk of malignancy in pancreatic cysts with cytology of high-grade epithelial atypia. Cancer Cytopathol. 2018 Sep;126(9):773–81. PMID:30257067

309. Hoda RS, Pitman MB. Pancreatic cytology. Surg Pathol Clin. 2018 Sep;11(3):563–88. PMID:30190141

310. Holmes BJ, Hruban RH, Wolfgang CL, et al. Fine needle aspirate of autoimmune pancreatitis (lymphoplasmacytic sclerosing pancreatitis): cytomorphologic characteristics and clinical correlates. Acta Cytol. 2012;56(3):228–32. PMID:22555522

311. Hong DS, DuBois SG, Kummar S, et al. Larotrectinib in patients with TRK fusion-positive solid tumours: a pooled analysis of three phase 1/2 clinical trials. Lancet Oncol. 2020 Apr;21(4):531–40. PMID:32105622

312. Hong SM, Vincent A, Kanda M, et al. Genome-wide somatic copy number alterations in low-grade PanINs and IPMNs from individuals with a family history of pancreatic cancer. Clin Cancer Res. 2012 Aug 15;18(16):4303–12. PMID:22723370

313. Hooper K, Mukhtar F, Li S, et al. Diagnostic error assessment and associated harm of endoscopic ultrasound-guided fine-needle aspiration of neuroendocrine neoplasms of the pancreas. Cancer Cytopathol. 2013 Nov;121(11):653–60. PMID:23839928

314. Hooper K, Tracht JM, Eldin-Eltoum IA. Cytologic criteria to reduce error in EUS-FNA of solid pseudopapillary neoplasms of the pancreas. J Am Soc Cytopathol. 2017 Nov-Dec;6(6):228–35. PMID:31043292

315. Hoorens A, Lemoine NR, McLellan E, et al. Pancreatic acinar cell carcinoma. An analysis of cell lineage markers, p53 expression, and Ki-ras mutation. Am J Pathol. 1993 Sep;143(3):685–98. PMID:8362971
316. Hopper KD, Abendroth CS, Sturtz KW, et al. Fine-needle aspiration biopsy for cytopathologic analysis: utility of syringe handles, automated guns, and the nonsuction method. Radiology. 1992 Dec;185(3):819–24. PMID:1438769
317. Horn AJ, Lele SM. Epidermoid cyst occurring within an intrapancreatic accessory spleen. A case report and review of the literature. JOP. 2011 May 6;12(3):279–82. PMID:21546709
318. Horwhat JD, Paulson EK, McGrath K, et al. A randomized comparison of EUS-guided FNA versus CT or US-guided FNA for the evaluation of pancreatic mass lesions. Gastrointest Endosc. 2006 Jun;63(7):966–75. PMID:16733111
319. Hoshimoto S, Matsui J, Miyata R, et al. Anaplastic carcinoma of the pancreas: case report and literature review of reported cases in Japan. World J Gastroenterol. 2016 Oct 14;22(38):8631–7. PMID:27784976
320. Hosoda W, Chianchiano P, Griffin JF, et al. Genetic analyses of isolated high-grade pancreatic intraepithelial neoplasia (HG-PanIN) reveal paucity of alterations in TP53 and SMAD4. J Pathol. 2017 May;242(1):16–23. PMID:28188630
321. Hosoda W, Sasaki E, Murakami Y, et al. BCL10 as a useful marker for pancreatic acinar cell carcinoma, especially using endoscopic ultrasound cytology specimens. Pathol Int. 2013 Mar;63(3):176–82. PMID:23530562
322. Hou T, Stewart JM, Lee JH, et al. Solid tumor metastases to the pancreas diagnosed using fine-needle aspiration. Am J Clin Pathol. 2020 Oct 13;154(5):692–9. PMID:32651950
323. Hou Y, Shen R, Tonkovich D, et al. Endoscopic ultrasound-guided fine-needle aspiration diagnosis of secondary tumors involving pancreas: an institution's experience. J Am Soc Cytopathol. 2018 Sep-Oct;7(5):261–7. PMID:31043285
324. Hruban RH, Adsay NV, Albores-Saavedra J, et al. Pancreatic intraepithelial neoplasia: a new nomenclature and classification system for pancreatic duct lesions. Am J Surg Pathol. 2001 May;25(5):579–86. PMID:11342768
325. Hruban RH, Maitra A, Goggins M. Update on pancreatic intraepithelial neoplasia. Int J Clin Exp Pathol. 2008 Jan 1;1(4):306–16. PMID:18787611
326. Hsu M, Sasaki M, Igarashi S, et al. KRAS and GNAS mutations and p53 overexpression in biliary intraepithelial neoplasia and intrahepatic cholangiocarcinomas. Cancer. 2013 May 1;119(9):1669–74. PMID:23335286
327. Hsu MY, Pan KT, Chu SY, et al. CT and MRI features of acinar cell carcinoma of the pancreas with pathological correlations. Clin Radiol. 2010 Mar;65(3):223–9. PMID:20152279
328. Hu ZI, Shia J, Stadler ZK, et al. Evaluating mismatch repair deficiency in pancreatic adenocarcinoma: challenges and recommendations. Clin Cancer Res. 2018 Mar 15;24(6):1326–36. PMID:29367431
329. Huang P, Staerkel G, Sneige N, et al. Fine-needle aspiration of pancreatic serous cystadenoma: cytologic features and diagnostic pitfalls. Cancer. 2006 Aug 25;108(4):239–49. PMID:16691573
330. Huang P, Zhang H, Zhang XF, et al. Evaluation of intraductal ultrasonography, endoscopic brush cytology and K-ras, p53 gene mutation in the early diagnosis of malignant bile duct stricture. Chin Med J (Engl). 2015 Jul 20;128(14):1887–92. PMID:26168827
331. Hutchinson CB, Canlas K, Evans JA, et al. Endoscopic ultrasound-guided fine needle aspiration biopsy of the intrapancreatic accessory spleen: a report of 2 cases. Acta Cytol. 2010 May-Jun;54(3):337–40. PMID:20518423
332. Hwang HS, Lee SS, Kim SC, et al. Intrapancreatic accessory spleen: clinicopathologic analysis of 12 cases. Pancreas. 2011 Aug;40(6):956–65. PMID:21562442
333. Iacobuzio-Donahue CA, Klimstra DS, Adsay NV, et al. Dpc-4 protein is expressed in virtually all human intraductal papillary mucinous neoplasms of the pancreas: comparison with conventional ductal adenocarcinomas. Am J Pathol. 2000 Sep;157(3):755–61. PMID:10980115
334. Igarashi H, Ito T, Nishimori I, et al. Pancreatic involvement in Japanese patients with von Hippel-Lindau disease: results of a nationwide survey. J Gastroenterol. 2014 Mar;49(3):511–6. PMID:23543325
335. Iglesias-Garcia J, de la Iglesia-Garcia D, Olmos-Martinez JM, et al. Differential diagnosis of solid pancreatic masses. Minerva Gastroenterol Dietol. 2020 Mar;66(1):70–81. PMID:31994370
336. Iglesias-Garcia J, Lariño-Noia J, Abdulkader I, et al. Rapid on-site evaluation of endoscopic-ultrasound-guided fine-needle aspiration diagnosis of pancreatic masses. World J Gastroenterol. 2014 Jul 28;20(28):9451–7. PMID:25071339
337. Ikeda K, Tate G, Suzuki T, et al. Comparison of immunocytochemical sensitivity between formalin-fixed and alcohol-fixed specimens reveals the diagnostic value of alcohol-fixed cytocentrifuged preparations in malignant effusion cytology. Am J Clin Pathol. 2011 Dec;136(6):934–42. PMID:22095380
338. Ikemura K, Yan L, Park JW. Follow-up of indeterminate cytologic diagnoses of solid pancreatic lesions: atypia versus suspicious (one institution's experience). J Am Soc Cytopathol. 2018 May-Jun;7(3):160–5. PMID:31043311
339. Inagaki Y, Xu H, Nakata M, et al. Clinicopathology of sialomucin: MUC1, particularly KL-6 mucin, in gastrointestinal, hepatic and pancreatic cancers. Biosci Trends. 2009 Dec;3(6):220–32. PMID:20103851
340. Ingkakul T, Warshaw AL, Fernández-Del Castillo C. Epidemiology of intraductal papillary mucinous neoplasms of the pancreas: sex differences between 3 geographic regions. Pancreas. 2011 Jul;40(5):779–80. PMID:21673537
341. Ioakim KJ, Sydney GI, Michaelides C, et al. Evaluation of metastases to the pancreas with fine needle aspiration: a case series from a single centre with review of the literature. Cytopathology. 2020 Mar;31(2):96–105. PMID:31788890
342. Ishii A, Kondo T, Oka T, et al. Granulocytic sarcoma of the pancreas on 18F-FDG PET/CT: a case report. Medicine (Baltimore). 2016 Dec;95(49):e5570. PMID:27930567
343. Ishii Y, Serikawa M, Tsuboi T, et al. Role of endoscopic ultrasonography and endoscopic retrograde cholangiopancreatography in the diagnosis of pancreatic cancer. Diagnostics (Basel). 2021 Feb 4;11(2):238. PMID:33557084
344. Ishikawa T, Haruta J, Yamaguchi T, et al. A case of mucinous cystic neoplasm of the pancreas misdiagnosed as a pancreatic pseudocyst at the initial exam and resected after a 2-year follow-up. J Med Ultrason (2001). 2015 Apr;42(2):257–65. PMID:26576582
345. Isobe T, Seki M, Yoshida K, et al. Integrated molecular characterization of the lethal pediatric cancer pancreatoblastoma. Cancer Res. 2018 Feb 15;78(4):865–76. PMID:29233928
346. Ito T, Sasano H, Tanaka M, et al. Epidemiological study of gastroenteropancreatic neuroendocrine tumors in Japan. J Gastroenterol. 2010 Feb;45(2):234–43. PMID:20058030
347. Jahng AW, Reicher S, Chung D, et al. Staining for p53 and Ki-67 increases the sensitivity of EUS-FNA to detect pancreatic malignancy. World J Gastrointest Endosc. 2010 Nov 16;2(11):362–8. PMID:21173913
348. Jain D, Roy-Chowdhuri S. Molecular pathology of lung cancer cytology specimens: a concise review. Arch Pathol Lab Med. 2018 Sep;142(9):1127–33. PMID:29547001
349. Jais B, Rebours V, Malleo G, et al. Serous cystic neoplasm of the pancreas: a multinational study of 2622 patients under the auspices of the International Association of Pancreatology and European Pancreatic Club (European Study Group on Cystic Tumors of the Pancreas). Gut. 2016 Feb;65(2):305–12. PMID:26045140
350. Janeway KA, Kim SY, Lodish M, et al. Defects in succinate dehydrogenase in gastrointestinal stromal tumors lacking KIT and PDGFRA mutations. Proc Natl Acad Sci U S A. 2011 Jan 4;108(1):314–8. PMID:21173220
351. Jang KT, Park SM, Basturk O, et al. Clinicopathologic characteristics of 29 invasive carcinomas arising in 178 pancreatic mucinous cystic neoplasms with ovarian-type stroma: implications for management and prognosis. Am J Surg Pathol. 2015 Feb;39(2):179–87. PMID:25517958
352. Jang S, Stevens T, Kou L, et al. Efficacy of digital single-operator cholangioscopy and factors affecting its accuracy in the evaluation of indeterminate biliary stricture. Gastrointest Endosc. 2020 Feb;91(2):385–393.e1. PMID:31541625
353. Jarboe EA, Layfield LJ. Cytologic features of pancreatic intraepithelial neoplasia and pancreatitis: potential pitfalls in the diagnosis of pancreatic ductal carcinoma. Diagn Cytopathol. 2011 Aug;39(8):575–81. PMID:20730891
354. Jhala D, Eloubeidi M, Chhieng DC, et al. Fine needle aspiration biopsy of the islet cell tumor of pancreas: a comparison between computerized axial tomography and endoscopic ultrasound-guided fine needle aspiration biopsy. Ann Diagn Pathol. 2002 Apr;6(2):106–12. PMID:12004358
355. Jhala N, Jhala D, Vickers SM, et al. Biomarkers in diagnosis of pancreatic carcinoma in fine-needle aspirates. Am J Clin Pathol. 2006 Oct;126(4):572–9. PMID:17019794
356. Jhala N, Srimunta P, Jhala D. Role of ancillary testing on endoscopic US-guided fine needle aspiration samples from cystic pancreatic neoplasms. Acta Cytol. 2020;64(1-2):124–35. PMID:31509835
357. Jhala NC, Jhala D, Eltoum I, et al. Endoscopic ultrasound-guided fine-needle aspiration biopsy: a powerful tool to obtain samples from small lesions. Cancer. 2004 Aug 25;102(4):239–46. PMID:15368316
358. Jhaveri KS, Hosseini-Nik H. MRI of cholangiocarcinoma. J Magn Reson Imaging. 2015 Nov;42(5):1165–79. PMID:25447417
359. Jiang Y, Xie J, Wang B, et al. TFE3 is a diagnostic marker for solid pseudopapillary neoplasms of the pancreas. Hum Pathol. 2018 Nov;81:166–75. PMID:30030118
360. Jiao Y, Shi C, Edil BH, et al. DAXX/ATRX, MEN1, and mTOR pathway genes are frequently altered in pancreatic neuroendocrine tumors. Science. 2011 Mar 4;331(6021):1199–203. PMID:21252315
361. Jin M, Roth R, Gayetsky V, et al. Grading pancreatic neuroendocrine neoplasms by Ki-67 staining on cytology cell blocks: manual count and digital image analysis of 58 cases. J Am Soc Cytopathol. 2016 Sep-Oct;5(5):286–95. PMID:31042505
362. Jin YH, Kim SH, Park CK. Diagnostic criteria for malignancy in bile cytology and its usefulness. J Korean Med Sci. 1999 Dec;14(6):643–7. PMID:10642942
363. Joensuu H, Rutkowski P, Nishida T, et al. KIT and PDGFRA mutations and the risk of GI stromal tumor recurrence. J Clin Oncol. 2015 Feb 20;33(6):634–42. PMID:25605837
364. Jones M, Zheng Z, Wang J, et al. Impact of next-generation sequencing on the clinical diagnosis of pancreatic cysts. Gastrointest Endosc. 2016 Jan;83(1):140–8. PMID:26253016
365. Jordan EJ, Lowery MA, Basturk O, et al. Brain metastases in pancreatic ductal adenocarcinoma: assessment of molecular genotype-phenotype features-an entity with an increasing incidence? Clin Colorectal Cancer. 2018 Jun;17(2):e315–21. PMID:29496399
366. Jovani M, Abidi WM, Lee LS. Novel fork-tip needles versus standard needles for EUS-guided tissue acquisition from solid masses of the upper GI tract: a matched cohort study. Scand J Gastroenterol. 2017 Jun-Jul;52(6-7):784–7. PMID:28355953
367. Jun SY, Hong SM. Nonductal pancreatic cancers. Surg Pathol Clin. 2016 Dec;9(4):581–93. PMID:27926361
368. Jurczyk MF, Zhu B, Villa C, et al. Cytomorphology of intraductal oncocytic papillary neoplasm of the liver. Diagn Cytopathol. 2014 Oct;42(10):895–8. PMID:24264957
369. Kalb B, Sarmiento JM, Kooby DA, et al. MR imaging of cystic lesions of the pancreas. Radiographics. 2009 Oct;29(6):1749–65. PMID:19959519
370. Kameta E, Sugimori K, Kaneko T, et al. Diagnosis of pancreatic lesions collected by endoscopic ultrasound-guided fine-needle aspiration using next-generation sequencing. Oncol Lett. 2016 Nov;12(5):3875–81. PMID:27895743
371. Kamisawa T, Chari ST, Giday SA, et al. Clinical profile of autoimmune pancreatitis and its histological subtypes: an international multicenter survey. Pancreas. 2011 Aug;40(6):809–14. PMID:21747310
372. Kamisawa T, Chari ST, Lerch MM, et al. Recent advances in autoimmune pancreatitis: type 1 and type 2. Gut. 2013 Sep;62(9):1373–80. PMID:23749606
373. Kamisawa T, Tsuruta K, Okamoto A, et al. Frequent and significant K-ras mutation in the pancreas, the bile duct, and the gallbladder in autoimmune pancreatitis. Pancreas. 2009 Nov;38(8):890–5. PMID:19752775
374. Kanda M, Matthaei H, Wu J, et al. Presence of somatic mutations in most early-stage pancreatic intraepithelial neoplasia. Gastroenterology. 2012 Apr;142(4):730–733.e9. PMID:22226782
375. Kane JR, Laskin WB, Matkowskyj KA, et al. Sarcomatoid (spindle cell) carcinoma of the pancreas: a case report and review of the literature. Oncol Lett. 2014 Jan;7(1):245–9. PMID:24348857
376. Kanno A, Ishida K, Hamada S, et al. Diagnosis of autoimmune pancreatitis by EUS-FNA by using a 22-gauge needle based on the International Consensus Diagnostic Criteria. Gastrointest Endosc. 2012 Sep;76(3):594–602. PMID:22898417
377. Kanno A, Masamune A, Fujishima F, et al. Diagnosis of autoimmune pancreatitis by EUS-guided FNA using a 22-gauge needle: a prospective multicenter study. Gastrointest Endosc. 2016 Nov;84(5):797–804.e1. PMID:27068878
378. Kanzawa M, Sanuki T, Onodera M, et al. Double immunostaining for maspin and p53 on cell blocks increases the diagnostic value of biliary brushing cytology. Pathol Int. 2017 Feb;67(2):91–8. PMID:28074620
379. Kapatia G, Gupta N, Saikia UN, et al. Fine needle aspiration cytology of primary and metastatic gastrointestinal stromal tumour. Cytopathology. 2020 Mar;31(2):136–43. PMID:31698512
380. Karajgikar J, Deshmukh S. Pancreatic lymphangioma: a case report and literature review. J Comput Assist Tomogr. 2019 Mar/Apr;43(2):242–4. PMID:30371621

381. Kardon DE, Thompson LD, Przygodzki RM, et al. Adenosquamous carcinoma of the pancreas: a clinicopathologic series of 25 cases. Mod Pathol. 2001 May;14(5):443–51. PMID:11353055
382. Katabathina VS, Dasyam AK, Dasyam N, et al. Adult bile duct strictures: role of MR imaging and MR cholangiopancreatography in characterization. Radiographics. 2014 May-Jun;34(3):565–86. PMID:24819781
383. Katabi N, Pillarisetty VG, DeMatteo R, et al. Choledochal cysts: a clinicopathologic study of 36 cases with emphasis on the morphologic and the immunohistochemical features of premalignant and malignant alterations. Hum Pathol. 2014 Oct;45(10):2107–14. PMID:25123074
384. Kato O, Hattori K, Matsuyama M, et al. Neurofibroma of the pancreas: differentiation from carcinoma. Am J Gastroenterol. 1982 Sep;77(9):630–2. PMID:7114026
385. Kato Y, Nakagouri T, Konishi M, et al. Intraductal oncocytic papillary neoplasm of the pancreas with strong accumulation on FDG-PET. Hepatogastroenterology. 2008 May-Jun;55(84):900–2. PMID:18705293
386. Kaura K, Sawas T, Bazerbachi F, et al. Cholangioscopy biopsies improve detection of cholangiocarcinoma when combined with cytology and FISH, but not in patients with PSC. Dig Dis Sci. 2020 May;65(5):1471–8. PMID:31571103
387. Kavuturu S, Sarwani NE, Ruggeiro FM, et al. Lymphoepithelial cysts of the pancreas. Can preoperative imaging distinguish this benign lesion from malignant or pre-malignant cystic pancreatic lesions? JOP. 2013 May 10;14(3):250–5. PMID:23669473
388. Kawa S, Kamisawa T, Notohara K, et al. Japanese clinical diagnostic criteria for autoimmune pancreatitis, 2018: revision of Japanese clinical diagnostic criteria for autoimmune pancreatitis, 2011. Pancreas. 2020 Jan;49(1):e13–4. PMID:31856100
389. Kawai Y, Nakamichi R, Kamata N, et al. A case of undifferentiated carcinoma of the pancreas mimicking main-duct intraductal papillary mucinous neoplasm (IPMN). Abdom Imaging. 2015 Mar;40(3):466–70. PMID:25526684
390. Kawamoto S, Johnson PT, Hall H, et al. Intrapancreatic accessory spleen: CT appearance and differential diagnosis. Abdom Imaging. 2012 Oct;37(5):812–27. PMID:22160284
391. Keppens C, Tack V, Hart N, et al. A stitch in time saves nine: external quality assessment rounds demonstrate improved quality of biomarker analysis in lung cancer. Oncotarget. 2018 Apr 17;9(29):20524–38. PMID:29755669
392. Kerr NJ, Chun YH, Yun K, et al. Pancreatoblastoma is associated with chromosome 11p loss of heterozygosity and IGF2 overexpression. Med Pediatr Oncol. 2002 Jul;39(1):52–4. PMID:12116082
393. Kerr NJ, Fukuzawa R, Reeve AE, et al. Beckwith-Wiedemann syndrome, pancreatoblastoma, and the wnt signaling pathway. Am J Pathol. 2002 Apr;160(4):1541–2. PMID:11943738
394. Kerr SE, Barr Fritcher EG, Campion MB, et al. Biliary dysplasia in primary sclerosing cholangitis harbors cytogenetic abnormalities similar to cholangiocarcinoma. Hum Pathol. 2014 Sep;45(9):1797–804. PMID:25027853
395. Khalid A, Dewitt J, Ohori NP, et al. EUS-FNA mutational analysis in differentiating autoimmune pancreatitis and pancreatic cancer. Pancreatology. 2011;11(5):482–6. PMID:21997479
396. Khan I, Baig M, Bandepalle T, et al. Utility of cyst fluid carcinoembryonic antigen in differentiating mucinous and non-mucinous pancreatic cysts: an updated meta-analysis. Dig Dis Sci. 2022 Sep;67(9):4541–8. PMID:34783970
397. Khorana AA, Mangu PB, Berlin J, et al. Potentially curable pancreatic cancer: American Society of Clinical Oncology clinical practice guideline. J Clin Oncol. 2016 Jul 20;34(21):2541–56. PMID:27247221
398. Khoshpouri P, Habibabadi RR, Hazhirkarzar B, et al. Imaging features of primary sclerosing cholangitis: from diagnosis to liver transplant follow-up. Radiographics. 2019 Nov-Dec;39(7):1938–64. PMID:31626561
399. Khoury T, Kadah A, Farraj M, et al. The role of rapid on-site evaluation on diagnostic accuracy of endoscopic ultrasound fine needle aspiration for pancreatic, submucosal upper gastrointestinal tract and adjacent lesions. Cytopathology. 2019 Sep;30(5):499–503. PMID:31034112
400. Kim EK, Jang M, Park M, et al. LEF1, TFE3, and AR are putative diagnostic markers of solid pseudopapillary neoplasms. Oncotarget. 2017 Oct 16;8(55):93404–13. PMID:29212159
401. Kim H, Park CY, Lee JH, et al. Ki-67 and p53 expression as a predictive marker for early postoperative recurrence in pancreatic head cancer. Ann Surg Treat Res. 2015 Apr;88(4):200–7. PMID:25844354
402. Kim JH, Park SW, Kim MK, et al. Meta-analysis for cyto-pathological outcomes in endoscopic ultrasonography-guided fine-needle aspiration with and without the stylet. Dig Dis Sci. 2016 Aug;61(8):2175–84. PMID:27010546
403. Kim JY, Brosnan-Cashman JA, An S, et al. Alternative lengthening of telomeres in primary pancreatic neuroendocrine tumors is associated with aggressive clinical behavior and poor survival. Clin Cancer Res. 2017 Mar 15;23(6):1598–606. PMID:27663587
404. Kim YS, Gum JR Jr, Crawley SC, et al. Mucin gene and antigen expression in biliopancreatic carcinogenesis. Ann Oncol. 1999;10 Suppl 4:51–5. PMID:10436785
405. Kim YS, Kim HG, Han J, et al. The significance of p53 and K-ras immunocytochemical staining in the diagnosis of malignant biliary obstruction by brush cytology during ERCP. Gut Liver. 2010 Jun;4(2):219–25. PMID:20559525
406. Kimura K, Yamanaka T, Ido K, et al. [Ultrasonically guided percutaneous fine needle aspiration biopsy of the pancreas –method and clinical significance in pancreatic cancer (author's transl)]. Nihon Shokakibyo Gakkai Zasshi. 1977 Dec;74(12):1743–52. Japanese. PMID:609129
407. Kimura W, Moriya T, Hirai I, et al. Multicenter study of serous cystic neoplasm of the Japan Pancreas Society. Pancreas. 2012 Apr;41(3):380–7. PMID:22415666
408. Kindblom LG, Remotti HE, Aldenborg F, et al. Gastrointestinal pacemaker cell tumor (GIPACT): gastrointestinal stromal tumors show phenotypic characteristics of the interstitial cells of Cajal. Am J Pathol. 1998 May;152(5):1259–69. PMID:9588894
409. Kinoshita M, Kubo S, Nakanuma Y, et al. Pathological spectrum of bile duct lesions from chronic bile duct injury to invasive cholangiocarcinoma corresponding to bile duct imaging findings of occupational cholangiocarcinoma. J Hepatobiliary Pancreat Sci. 2016 Feb;23(2):92–101. PMID:26580863
410. Kipp BR, Barr Fritcher EG, Pettengill JE, et al. Improving the accuracy of pancreatobiliary tract cytology with fluorescence in situ hybridization: a molecular test with proven clinical success. Cancer Cytopathol. 2013 Nov;121(11):610–9. PMID:23633236
411. Kipp BR, Stadheim LM, Halling SA, et al. A comparison of routine cytology and fluorescence in situ hybridization for the detection of malignant bile duct strictures. Am J Gastroenterol. 2004 Sep;99(9):1675–81. PMID:15330900
412. Kirkegård J, Mortensen FV, Cronin-Fenton D. Chronic pancreatitis and pancreatic cancer risk: a systematic review and meta-analysis. Am J Gastroenterol. 2017 Sep;112(9):1366–72. PMID:28762376
413. Kissane JM. Carcinoma of the exocrine pancreas: pathologic aspects. J Surg Oncol. 1975;7(2):167–74. PMID:168438
414. Kitano M, Gress TM, Garg PK, et al. International consensus guidelines on interventional endoscopy in chronic pancreatitis. Recommendations from the working group for the international consensus guidelines for chronic pancreatitis in collaboration with the International Association of Pancreatology, the American Pancreatic Association, the Japan Pancreas Society, and European Pancreatic Club. Pancreatology. 2020 Sep;20(6):1045–55. PMID:32792253
415. Kitano M, Yoshida T, Itonaga M, et al. Impact of endoscopic ultrasonography on diagnosis of pancreatic cancer. J Gastroenterol. 2019 Jan;54(1):19–32. PMID:30406288
416. Kleeff J, Korc M, Apte M, et al. Pancreatic cancer. Nat Rev Dis Primers. 2016 Apr 21;2:16022. PMID:27158978
417. Klimstra DS. Nonductal neoplasms of the pancreas. Mod Pathol. 2007 Feb;20 Suppl 1:S94–112. PMID:17486055
418. Klimstra DS, Adsay V. Acinar neoplasms of the pancreas-a summary of 25 years of research. Semin Diagn Pathol. 2016 Sep;33(5):307–18. PMID:27320062
419. Klimstra DS, Heffess CS, Oertel JE, et al. Acinar cell carcinoma of the pancreas. A clinicopathologic study of 28 cases. Am J Surg Pathol. 1992 Sep;16(9):815–37. PMID:1384374
420. Klimstra DS, Modlin IR, Adsay NV, et al. Pathology reporting of neuroendocrine tumors: application of the Delphic consensus process to the development of a minimum pathology data set. Am J Surg Pathol. 2010 Mar;34(3):300–13. PMID:20118772
421. Klimstra DS, Wenig BM, Adair CF, et al. Pancreatoblastoma. A clinicopathologic study and review of the literature. Am J Surg Pathol. 1995 Dec;19(12):1371–89. PMID:7503360
422. Klöppel G. Chronic pancreatitis, pseudotumors and other tumor-like lesions. Mod Pathol. 2007 Feb;20 Suppl 1:S113–31. PMID:17486047
423. Klöppel G. Clinicopathologic view of intraductal papillary-mucinous tumor of the pancreas. Hepatogastroenterology. 1998 Nov-Dec;45(24):1981–5. PMID:9951851
424. Klöppel G, Basturk O, Schlitter AM, et al. Intraductal neoplasms of the pancreas. Semin Diagn Pathol. 2014 Nov;31(6):452–66. PMID:25282472
425. Klöppel G, Lüttges J. WHO-classification 2000: exocrine pancreatic tumors. Verh Dtsch Ges Pathol. 2001;85:219–28. PMID:11894402
426. Klöppel G, Morohoshi T, John HD, et al. Solid and cystic acinar cell tumour of the pancreas. A tumour in young women with favourable prognosis. Virchows Arch A Pathol Anat Histol. 1981;392(2):171–83. PMID:7281507
427. Kocjan G, Rode J, Lees WR. Percutaneous fine needle aspiration cytology of the pancreas: advantages and pitfalls. J Clin Pathol. 1989 Apr;42(4):341–7. PMID:2541174
428. Komforti MK, Sokolovskaya E, D'Agostino CA, et al. Extra-osseous Ewing sarcoma of the pancreas: case report with radiologic, pathologic, and molecular correlation, and brief review of the literature. Virchows Arch. 2018 Sep;473(3):361–9. PMID:29611053
429. Komori T, Inoue D, Zen Y, et al. CT imaging comparison between intraductal papillary neoplasms of the bile duct and papillary cholangiocarcinomas. Eur Radiol. 2019 Jun;29(6):3132–40. PMID:30519930
430. Kong F, Zhu J, Kong X, et al. Rapid on-site evaluation does not improve endoscopic ultrasound-guided fine needle aspiration adequacy in pancreatic masses: a meta-analysis and systematic review. PLoS One. 2016 Sep 22;11(9):e0163056. PMID:27657529
431. Königsrainer I, Glatzle J, Klöppel G, et al. Intraductal and cystic tubulopapillary adenocarcinoma of the pancreas–a possible variant of intraductal tubular carcinoma. Pancreas. 2008 Jan;36(1):92–5. PMID:18192889
432. Konukiewitz B, Jesinghaus M, Steiger K, et al. Pancreatic neuroendocrine carcinomas reveal a closer relationship to ductal adenocarcinomas than to neuroendocrine tumors G3. Hum Pathol. 2018 Jul;77:70–9. PMID:29596894
433. Kosmahl M, Pauser U, Peters K, et al. Cystic neoplasms of the pancreas and tumor-like lesions with cystic features: a review of 418 cases and a classification proposal. Virchows Arch. 2004 Aug;445(2):168–78. PMID:15185076
434. Koul A, Baxi AC, Shang R, et al. The efficacy of rapid on-site evaluation during endoscopic ultrasound-guided fine needle aspiration of pancreatic masses. Gastroenterol Rep (Oxf). 2018 Feb;6(1):45–8. PMID:29479442
435. Krepline A, Tsai S. Has personalized medicine for pancreatic cancer arrived? Adv Surg. 2019 Sep;53:103–15. PMID:31327440
436. Kriger AG, Gorin DS, Kaldarov AR, et al. [Intrapancreatic accessory spleen]. Khirurgiia (Mosk). 2018;(8):68–71. Russian. PMID:30113596
437. Krishna SG, Bhattacharya A, Ross WA, et al. Pretest prediction and diagnosis of metastatic lesions to the pancreas by endoscopic ultrasound-guided fine needle aspiration. J Gastroenterol Hepatol. 2015 Oct;30(10):1552–60. PMID:25867963
438. Krishna SG, Li F, Bhattacharya A, et al. Differentiation of pancreatic ductal adenocarcinoma from other neoplastic solid pancreatic lesions: a tertiary oncology center experience. Gastrointest Endosc. 2015 Feb;81(2):370–9. PMID:25442085
439. Kroft SH, Sever CE, Bagg A, et al. Laboratory workup of lymphoma in adults: guideline from the American Society for Clinical Pathology and the College of American Pathologists. Arch Pathol Lab Med. 2021 Mar 1;145(3):269–90. PMID:33175094
440. Kuboki Y, Shimizu K, Hatori T, et al. Molecular biomarkers for progression of intraductal papillary mucinous neoplasm of the pancreas. Pancreas. 2015 Mar;44(2):227–35. PMID:25423558
441. Kubota K, Jang JY, Nakanuma Y, et al. Clinicopathological characteristics of intraductal papillary neoplasm of the bile duct: a Japan-Korea collaborative study. J Hepatobiliary Pancreat Sci. 2020 Sep;27(9):581–97. PMID:32511838
442. Kumar N, Singhal P, Agarwal A, et al. Cytopathological diagnosis of gallbladder mass and mural thickening based on imaging findings: a prospective study of 51 cases. J Cytol. 2015 Oct-Dec;32(4):234–7. PMID:26811570
443. Kumar R, Srinivasan R, Gupta N, et al. Spectrum of gallbladder malignancies on fine-needle aspiration cytology: 5 years retrospective single institutional study with emphasis on uncommon variants. Diagn Cytopathol. 2017 Jan;45(1):36–42. PMID:27873474
444. Kurita A, Yasukawa S, Zen Y, et al. Comparison of a 22-gauge Franseen-tip needle with a 20-gauge forward-bevel needle for the diagnosis of type 1 autoimmune pancreatitis: a prospective, randomized, controlled, multicenter study (COMPAS study). Gastrointest Endosc. 2020 Feb;91(2):373–381.e2. PMID:31654634

445. Kurtycz DF, Field A, Tabatabai L, et al. Post-brushing and fine-needle aspiration biopsy follow-up and treatment options for patients with pancreatobiliary lesions: the Papanicolaou Society of Cytopathology guidelines. Cytojournal. 2014 Jun 2;11(Suppl 1):5. PMID:25191519
446. Kurzawa P, Mullen JT, Chen YL, et al. Prognostic value of myogenic differentiation in dedifferentiated liposarcoma. Am J Surg Pathol. 2020 Jun;44(6):799–804. PMID:31985499
447. Kushnir VM, Mullady DK, Das K, et al. The diagnostic yield of malignancy comparing cytology, FISH, and molecular analysis of cell free cytology brush supernatant in patients with biliary strictures undergoing endoscopic retrograde cholangiography (ERC): a prospective study. J Clin Gastroenterol. 2019 Oct;53(9):686–92. PMID:30106834
448. Kwon MJ, Jeon JY, Park HR, et al. Low frequency of KRAS mutation in pancreatic ductal adenocarcinomas in Korean patients and its prognostic value. Pancreas. 2015 Apr;44(3):484–92. PMID:25513781
449. Kwon MS, Koh JS, Lee SS, et al. Fine needle aspiration cytology (FNAC) of gastrointestinal stromal tumor: an emphasis on diagnostic role of FNAC, cell block, and immunohistochemistry. J Korean Med Sci. 2002 Jun;17(3):353–9. PMID:12068139
450. La Rosa S, Adsay V, Albarello L, et al. Clinicopathologic study of 62 acinar cell carcinomas of the pancreas: insights into the morphology and immunophenotype and search for prognostic markers. Am J Surg Pathol. 2012 Dec;36(12):1782–95. PMID:23026929
451. La Rosa S, Franzi F, Marchet S, et al. The monoclonal anti-BCL10 antibody (clone 331.1) is a sensitive and specific marker of pancreatic acinar cell carcinoma and pancreatic metaplasia. Virchows Arch. 2009 Feb;454(2):133–42. PMID:19066953
452. Lai A, Davis-Yadley A, Lipka S, et al. The use of a stylet in endoscopic ultrasound with fine-needle aspiration: a systematic review and meta-analysis. J Clin Gastroenterol. 2019 Jan;53(1):1–8. PMID:28644309
453. Landsman MK. The patient with chronic renal failure: a marginal man. Ann Intern Med. 1975 Feb;82(2):268–70. PMID:1115449
454. Laquière AE, Lagarde A, Napoléon B, et al. Genomic profile concordance between pancreatic cyst fluid and neoplastic tissue. World J Gastroenterol. 2019 Sep 28;25(36):5530–42. PMID:31576098
455. La Rosa S, Bongiovanni M. Pancreatic solid pseudopapillary neoplasm: key pathologic and genetic features. Arch Pathol Lab Med. 2020 Jul 1;144(7):829–37. PMID:31958381
456. Larsen AK, Krag C, Geertsen P, et al. Isolated malignant melanoma metastasis to the pancreas. Plast Reconstr Surg Glob Open. 2013 Dec 6;1(8):e74. PMID:25289269
457. Lavu H, Yeo CJ. Metastatic renal cell carcinoma to the pancreas. Gastroenterol Hepatol (N Y). 2011 Oct;7(10):699–700. PMID:22298967
458. Law JK, Ahmed A, Singh VK, et al. A systematic review of solid-pseudopapillary neoplasms: Are these rare lesions? Pancreas. 2014 Apr;43(3):331–7. PMID:24622060
459. Layfield L. Role of ancillary techniques in biliary cytopathology specimens. Acta Cytol. 2020;64(1-2):175–81. PMID:31121596
460. Layfield LJ, Bentz JS, Gopez EV. Immediate on-site interpretation of fine-needle aspiration smears: a cost and compensation analysis. Cancer. 2001 Oct 25;93(5):319–22. PMID:11668466
461. Layfield LJ, Dodd L, Factor R, et al. Malignancy risk associated with diagnostic categories defined by the Papanicolaou Society of Cytopathology pancreaticobiliary guidelines. Cancer Cytopathol. 2014 Jun;122(6):420–7. PMID:24339321
462. Layfield LJ, Ehya H, Filie AC, et al. Utilization of ancillary studies in the cytologic diagnosis of biliary and pancreatic lesions: the Papanicolaou Society of Cytopathology guidelines for pancreatobiliary cytology. Diagn Cytopathol. 2014 Apr;42(4):351–62. PMID:24639398
463. Layfield LJ, Ehya H, Filie AC, et al. Utilization of ancillary studies in the cytologic diagnosis of biliary and pancreatic lesions: the Papanicolaou Society of Cytopathology guidelines. Cytojournal. 2014 Jun 2;11(Suppl 1):4. PMID:25191518
464. Layfield LJ, Hirschowitz SL, Adler DG. Metastatic disease to the pancreas documented by endoscopic ultrasound guided fine-needle aspiration: a seven-year experience. Diagn Cytopathol. 2012 Mar;40(3):228–33. PMID:22334524
465. Layfield LJ, Jarboe EA. Cytopathology of the pancreas: neoplastic and nonneoplastic entities. Ann Diagn Pathol. 2010 Apr;14(2):140–51. PMID:20227021
466. Layfield LJ, Schmidt RL, Chadwick BE, et al. Interobserver reproducibility and agreement with original diagnosis in the categories "atypical" and "suspicious for malignancy" for bile and pancreatic duct brushings. Diagn Cytopathol. 2015 Oct;43(10):797–801. PMID:26153872
467. Layfield LJ, Wax TD, Lee JG, et al. Accuracy and morphologic aspects of pancreatic and biliary duct brushings. Acta Cytol. 1995 Jan-Feb;39(1):11–8. PMID:7846997
468. Layfield LJ, Zhang T, Esebua M. Diagnostic sensitivity and risk of malignancy for bile duct brushings categorized by the Papanicolaou Society of Cytopathology System for reporting pancreaticobiliary cytopathology. Diagn Cytopathol. 2022 Jan;50(1):24–7. PMID:34800330
469. Le DT, Durham JN, Smith KN, et al. Mismatch repair deficiency predicts response of solid tumors to PD-1 blockade. Science. 2017 Jul 28;357(6349):409–13. PMID:28596308
470. Le DT, Uram JN, Wang H, et al. PD-1 blockade in tumors with mismatch-repair deficiency. N Engl J Med. 2015 Jun 25;372(26):2509–20. PMID:26028255
471. Le Borgne J, de Calan L, Partensky C, et al. Cystadenomas and cystadenocarcinomas of the pancreas: a multiinstitutional retrospective study of 398 cases. Ann Surg. 1999 Aug;230(2):152–61. PMID:10450728
472. Lee A, Kadiyala V, Lee LS. Evaluation of AGA and Fukuoka Guidelines for EUS and surgical resection of incidental pancreatic cysts. Endosc Int Open. 2017 Feb;5(2):E116–22. PMID:28210708
473. Lee BS, Nguyen AK, Tekeste TF, et al. Long-term follow-up of branch-duct intraductal papillary mucinous neoplasms with no change in first 5 years of diagnosis. Pancreatology. 2021 Jan;21(1):144–54. PMID:33309223
474. Lee JK, Lee KT, Choi ER, et al. A prospective, randomized trial comparing 25-gauge and 22-gauge needles for endoscopic ultrasound-guided fine needle aspiration of pancreatic masses. Scand J Gastroenterol. 2013 Jun;48(6):752–7. PMID:23600919
475. Lee KY, Cho HD, Hwangbo Y, et al. Efficacy of 3 fine-needle biopsy techniques for suspected pancreatic malignancies in the absence of an on-site cytopathologist. Gastrointest Endosc. 2019 Apr;89(4):825–831.e1. PMID:30403966
476. Lee LS, Andersen DK, Ashida R, et al. EUS and related technologies for the diagnosis and treatment of pancreatic disease: research gaps and opportunities-summary of a National Institute of Diabetes and Digestive and Kidney Diseases workshop. Gastrointest Endosc. 2017 Nov;86(5):768–78. PMID:28941651
477. Lee PJ, Owens CL, Hutchinson L, et al. Intranuclear cytoplasmic inclusions are a specific feature of intraductal papillary mucinous neoplasms that distinguish contaminating gastric epithelium. J Am Soc Cytopathol. 2014 Mar-Apr;3(2):108–13. PMID:31051700
478. Lee WY, Tzeng CC, Chen RM, et al. Papillary cystic tumors of the pancreas: assessment of malignant potential by analysis of progesterone receptor, flow cytometry, and ras oncogene mutation. Anticancer Res. 1997 Jul-Aug;17 4A:2587–91. PMID:9252685
479. Leung SW, Bédard YC. Immunocytochemical staining on ThinPrep processed smears. Mod Pathol. 1996 Mar;9(3):304–6. PMID:8685232
480. Levenick JM, Gordon SR, Sutton JE, et al. A comprehensive, case-based review of groove pancreatitis. Pancreas. 2009 Aug;38(6):e169–75. PMID:19629001
481. Levy C, Lymp J, Angulo P, et al. The value of serum CA 19-9 in predicting cholangiocarcinomas in patients with primary sclerosing cholangitis. Dig Dis Sci. 2005 Sep;50(9):1734–40. PMID:16133981
482. Levy M, Lin F, Xu H, et al. S100P, von Hippel-Lindau gene product, and IMP3 serve as a useful immunohistochemical panel in the diagnosis of adenocarcinoma on endoscopic bile duct biopsy. Hum Pathol. 2010 Sep;41(9):1210–9. PMID:20382408
483. Levy MJ, Baron TH, Clayton AC, et al. Prospective evaluation of advanced molecular markers and imaging techniques in patients with indeterminate bile duct strictures. Am J Gastroenterol. 2008 May;103(5):1263–73. PMID:18477350
484. Li L, Liu X, Chen J, et al. Laparoscopic spleen-preserving pancreatic resection for intrapancreatic accessory spleen: case report. Medicine (Baltimore). 2019 Aug;98(31):e16488. PMID:31374010
485. Li S, Ai SZ, Owens C, et al. Intrapancreatic schwannoma diagnosed by endoscopic ultrasound-guided fine-needle aspiration cytology. Diagn Cytopathol. 2009 Feb;37(2):132–5. PMID:19031416
486. Li XO, Li ZP, Wang P, et al. Pancreatic metastasis of papillary thyroid carcinoma: a case report with review of the literature. Int J Clin Exp Pathol. 2014 Jan 15;7(2):819–22. PMID:24551310
487. Liang W, He W, Li Z. Extranodal follicular dendritic cell sarcoma originating in the pancreas: a case report. Medicine (Baltimore). 2016 Apr;95(15):e3377. PMID:27082603
488. Liau JY, Tsai JH, Jeng YM, et al. The diagnostic utility of PAX8 for neuroendocrine tumors: an immunohistochemical reappraisal. Appl Immunohistochem Mol Morphol. 2016 Jan;24(1):57–63. PMID:25710581
489. Liew ZH, Loh TJ, Lim TKH, et al. Role of fluorescence in situ hybridization in diagnosing cholangiocarcinoma in indeterminate biliary strictures. J Gastroenterol Hepatol. 2018 Jan;33(1):315–9. PMID:28543841
490. Lightdale CJ. Indications, contraindications, and complications of endoscopic ultrasonography. Gastrointest Endosc. 1996 Feb;43(2 Pt 2):S15–9. PMID:8929801
491. Lilo MT, VandenBussche CJ, Allison DB, et al. Serous cystadenoma of the pancreas: potentials and pitfalls of a preoperative cytopathologic diagnosis. Acta Cytol. 2017;61(1):27–33. PMID:27889754
492. Lin F, Shi J, Liu H, et al. Diagnostic utility of S100P and von Hippel-Lindau gene product (pVHL) in pancreatic adenocarcinoma-with implication of their roles in early tumorigenesis. Am J Surg Pathol. 2008 Jan;32(1):78–91. PMID:18162774
493. Lin F, Staerkel G. Cytologic criteria for well differentiated adenocarcinoma of the pancreas in fine-needle aspiration biopsy specimens. Cancer. 2003 Feb 25;99(1):44–50. PMID:12589645
494. Lindeman NI, Cagle PT, Aisner DL, et al. Updated molecular testing guideline for the selection of lung cancer patients for treatment with targeted tyrosine kinase inhibitors: guideline from the College of American Pathologists, the International Association for the Study of Lung Cancer, and the Association for Molecular Pathology. J Thorac Oncol. 2018 Mar;13(3):323–58. PMID:29396253
495. Liu H, Shi J, Anandan V, et al. Reevaluation and identification of the best immunohistochemical panel (pVHL, maspin, S100P, IMP-3) for ductal adenocarcinoma of the pancreas. Arch Pathol Lab Med. 2012 Jun;136(6):601–9. PMID:22646265
496. Liu X, Rauch TM, Siegal GP, et al. Solid-pseudopapillary neoplasm of the pancreas: three cases with a literature review. Appl Immunohistochem Mol Morphol. 2006 Dec;14(4):445–53. PMID:17122644
497. Lloyd RV. Practical markers used in the diagnosis of neuroendocrine tumors. Endocr Pathol. 2003 Winter;14(4):293–301. PMID:14739487
498. Logrono R, Kurtycz DF, Molina CP, et al. Analysis of false-negative diagnoses on endoscopic brush cytology of biliary and pancreatic duct strictures: the experience at 2 university hospitals. Arch Pathol Lab Med. 2000 Mar;124(3):387–92. PMID:10705391
499. Lok T, Chen L, Lin F, et al. Immunohistochemical distinction between intrahepatic cholangiocarcinoma and pancreatic ductal adenocarcinoma. Hum Pathol. 2014 Feb;45(2):394–400. PMID:24439226
501. Lopes CV. Cyst fluid glucose: an alternative to carcinoembryonic antigen for pancreatic mucinous cysts. World J Gastroenterol. 2019 May 21;25(19):2271–8. PMID:31148899
502. López-Ramírez AN, Villegas-González LF, Serrano-Arévalo ML, et al. Reclassification of lesions in biopsies by fine-needle aspiration of pancreas and biliary tree using Papanicolaou classification. J Gastrointest Oncol. 2018 Oct;9(5):847–52. PMID:30505584
503. Lozano MD, Echeveste JI, Abengozar M, et al. Cytology smears in the era of molecular biomarkers in non-small cell lung cancer: doing more with less. Arch Pathol Lab Med. 2018 Mar;142(3):291–8. PMID:29494220
504. Lu T, Pu H, Zhao G. Primary pancreatic plasmacytoma: a rare case report. BMC Gastroenterol. 2017 Dec 20;17(1):167. PMID:29262780
505. Luong-Player A, Liu H, Wang HL, et al. Immunohistochemical reevaluation of carbonic anhydrase IX (CA IX) expression in tumors and normal tissues. Am J Clin Pathol. 2014 Feb;141(2):219–25. PMID:24436269
506. Ma Y, Shen B, Jia Y, et al. Pancreatic schwannoma: a case report and an updated 40-year review of the literature yielding 68 cases. BMC Cancer. 2017 Dec 14;17(1):853. PMID:29241452
507. Macdonald F, Downing R, Allum WH. Expression of CA125 in pancreatic carcinoma and chronic pancreatitis. Br J Cancer. 1988 Oct;58(4):505–6. PMID:3207606
508. Macgregor-Das AM, Iacobuzio-Donahue CA. Molecular pathways in pancreatic carcinogenesis. J Surg Oncol. 2013 Jan;107(1):8–14. PMID:22806689
509. Machado I, López-Soto MV, Pérez-López AS, et al. Hyaline globules and papillary fragments in cytologic smears from two intra-abdominal tumors (ovarian and hepatic) in female patients: a diagnostic pitfall with histologic correlation. Diagn Cytopathol. 2016 Nov;44(11):935–43. PMID:27407028
510. Machairas N, Paspala A, Schizas D, et al. Metastatic squamous cell carcinoma to the pancreas: report of an extremely rare case. Mol Clin Oncol. 2019 Jan;10(1):144–6. PMID:30655990

511. Macin G, Hekimoglu K, Uner H, et al. Pancreatic cystic lymphangioma: diagnostic approach with MDCT and MR imaging. JBR-BTR. 2014 Mar-Apr;97(2):97–9. PMID:25073240
512. Madan R, Khan E, Cuka N, et al. Pancreatic cystic lesions without overt cytologic atypia: proposed diagnostic categories for endoscopic ultrasound-guided fine-needle aspiration cytology with utilization of fluid carcinoembryonic antigen level. Acta Cytol. 2012;56(1):34–40. PMID:22236743
513. Maitra A, Adsay NV, Argani P, et al. Multicomponent analysis of the pancreatic adenocarcinoma progression model using a pancreatic intraepithelial neoplasia tissue microarray. Mod Pathol. 2003 Sep;16(9):902–12. PMID:13679454
514. Majeed A, Castedal M, Arnelo U, et al. Optimizing the detection of biliary dysplasia in primary sclerosing cholangitis before liver transplantation. Scand J Gastroenterol. 2018 Jan;53(1):56–63. PMID:28990806
515. Majumder S, Chari ST. EUS-guided FNA for diagnosing autoimmune pancreatitis: Does it enhance existing consensus criteria? Gastrointest Endosc. 2016 Nov;84(5):805–7. PMID:27742043
516. Majumder S, Takahashi N, Chari ST. Autoimmune pancreatitis. Dig Dis Sci. 2017 Jul;62(7):1762–9. PMID:28365915
517. Makovitzky J. The distribution and localization of the monoclonal antibody-defined antigen 19-9 (CA19-9) in chronic pancreatitis and pancreatic carcinoma. An immunohistochemical study. Virchows Arch B Cell Pathol Incl Mol Pathol. 1986;51(6):535–44. PMID:2878526
518. Malapelle U, Mayo-de-Las-Casas C, Molina-Vila MA, et al. Consistency and reproducibility of next-generation sequencing and other multigene mutational assays: a worldwide ring trial study on quantitative cytological molecular reference specimens. Cancer Cytopathol. 2017 Aug;125(8):615–26. PMID:28475299
519. Manning MA, Paal EE, Srivastava A, et al. Nonepithelial neoplasms of the pancreas, part 2: malignant tumors and tumors of uncertain malignant potential from the Radiologic Pathology Archives. Radiographics. 2018 Jul-Aug;38(4):1047–72. PMID:29787363
520. Manning MA, Srivastava A, Paal EE, et al. Nonepithelial neoplasms of the pancreas: radiologic-pathologic correlation, part 1–benign tumors: from the Radiologic Pathology Archives. Radiographics. 2016 Jan-Feb;36(1):123–41. PMID:26761535
521. Mantese G. Gastrointestinal stromal tumor: epidemiology, diagnosis, and treatment. Curr Opin Gastroenterol. 2019 Nov;35(6):555–9. PMID:31577561
522. Marchegiani G, Andrianello S, Massignani M, et al. Solid pseudopapillary tumors of the pancreas: specific pathological features predict the likelihood of postoperative recurrence. J Surg Oncol. 2016 Oct;114(5):597–601. PMID:27471041
523. Marchegiani G, Mino-Kenudson M, Ferrone CR, et al. Oncocytic-type intraductal papillary mucinous neoplasms: a unique malignant pancreatic tumor with good long-term prognosis. J Am Coll Surg. 2015 May;220(5):839–44. PMID:25840549
524. Marchetti A, Barberis M, Papotti M, et al. ALK rearrangement testing by FISH analysis in non-small-cell lung cancer patients: results of the first Italian external quality assurance scheme. J Thorac Oncol. 2014 Oct;9(10):1470–6. PMID:25170637
525. Marinoni I, Kurrer AS, Vassella E, et al. Loss of DAXX and ATRX are associated with chromosome instability and reduced survival of patients with pancreatic neuroendocrine tumors. Gastroenterology. 2014 Feb;146(2):453–60.e5. PMID:24148618
526. Martin HE, Ellis EB. Biopsy by needle puncture and aspiration. Ann Surg. 1930 Aug;92(2):169–81. PMID:17866350
527. Massironi S, Rossi RE, Zilli A, et al. A wait-and-watch approach to small pancreatic neuroendocrine tumors: prognosis and survival. Oncotarget. 2016 Apr 5;7(14):18978–83. PMID:26959887
528. Matsuda Y, Furukawa T, Yachida S, et al. The prevalence and clinicopathological characteristics of high-grade pancreatic intraepithelial neoplasia: autopsy study evaluating the entire pancreatic parenchyma. Pancreas. 2017 May/Jun;46(5):658–64. PMID:28196020
529. Matter MS, Chijioke O, Savic S, et al. Narrative review of molecular pathways of kinase fusions and diagnostic approaches for their detection in non-small cell lung carcinomas. Transl Lung Cancer Res. 2020 Dec;9(6):2645–55. PMID:33489824
530. Matthaei H, Norris AL, Tsiatis AC, et al. Clinicopathological characteristics and molecular analyses of multifocal intraductal papillary mucinous neoplasms of the pancreas. Ann Surg. 2012 Feb;255(2):326–33. PMID:22167000
531. McCall CM, Shi C, Cornish TC, et al. Grading of well-differentiated pancreatic neuroendocrine tumors is improved by the inclusion of both Ki67 proliferative index and mitotic rate. Am J Surg Pathol. 2013 Nov;37(11):1671–7. PMID:24121170
532. McGuigan A, Kelly P, Turkington RC, et al. Pancreatic cancer: a review of clinical diagnosis, epidemiology, treatment and outcomes. World J Gastroenterol. 2018 Nov 21;24(43):4846–61. PMID:30487695
533. McHugh KE, Mukhopadhyay S, Doxtader EE, et al. INSM1 is a highly specific marker of neuroendocrine differentiation in primary neoplasms of the gastrointestinal tract, appendix, and pancreas. Am J Clin Pathol. 2020 May 5;153(6):811–20. PMID:32128564
534. McHugh KE, Stelow EB, Harrison GP, et al. The usefulness of lymphoid enhancer-binding factor 1 and androgen receptor in diagnosing solid pseudopapillary neoplasm of the pancreas on cytopathology. Cancer Cytopathol. 2019 Nov;127(11):700–7. PMID:31584754
535. McKinley M, Newman M. Observations on the application of the Papanicolaou Society of Cytopathology standardised terminology and nomenclature for pancreaticobiliary cytology. Pathology. 2016 Jun;48(4):353–6. PMID:27114371
536. Mechtersheimer G, Staudter M, Möller P. Expression of the natural killer cell-associated antigens CD56 and CD57 in human neural and striated muscle cells and in their tumors. Cancer Res. 1991 Feb 15;51(4):1300–7. PMID:1705171
537. Megibow AJ, Baker ME, Morgan DE, et al. Management of incidental pancreatic cysts: a white paper of the ACR Incidental Findings Committee. J Am Coll Radiol. 2017 Jul;14(7):911–23. PMID:28533111
538. Mehmood S, Loya A, Yusuf MA. Biliary brush cytology revisited. Acta Cytol. 2016;60(2):167–72. PMID:27221813
539. Mehta N, Modi L, Patel T, et al. Study of cytomorphology of solid pseudopapillary tumor of pancreas and its differential diagnosis. J Cytol. 2010 Oct;27(4):118–22. PMID:21157561
540. Menges M, Lerch MM, Zeitz M. The double duct sign in patients with malignant and benign pancreatic lesions. Gastrointest Endosc. 2000 Jul;52(1):74–7. PMID:10882966
541. Meriden Z, Shi C, Edil BH, et al. Hyaline globules in neuroendocrine and solid-pseudopapillary neoplasms of the pancreas: a clue to the diagnosis. Am J Surg Pathol. 2011 Jul;35(7):981–8. PMID:21677537
542. Mesa H, Stelow EB, Stanley MW, et al. Diagnosis of nonprimary pancreatic neoplasms by endoscopic ultrasound-guided fine-needle aspiration. Diagn Cytopathol. 2004 Nov;31(5):313–8. PMID:15468134
543. Michaels PJ, Brachtel EF, Bounds BC, et al. Intraductal papillary mucinous neoplasm of the pancreas: cytologic features predict histologic grade. Cancer. 2006 Jun 25;108(3):163–73. PMID:16550572
544. Miller DL, Roy-Chowdhuri S, Illei P, et al. Primary pancreatic Ewing sarcoma: a cytomorphologic and histopathologic study of 13 cases. J Am Soc Cytopathol. 2020 Nov-Dec;9(6):502–12. PMID:32536453
545. Miller RT. Avoiding pitfalls in diagnostic immunohistochemistry-important technical aspects that every pathologist should know. Semin Diagn Pathol. 2019 Sep;36(5):312–35. PMID:31227425
546. Minni F, Casadei R, Perenze B, et al. Pancreatic metastases: observations of three cases and review of the literature. Pancreatology. 2004;4(6):509–20. PMID:15316227
547. Mino-Kenudson M, Fernández-del Castillo C, Baba Y, et al. Prognosis of invasive intraductal papillary mucinous neoplasm depends on histological and precursor epithelial subtypes. Gut. 2011 Dec;60(12):1712–20. PMID:21508421
548. Miranda C, Nucifora M, Molinari F, et al. KRAS and BRAF mutations predict primary resistance to imatinib in gastrointestinal stromal tumors. Clin Cancer Res. 2012 Mar 15;18(6):1769–76. PMID:22282465
549. Misdraji J, Centeno BA, Pitman MB. Ancillary tests in the diagnosis of liver and pancreatic neoplasms. Cancer Cytopathol. 2018 Aug;126 Suppl 8:672–90. PMID:30156777
550. Misra S, Saran RK, Srivastava S, et al. Utility of cytomorphology in distinguishing solid pseudopapillary neoplasm of pancreas from pancreatic neuroendocrine tumor with emphasis on nuclear folds and nuclear grooves. Diagn Cytopathol. 2019 Jun;47(6):531–40. PMID:30677247
551. Mitchell RA, Stanger D, Shuster C, et al. Repeat endoscopic ultrasound-guided fine-needle aspiration in patients with suspected pancreatic cancer: diagnostic yield and associated change in access to appropriate care. Can J Gastroenterol Hepatol. 2016;2016:7678403. PMID:27648440
552. Mittal PK, Harri P, Nandwana S, et al. Paraduodenal pancreatitis: benign and malignant mimics at MRI. Abdom Radiol (NY). 2017 Nov;42(11):2652–74. PMID:28660333
553. Mizrahi JD, Surana R, Valle JW, et al. Pancreatic cancer. Lancet. 2020 Jun 27;395(10242):2008–20. PMID:32593337
554. Mograbi M, Stump MS, Luyimbazi DT, et al. Pancreatic inflammatory pseudotumor-like follicular dendritic cell tumor. Case Rep Pathol. 2019 Dec 5;2019:2648123. PMID:31885993
555. Mohan BP, Madhu D, Khan SR, et al. Intracystic glucose levels in differentiating mucinous from nonmucinous pancreatic cysts: a systematic review and meta-analysis. J Clin Gastroenterol. 2022 Feb 1;56(2):e131–6. PMID:33731599
557. Mondal U, Henkes N, Henkes D, et al. Cavernous hemangioma of adult pancreas: a case report and literature review. World J Gastroenterol. 2015 Sep 7;21(33):9793–802. PMID:26361427
558. Montemarano H, Lonergan GJ, Bulas DI, et al. Pancreatoblastoma: imaging findings in 10 patients and review of the literature. Radiology. 2000 Feb;214(2):476–82. PMID:10671596
559. Monzen M, Shimizu K, Hatori T, et al. Usefulness of cell block cytology for preoperative grading and typing of intraductal papillary mucinous neoplasms. Pancreatology. 2013 Jul-Aug;13(4):369–78. PMID:23890135
560. Moon SH, Kim MH, Park DH, et al. Is a 2-week steroid trial after initial negative investigation for malignancy useful in differentiating autoimmune pancreatitis from pancreatic cancer? A prospective outcome study. Gut. 2008 Dec;57(12):1704–12. PMID:18583399
561. Moore PS, Zamboni G, Brighenti A, et al. Molecular characterization of pancreatic serous microcystic adenomas: evidence for a tumor suppressor gene on chromosome 10q. Am J Pathol. 2001 Jan;158(1):317–21. PMID:11141506
562. Morales-Oyarvide V, Yoon WJ, Ingkakul T, et al. Cystic pancreatic neuroendocrine tumors: the value of cytology in preoperative diagnosis. Cancer Cytopathol. 2014 Jun;122(6):435–44. PMID:24591417
563. Moreno Luna LE, Kipp B, Halling KC, et al. Advanced cytologic techniques for the detection of malignant pancreatobiliary strictures. Gastroenterology. 2006 Oct;131(4):1064–72. PMID:17030177
564. Moris M, Raimondo M, Woodward TA, et al. Diagnostic accuracy of endoscopic ultrasound-guided fine-needle aspiration cytology, carcinoembryonic antigen, and amylase in intraductal papillary mucinous neoplasm. Pancreas. 2016 Jul;45(6):870–5. PMID:26646270
565. Morishima T, Kawashima H, Ohno E, et al. Prospective multicenter study on the usefulness of EUS-guided FNA biopsy for the diagnosis of autoimmune pancreatitis. Gastrointest Endosc. 2016 Aug;84(2):241–8. PMID:26777565
566. Moriya T, Kimura W, Hirai I, et al. Pancreatic schwannoma: case report and an updated 30-year review of the literature yielding 47 cases. World J Gastroenterol. 2012 Apr 7;18(13):1538–44. PMID:22509087
567. Moskaluk CA, Hruban RH, Kern SE. p16 and K-ras gene mutations in the intraductal precursors of human pancreatic adenocarcinoma. Cancer Res. 1997 Jun 1;57(11):2140–3. PMID:9187111
568. Mostafa ME, Erbarut-Seven I, Pehlivanoglu B, et al. Pathologic classification of "pancreatic cancers": current concepts and challenges. Chin Clin Oncol. 2017 Dec;6(6):59. PMID:29307199
569. Motosugi U, Yamaguchi H, Furukawa T, et al. Imaging studies of intraductal tubulopapillary neoplasms of the pancreas: 2-tone duct sign and cork-of-wine-bottle sign as indicators of intraductal tumor growth. J Comput Assist Tomogr. 2012 Nov-Dec;36(6):710–7. PMID:23192209
570. Mullick SS, Mody DR. "Osteoclastic" giant cell carcinoma of the pancreas. Report of a case with aspiration cytology. Acta Cytol. 1996 Sep-Oct;40(5):975–9. PMID:8842177
571. Muraki T, Kim GE, Reid MD, et al. Paraduodenal pancreatitis: imaging and pathologic correlation of 47 cases elucidates distinct subtypes and the factors involved in its etiopathogenesis. Am J Surg Pathol. 2017 Oct;41(10):1347–63. PMID:28795998
572. Muraki T, Reid MD, Basturk O, et al. Undifferentiated carcinoma with osteoclastic giant cells of the pancreas: clinicopathologic analysis of 38 cases highlights a more protracted clinical course than currently appreciated. Am J Surg Pathol. 2016 Sep;40(9):1203–16. PMID:27508975
573. Muraki T, Uehara T, Sano K, et al. A case of MUC5AC-positive intraductal neoplasm of the pancreas classified as an intraductal tubulopapillary neoplasm? Pathol Res Pract. 2015 Dec;211(12):1034–9. PMID:26586167
574. Nabae T, Yamaguchi K, Takahata S, et al. Adenosquamous carcinoma of the pancreas: report of two cases. Am J Gastroenterol. 1998 Jul;93(7):1167–70. PMID:9672355

575. Nagata K, Horinouchi M, Saitou M, et al. Mucin expression profile in pancreatic cancer and the precursor lesions. J Hepatobiliary Pancreat Surg. 2007;14(3):243–54. PMID:17520199
576. Nagino M, Hirano S, Yoshitomi H, et al. Clinical practice guidelines for the management of biliary tract cancers 2019: the 3rd English edition. J Hepatobiliary Pancreat Sci. 2021 Jan;28(1):26–54. PMID:33259690
577. Nagle JA, Wilbur DC, Pitman MB. Cytomorphology of gastric and duodenal epithelium and reactivity to B72.3: a baseline for comparison to pancreatic lesions aspirated by EUS-FNAB. Diagn Cytopathol. 2005 Dec;33(6):381–6. PMID:16299750
578. Nakai Y, Isayama H, Wang HP, et al. International consensus statements for endoscopic management of distal biliary stricture. J Gastroenterol Hepatol. 2020 Jun;35(6):967–79. PMID:31802537
579. Nakajima T, Tajima Y, Sugano I, et al. Multivariate statistical analysis of bile cytology. Acta Cytol. 1994 Jan-Feb;38(1):51–5. PMID:8291355
580. Nakamura H, Arai Y, Totoki Y, et al. Genomic spectra of biliary tract cancer. Nat Genet. 2015 Sep;47(9):1003–10. PMID:26258846
581. Nakanishi Y, Zen Y, Kondo S, et al. Expression of cell cycle-related molecules in biliary premalignant lesions: biliary intraepithelial neoplasia and biliary intraductal papillary neoplasm. Hum Pathol. 2008 Aug;39(8):1153–61. PMID:18495210
582. Nakanuma Y, Sudo Y. Biliary tumors with pancreatic counterparts. Semin Diagn Pathol. 2017 Mar;34(2):167–75. PMID:28109714
583. Nakanuma Y, Uesaka K, Kakuda Y, et al. Intraductal papillary neoplasm of bile duct: updated clinicopathological characteristics and molecular and genetic alterations. J Clin Med. 2020 Dec 9;9(12):3991. PMID:33317146
584. Nakanuma Y, Uesaka K, Okamura Y, et al. Reappraisal of pathological features of intraductal papillary neoplasm of bile duct with respect to the type 1 and 2 subclassifications. Hum Pathol. 2021 May;111:21–35. PMID:33508254
585. Nanda A, Brown JM, Berger SH, et al. Triple modality testing by endoscopic retrograde cholangiopancreatography for the diagnosis of cholangiocarcinoma. Therap Adv Gastroenterol. 2015 Mar;8(2):56–65. PMID:25729431
586. Nasr J, Sanders M, Fasanella K, et al. Lymphoepithelial cysts of the pancreas: an EUS case series. Gastrointest Endosc. 2008 Jul;68(1):170–3. PMID:18513719
587. National Comprehensive Cancer Network (NCCN). NCCN clinical practice guidelines in oncology (NCCN guidelines): Hepatobiliary cancers. Version 3.2021. Fort Washington (PA): NCCN; 2021. Available from: https://www.nccn.org/professionals/physician_gls/default.aspx.
588. Navaneethan U, Hasan MK, Lourdusamy V, et al. Single-operator cholangioscopy and targeted biopsies in the diagnosis of indeterminate biliary strictures: a systematic review. Gastrointest Endosc. 2015 Oct;82(4):608–14.e2. PMID:26071061
589. Navaneethan U, Njei B, Lourdusamy V, et al. Comparative effectiveness of biliary brush cytology and intraductal biopsy for detection of malignant biliary strictures: a systematic review and meta-analysis. Gastrointest Endosc. 2015 Jan;81(1):168–76. PMID:25440678
590. Nawgiri RS, Nagle JA, Wilbur DC, et al. Cytomorphology and B72.3 labeling of benign and malignant ductal epithelium in pancreatic lesions compared to gastrointestinal epithelium. Diagn Cytopathol. 2007 May;35(5):300–5. PMID:17427224
591. Nayer H, Weir EG, Sheth S, et al. Primary pancreatic lymphomas: a cytopathologic analysis of a rare malignancy. Cancer. 2004 Oct 25;102(5):315–21. PMID:15386314
592. Nesi G, Pantalone D, Ragionieri I, et al. Primary leiomyosarcoma of the pancreas: a case report and review of literature. Arch Pathol Lab Med. 2001 Jan;125(1):152–5. PMID:11151070
593. Nevala-Plagemann C, Hidalgo M, Garrido-Laguna I. From state-of-the-art treatments to novel therapies for advanced-stage pancreatic cancer. Nat Rev Clin Oncol. 2020 Feb;17(2):108–23. PMID:31705130
594. Nguyen NQ, Johns AL, Gill AJ, et al. Clinical and immunohistochemical features of 34 solid pseudopapillary tumors of the pancreas. J Gastroenterol Hepatol. 2011 Feb;26(2):267–74. PMID:21261715
595. Nikas IP, Proctor T, Seide S, et al. Diagnostic performance of pancreatic cytology with the Papanicolaou Society of Cytopathology System: a systematic review, before shifting into the upcoming WHO international system. Int J Mol Sci. 2022 Jan 31;23(3):1650. PMID:35163571
596. Nishizawa N, Kumamoto Y, Igarashi K, et al. A peripheral primitive neuroectodermal tumor originating from the pancreas: a case report and review of the literature. Surg Case Rep. 2015 Sep 11;1:80. PMID:26380804
597. Noë M, Niknafs N, Fischer CG, et al. Genomic characterization of malignant progression in neoplastic pancreatic cysts. Nat Commun. 2020 Aug 14;11(1):4085. PMID:32796935
598. Noh KW, Wallace MB. Endoscopic ultrasound-guided fine-needle aspiration in the diagnosis and staging of pancreatic adenocarcinoma. MedGenMed. 2005 May 25;7(2):15. PMID:16369394
599. Notohara K, Burgart LJ, Yadav D, et al. Idiopathic chronic pancreatitis with periductal lymphoplasmacytic infiltration: clinicopathologic features of 35 cases. Am J Surg Pathol. 2003 Aug;27(8):1119–27. PMID:12883244
600. Notohara K, Kamisawa T, Fukushima N, et al. Guidance for diagnosing autoimmune pancreatitis with biopsy tissues. Pathol Int. 2020 Oct;70(10):699–711. PMID:32767550
601. Notohara K, Kamisawa T, Kanno A, et al. Efficacy and limitations of the histological diagnosis of type 1 autoimmune pancreatitis with endoscopic ultrasound-guided fine needle biopsy with large tissue amounts. Pancreatology. 2020 Jul;20(5):834–43. PMID:32624418
602. Notohara K, Nishimori I, Mizuno N, et al. Clinicopathological features of type 2 autoimmune pancreatitis in Japan: results of a multicenter survey. Pancreas. 2015 Oct;44(7):1072–7. PMID:26335013
603. Novikov A, Kowalski TE, Loren DE. Practical management of indeterminate biliary strictures. Gastrointest Endosc Clin N Am. 2019 Apr;29(2):205–14. PMID:30846149
604. Ogura T, Yamao K, Sawaki A, et al. Clinical impact of K-ras mutation analysis in EUS-guided FNA specimens from pancreatic masses. Gastrointest Endosc. 2012 Apr;75(4):769–74. PMID:22284089
605. Oh HC, Kang H, Brugge WR. Cyst fluid amylase and CEA levels in the differential diagnosis of pancreatic cysts: a single-center experience with histologically proven cysts. Dig Dis Sci. 2014 Dec;59(12):3111–6. PMID:24965184
606. Ohaki Y, Misugi K, Fukuda J, et al. Immunohistochemical study of pancreatoblastoma. Acta Pathol Jpn. 1987 Oct;37(10):1581–90. PMID:2449037
607. Ohara Y, Oda T, Hashimoto S, et al. Pancreatic neuroendocrine tumor and solid-pseudopapillary neoplasm: key immunohistochemical profiles for differential diagnosis. World J Gastroenterol. 2016 Oct 14;22(38):8596–604. PMID:27784972
608. Ohmoto T, Yoshitani N, Nishitsuji K, et al. CD44-expressing undifferentiated carcinoma with rhabdoid features of the pancreas: molecular analysis of aggressive invasion and metastasis. Pathol Int. 2015 May;65(5):264–70. PMID:25753521
609. Okasha HH, Naga MI, Esmat S, et al. Endoscopic ultrasound-guided fine needle aspiration versus percutaneous ultrasound-guided fine needle aspiration in diagnosis of focal pancreatic masses. Endosc Ultrasound. 2013 Oct;2(4):190–3. PMID:24949394
610. Olofson AM, Biernacka A, Li Z, et al. Indeterminate diagnoses in EUS-guided FNA of the pancreas: analysis of cytologist and clinician perceptions, cytologic features, and clinical outcomes. J Am Soc Cytopathol. 2018 Sep-Oct;7(5):274–81. PMID:31043287
611. Olson MT, Siddiqui MT, Ali SZ. The differential diagnosis of squamous cells in pancreatic aspirates: from contamination to adenosquamous carcinoma. Acta Cytol. 2013;57(2):139–46. PMID:23406837
612. Olson MT, Wakely PE Jr, Ali SZ. Metastases to the pancreas diagnosed by fine-needle aspiration. Acta Cytol. 2013;57(5):473–80. PMID:24021904
613. Omiyale AO. Clinicopathological review of pancreatoblastoma in adults. Gland Surg. 2015 Aug;4(4):322–8. PMID:26312218
614. Onoyama T, Takeda Y, Kawata S, et al. Adequate tissue acquisition rate of peroral cholangioscopy-guided forceps biopsy. Ann Transl Med. 2020 Sep;8(17):1073. PMID:33145292
615. Orcutt ST, Coppola D, Hodul PJ. Colloid carcinoma of the pancreas: case report and review of the literature. Case Rep Pancreat Cancer. 2016 Jun 1;2(1):40–5. PMID:30631814
616. O'Reilly EM, Hechtman JF. Tumour response to TRK inhibition in a patient with pancreatic adenocarcinoma harbouring an NTRK gene fusion. Ann Oncol. 2019 Nov 1;30(Suppl_8):viii36–viii40. PMID:31605106
617. Oscarson J, Stormby N, Sundgren R. Selective angiography in fine-needle aspiration cytodiagnosis of gastric and pancreatic tumours. Acta Radiol Diagn (Stockh). 1972 Nov;12(6):737–50. PMID:4651749
618. Ozcan A, Shen SS, Hamilton C, et al. PAX 8 expression in non-neoplastic tissues, primary tumors, and metastatic tumors: a comprehensive immunohistochemical study. Mod Pathol. 2011 Jun;24(6):751–64. PMID:21317881
619. Ozretić L, Simonović AV, Rathbone ML, et al. The benefits of the Papanicolaou Society of Cytopathology System for reporting pancreatobiliary cytology: a 2-year review from a single academic institution. Cytopathology. 2021 Mar;32(2):227–32. PMID:33415845
620. Paal E, Thompson LD, Frommelt RA, et al. A clinicopathologic and immunohistochemical study of 35 anaplastic carcinomas of the pancreas with a review of the literature. Ann Diagn Pathol. 2001 Jun;5(3):129–40. PMID:11436166
621. Paal E, Thompson LD, Heffess CS. A clinicopathologic and immunohistochemical study of ten pancreatic lymphangiomas and a review of the literature. Cancer. 1998 Jun 1;82(11):2150–8. PMID:9610694
622. Pais SA, Al-Haddad M, Mohamadnejad M, et al. EUS for pancreatic neuroendocrine tumors: a single-center, 11-year experience. Gastrointest Endosc. 2010 Jun;71(7):1185–93. PMID:20304401
623. Pang JC, Roh MH. Metastases to the pancreas encountered on endoscopic ultrasound-guided, fine-needle aspiration. Arch Pathol Lab Med. 2015 Oct;139(10):1248–52. PMID:26414469
624. Park HJ, Kim SY, Kim HJ, et al. Intraductal papillary neoplasm of the bile duct: clinical, imaging, and pathologic features. AJR Am J Roentgenol. 2018 Jul;211(1):67–75. PMID:29629808
625. Park JK, Lee YJ, Lee JK, et al. KRAS mutation analysis of washing fluid from endoscopic ultrasound-guided fine needle aspiration improves cytologic diagnosis of pancreatic ductal adenocarcinoma. Oncotarget. 2017 Jan 10;8(2):3519–27. PMID:27974679
626. Park JK, Paik WH, Song BJ, et al. Additional K-ras mutation analysis and plectin-1 staining improve the diagnostic accuracy of pancreatic solid mass in EUS-guided fine needle aspiration. Oncotarget. 2017 Mar 11;8(38):64440–8. PMID:28969083
627. Park JY, Hong SM, Klimstra DS, et al. Pdx1 expression in pancreatic precursor lesions and neoplasms. Appl Immunohistochem Mol Morphol. 2011 Oct;19(5):444–9. PMID:21297446
628. Park WG, Mascarenhas R, Palaez-Luna M, et al. Diagnostic performance of cyst fluid carcinoembryonic antigen and amylase in histologically confirmed pancreatic cysts. Pancreas. 2011 Jan;40(1):42–5. PMID:20966811
629. Párniczky A, Kui B, Szentesi A, et al. Prospective, multicentre, nationwide clinical data from 600 cases of acute pancreatitis. PLoS One. 2016 Oct 31;11(10):e0165309. PMID:27798670
630. Pelosi G, Iannucci A, Zamboni G, et al. Solid and cystic papillary neoplasm of the pancreas: a clinico-cytopathologic and immunocytochemical study of five new cases diagnosed by fine-needle aspiration cytology and a review of the literature. Diagn Cytopathol. 1995 Oct;13(3):233–46. PMID:8575283
631. Pereira P, Morais R, Vilas-Boas F, et al. Brush cytology performance for the assessment of biliopancreatic strictures. Acta Cytol. 2020;64(4):344–51. PMID:31550713
632. Pérez-Cuadrado-Robles E, Deprez PH. Indications for single-operator cholangioscopy and pancreatoscopy: an expert review. Curr Treat Options Gastroenterol. 2019 Sep;17(3):408–19. PMID:31165382
633. Perez-Machado MA. Pancreatic cytology: standardised terminology and nomenclature. Cytopathology. 2016 Jun;27(3):157–60. PMID:27221751
634. Pettinato G, Di Vizio D, Manivel JC, et al. Solid-pseudopapillary tumor of the pancreas: a neoplasm with distinct and highly characteristic cytological features. Diagn Cytopathol. 2002 Dec;27(6):325–34. PMID:12451561
635. Pezzilli R, Buscarini E, Pollini T, et al. Epidemiology, clinical features and diagnostic work-up of cystic neoplasms of the pancreas: interim analysis of the prospective PANCY survey. Dig Liver Dis. 2020 May;52(5):547–54. PMID:32122771
636. Pham A, Forsmark C. Chronic pancreatitis: review and update of etiology, risk factors, and management. F1000Res. 2018 May 17;7:F1000 Faculty Rev-607. PMID:29946424
637. Pileri SA, Ascani S, Cox MC, et al. Myeloid sarcoma: clinico-pathologic, phenotypic and cytogenetic analysis of 92 adult patients. Leukemia. 2007 Feb;21(2):340–50. PMID:17170724
638. Pisapia P, Lozano MD, Vigliar E, et al. ALK and ROS1 testing on lung cancer cytologic samples: perspectives. Cancer Cytopathol. 2017 Nov;125(11):817–30. PMID:28743163
639. Pisapia P, Malapelle U, Roma G, et al. Consistency and reproducibility of next-generation sequencing in cytopathology: a second worldwide ring trial study on improved cytological molecular reference specimens. Cancer Cytopathol. 2019 May;127(5):285–96. PMID:31021538
640. Pitman MB. Pancreatic cyst fluid triage: a critical component of the preoperative evaluation of pancreatic cysts. Cancer Cytopathol. 2013 Feb;121(2):57–60. PMID:22961913

641. Pitman MB, Brugge WR, Warshaw AL. The value of cyst fluid analysis in the pre-operative evaluation of pancreatic cysts. J Gastrointest Oncol. 2011 Dec;2(4):195–8. PMID:22811850
642. Pitman MB, Centeno BA, Ali SZ, et al. Standardized terminology and nomenclature for pancreatobiliary cytology: the Papanicolaou Society of Cytopathology guidelines. Cytojournal. 2014 Jun 2;11(Suppl 1):3. PMID:25191517
643. Pitman MB, Centeno BA, Ali SZ, et al. Standardized terminology and nomenclature for pancreatobiliary cytology: the Papanicolaou Society of Cytopathology guidelines. Diagn Cytopathol. 2014 Apr;42(4):338–50. PMID:24554455
644. Pitman MB, Centeno BA, Daglilar ES, et al. Cytological criteria of high-grade epithelial atypia in the cyst fluid of pancreatic intraductal papillary mucinous neoplasms. Cancer Cytopathol. 2014 Jan;122(1):40–7. PMID:23939829
645. Pitman MB, Centeno BA, Genevay M, et al. Grading epithelial atypia in endoscopic ultrasound-guided fine-needle aspiration of intraductal papillary mucinous neoplasms: an international interobserver concordance study. Cancer Cytopathol. 2013 Dec;121(12):729–36. PMID:23881863
646. Pitman MB, Deshpande V. Endoscopic ultrasound-guided fine needle aspiration cytology of the pancreas: a morphological and multimodal approach to the diagnosis of solid and cystic mass lesions. Cytopathology. 2007 Dec;18(6):331–47. PMID:17559566
647. Pitman MB, Faquin WC. The fine-needle aspiration biopsy cytology of pancreatoblastoma. Diagn Cytopathol. 2004 Dec;31(6):402–6. PMID:15540188
648. Pitman MB, Genevay M, Yaeger K, et al. High-grade atypical epithelial cells in pancreatic mucinous cysts are a more accurate predictor of malignancy than "positive" cytology. Cancer Cytopathol. 2010 Dec 25;118(6):434–40. PMID:20931638
649. Pitman MB, Layfield LJ. Guidelines for pancreaticobiliary cytology from the Papanicolaou Society of Cytopathology: a review. Cancer Cytopathol. 2014 Jun;122(6):399–411. PMID:24777782
650. Pitman MB, Layfield LJ, editors. The Papanicolaou Society of Cytopathology System for Reporting Pancreaticobiliary Cytology: definitions, criteria, and explanatory notes. Cham (Switzerland): Springer; 2015.
651. Pitman MB, Lewandrowski K, Shen J, et al. Pancreatic cysts: preoperative diagnosis and clinical management. Cancer Cytopathol. 2010 Feb 25;118(1):1–13. PMID:20043327
652. Pitman MB, Yaeger KA, Brugge WR, et al. Prospective analysis of atypical epithelial cells as a high-risk cytologic feature for malignancy in pancreatic cysts. Cancer Cytopathol. 2013 Jan;121(1):29–36. PMID:23132817
653. Pitman MB. Chapter 14: Pancreas and biliary tree. In: Cibas ES, Ducatman BS, editors. Cytology: diagnostic principles and clinical correlates. 5th ed. New York (NY): Elsevier; 2019.
654. Pittman ME, Rao R, Hruban RH. Classification, morphology, molecular pathogenesis, and outcome of premalignant lesions of the pancreas. Arch Pathol Lab Med. 2017 Dec;141(12):1606–14. PMID:29189063
655. Plougmann JI, Klausen P, Toxvaerd A, et al. DNA sequencing of cytopathologically inconclusive EUS-FNA from solid pancreatic lesions suspicious for malignancy confirms EUS diagnosis. Endosc Ultrasound. 2020 Jan-Feb;9(1):37–44. PMID:31552911
656. Policarpio-Nicolas MLC, McHugh KE, Sae-Ow W, et al. Pleomorphic and atypical multinucleated giant cells in solid pseudopapillary neoplasm of pancreas: a diagnostic pitfall in cytology and a review of the literature. Diagn Cytopathol. 2019 May;47(5):488–93. PMID:30552752
657. Polkowski M, Jenssen C, Kaye P, et al. Technical aspects of endoscopic ultrasound (EUS)-guided sampling in gastroenterology: European Society of Gastrointestinal Endoscopy (ESGE) Technical Guideline - March 2017. Endoscopy. 2017 Oct;49(10):989–1006. PMID:28898917
658. Poller DN, Schmitt F. Should uncertainty concerning the risk of malignancy be included in diagnostic (nongynecologic) cytopathology reports? Cancer Cytopathol. 2021 Jan;129(1):16–21. PMID:32649050
659. Proietti A, Ali G, Pelliccioni S, et al. Anaplastic lymphoma kinase gene rearrangements in cytological samples of non-small cell lung cancer: comparison with histological assessment. Cancer Cytopathol. 2014 Jun;122(6):445–53. PMID:24648382
660. Puli SR, Bechtold ML, Buxbaum JL, et al. How good is endoscopic ultrasound-guided fine-needle aspiration in diagnosing the correct etiology for a solid pancreatic mass?: A meta-analysis and systematic review. Pancreas. 2013 Jan;42(1):20–6. PMID:23254913
661. Rahemtullah A, Misdraji J, Pitman MB. Adenosquamous carcinoma of the pancreas: cytologic features in 14 cases. Cancer. 2003 Dec 25;99(6):372–8. PMID:14681946
662. Rainone M, Singh I, Salo-Mullen EE, et al. An emerging paradigm for germline testing in pancreatic ductal adenocarcinoma and immediate implications for clinical practice: a review. JAMA Oncol. 2020 May 1;6(5):764–71. PMID:32053139
663. Ramani NS, Chen H, Broaddus RR, et al. Utilization of cytology smears improves success rates of RNA-based next-generation sequencing gene fusion assays for clinically relevant predictive biomarkers. Cancer Cytopathol. 2021 May;129(5):374–82. PMID:33119213
664. Rangarajan K, Pucher PH, Armstrong T, et al. Systemic neoadjuvant chemotherapy in modern pancreatic cancer treatment: a systematic review and meta-analysis. Ann R Coll Surg Engl. 2019 Sep;101(7):453–62. PMID:31304767
665. Rao RN, Vij M, Singla N, et al. Malignant pancreatic extra-gastrointestinal stromal tumor diagnosed by ultrasound guided fine needle aspiration cytology. A case report with a review of the literature. JOP. 2011 May 6;12(3):283–6. PMID:21546710
666. Rasmussen SN, Holm HH, Kristensen JK, et al. Ultrasonically-guided liver biopsy. Br Med J. 1972 May 27;2(5812):500–2. PMID:5031210
667. Raut CP, Fernandez-del Castillo C. Giant lipoma of the pancreas: case report and review of lipomatous lesions of the pancreas. Pancreas. 2003 Jan;26(1):97–9. PMID:12499926
668. Raval JS, Zeh HJ, Moser AJ, et al. Pancreatic lymphoepithelial cysts express CEA and can contain mucous cells: potential pitfalls in the preoperative diagnosis. Mod Pathol. 2010 Nov;23(11):1467–76. PMID:20802468
669. Ray S, Lu Z, Rajendiran S. Clear cell ductal adenocarcinoma of pancreas: a case report and review of the literature. Arch Pathol Lab Med. 2004 Jun;128(6):693–6. PMID:15163226
670. Raymond SLT, Yugawa D, Chang KHF, et al. Metastatic neoplasms to the pancreas diagnosed by fine-needle aspiration/biopsy cytology: a 15-year retrospective analysis. Diagn Cytopathol. 2017 Sep;45(9):771–83. PMID:28603895
671. Real FX, Vilá MR, Skoudy A, et al. Intermediate filaments as differentiation markers of exocrine pancreas. II. Expression of cytokeratins of complex and stratified epithelia in normal pancreas and in pancreas cancer. Int J Cancer. 1993 Jul 9;54(5):720–7. PMID:7686885
672. Rebours V, Lévy P, Mosnier JF, et al. Pathology analysis reveals that dysplastic pancreatic ductal lesions are frequent in patients with hereditary pancreatitis. Clin Gastroenterol Hepatol. 2010 Feb;8(2):206–12. PMID:19765677
673. Recavarren C, Labow DM, Liang J, et al. Histologic characteristics of pancreatic intraepithelial neoplasia associated with different pancreatic lesions. Hum Pathol. 2011 Jan;42(1):18–24. PMID:21056895
674. Redelman M, Cramer HM, Wu HH. Pancreatic fine-needle aspiration cytology in patients < 35-years of age: a retrospective review of 174 cases spanning a 17-year period. Diagn Cytopathol. 2014 Apr;42(4):297–301. PMID:24273058
675. Reid MD. Cytologic assessment of cystic/intraductal lesions of the pancreatobiliary tract. Arch Pathol Lab Med. 2022 Mar 1;146(3):280–97. PMID:33836534
676. Reid MD, Bagci P, Adsay NV. Histopathologic assessment of pancreatic cancer: Does one size fit all? J Surg Oncol. 2013 Jan;107(1):67–77. PMID:22711682
677. Reid MD, Bagci P, Ohike N, et al. Calculation of the Ki67 index in pancreatic neuroendocrine tumors: a comparative analysis of four counting methodologies. Mod Pathol. 2015 May;28(5):686–94. PMID:25412850
678. Reid MD, Balci S, Saka B, et al. Neuroendocrine tumors of the pancreas: current concepts and controversies. Endocr Pathol. 2014 Mar;25(1):65–79. PMID:24430597
679. Reid MD, Bhattarai S, Graham RP, et al. Pancreatoblastoma: cytologic and histologic analysis of 12 adult cases reveals helpful criteria in their diagnosis and distinction from common mimics. Cancer Cytopathol. 2019 Nov;127(11):708–19. PMID:31581358
680. Reid MD, Choi HJ, Memis B, et al. Serous neoplasms of the pancreas: a clinicopathologic analysis of 193 cases and literature review with new insights on macrocystic and solid variants and critical reappraisal of so-called "serous cystadenocarcinoma". Am J Surg Pathol. 2015 Dec;39(12):1597–610. PMID:26559376
681. Reid MD, Lewis MM, Willingham FF, et al. The evolving role of pathology in new developments, classification, terminology, and diagnosis of pancreatobiliary neoplasms. Arch Pathol Lab Med. 2017 Mar;141(3):366–80. PMID:28055239
682. Reid MD, Muraki T, HooKim K, et al. Cytologic features and clinical implications of undifferentiated carcinoma with osteoclastic giant cells of the pancreas: an analysis of 15 cases. Cancer Cytopathol. 2017 Jul;125(7):563–75. PMID:28371566
683. Reid MD, Stallworth CR, Lewis MM, et al. Cytopathologic diagnosis of oncocytic type intraductal papillary mucinous neoplasm: criteria and clinical implications of accurate diagnosis. Cancer Cytopathol. 2016 Feb;124(2):122–34. PMID:26415076
684. Renno A, Hill M, Abdel-Aziz Y, et al. Diagnosis of intrapancreatic accessory spleen by endoscopic ultrasound-guided fine-needle aspiration mimicking a pancreatic neoplasm: a case report and review of literature. Clin J Gastroenterol. 2020 Apr;13(2):287–97. PMID:31549337
685. Renshaw AA, Madge R, Jiroutek M, et al. Bile duct brushing cytology: statistical analysis of proposed diagnostic criteria. Am J Clin Pathol. 1998 Nov;110(5):635–40. PMID:9802349
686. Reyes MC, Huang X, Bain A, et al. Primary pancreatic leiomyosarcoma with metastasis to the liver diagnosed by endoscopic ultrasound-guided fine needle aspiration and fine needle biopsy: a case report and review of literature. Diagn Cytopathol. 2016 Dec;44(12):1070–3. PMID:27455910
687. Ribaldone DG, Bruno M, Gaia S, et al. Differential diagnosis of pancreatic cysts: a prospective study on the role of intra-cystic glucose concentration. Dig Liver Dis. 2020 Sep;52(9):1026–32. PMID:32675041
688. Richardson SO, Huibers MMH, de Weger RA, et al. One-fits-all pretreatment protocol facilitating fluorescence in situ hybridization on formalin-fixed paraffin-embedded, fresh frozen and cytological slides. Mol Cytogenet. 2019 Jun 17;12:27. PMID:31236139
689. Rizvi S, Eaton JE, Gores GJ. Primary sclerosing cholangitis as a premalignant biliary tract disease: surveillance and management. Clin Gastroenterol Hepatol. 2015 Nov;13(12):2152–65. PMID:26051390
690. Rizvi S, Khan SA, Hallemeier CL, et al. Cholangiocarcinoma - evolving concepts and therapeutic strategies. Nat Rev Clin Oncol. 2018 Feb;15(2):95–111. PMID:28994423
691. Robins DB, Katz RL, Evans DB, et al. Fine needle aspiration of the pancreas. In quest of accuracy. Acta Cytol. 1995 Jan-Feb;39(1):1–10. PMID:7846994
692. Robison LS, Canon CL, Varadarajulu S, et al. Autoimmune pancreatitis mimicking pancreatic cancer. J Hepatobiliary Pancreat Sci. 2011 Mar;18(2):162–9. PMID:20811916
693. Rodriguez E, Netto G, Li QK. Intrapancreatic accessory spleen: a case report and review of literature. Diagn Cytopathol. 2013 May;41(5):466–9. PMID:22241738
694. Rodriguez-Matta E, Hemmerich A, Starr J, et al. Molecular genetic changes in solid pseudopapillary neoplasms (SPN) of the pancreas. Acta Oncol. 2020 Sep;59(9):1024–7. PMID:32672484
695. Rogers C, Samore W, Pitman MB, et al. Solitary fibrous tumor involving the pancreas: report of the cytologic features and first report of a primary pancreatic solitary fibrous tumor diagnosed by fine-needle aspiration biopsy. J Am Soc Cytopathol. 2020 Jul-Aug;9(4):272–7. PMID:32423685
696. Roh MH. The utilization of cytologic and small biopsy samples for ancillary molecular testing. Mod Pathol. 2019 Jan;32(Suppl 1):77–85. PMID:30600323
697. Roh YH, Hwang SY, Lee SM, et al. Extramedullary plasmacytoma of the pancreas diagnosed using endoscopic ultrasonography-guided fine needle aspiration. Clin Endosc. 2014 Jan;47(1):115–8. PMID:24570894
698. Rooney SL, Shi J. Intraductal tubulopapillary neoplasm of the pancreas: an update from a pathologist's perspective. Arch Pathol Lab Med. 2016 Oct;140(10):1068–73. PMID:27684978
699. Rosenbaum MW, Arpin R, Limbocker J, et al. Cytomorphologic characteristics of next-generation sequencing-positive bile duct brushing specimens. J Am Soc Cytopathol. 2020 Nov-Dec;9(6):520–7. PMID:32839152
700. Rosenbaum MW, Jones M, Dudley JC, et al. Next-generation sequencing adds value to the preoperative diagnosis of pancreatic cysts. Cancer Cytopathol. 2017 Jan;125(1):41–7. PMID:27647802
701. Roy S, LaFramboise WA, Liu TC, et al. Loss of chromatin-remodeling proteins and/or CDKN2A associates with metastasis of pancreatic neuroendocrine tumors and reduced patient survival times. Gastroenterology. 2018 Jun;154(8):2060–2063.e8. PMID:29486199
702. Roy-Chowdhuri S, Stewart J. Preanalytic variables in cytology: lessons learned from next-generation sequencing-the MD Anderson experience. Arch Pathol Lab Med. 2016 Nov;140(11):1191–9. PMID:27333361
703. Roy-Chowdhuri S, VanderLaan PA, Stewart JM, et al., editors. Molecular diagnostics in cytopathology: a practical handbook for the practicing pathologist. Cham (Switzerland): Springer; 2019.
704. Russell-Goldman E, Hornick JL, Qian X, et al. NKX2.2 immunohistochemistry in the distinction of Ewing sarcoma from cytomorphologic mimics: diagnostic utility and pitfalls. Cancer Cytopathol. 2018 Nov;126(11):942–9. PMID:30376220

705. Sadakari Y, Kanda M, Maitani K, et al. Mutant KRAS and GNAS DNA concentrations in secretin-stimulated pancreatic fluid collected from the pancreatic duct and the duodenal lumen. Clin Transl Gastroenterol. 2014 Nov 13;5(11):e62. PMID:25393586

706. Sagami R, Yamao K, Nakahodo J, et al. Pre-operative imaging and pathological diagnosis of localized high-grade pancreatic intra-epithelial neoplasia without invasive carcinoma. Cancers (Basel). 2021 Feb 24;13(5):945. PMID:33668239

707. Sah RP, Chari ST, Pannala R, et al. Differences in clinical profile and relapse rate of type 1 versus type 2 autoimmune pancreatitis. Gastroenterology. 2010 Jul;139(1):140–8. PMID:20353791

708. Sah RP, Garg P, Saluja AK. Pathogenic mechanisms of acute pancreatitis. Curr Opin Gastroenterol. 2012 Sep;28(5):507–15. PMID:22885948

709. Sahu KK, Rau AR, Bhat N, et al. Imprint cytology of pancreatoblastoma: a case report and review of the literature. Diagn Cytopathol. 2009 Apr;37(4):290–2. PMID:19229998

710. Saieg M. Implementing the Papanicolaou Society of Cytopathology terminology system for reporting pancreaticobiliary cytology refines risk of malignancy in pancreatic specimens. J Am Soc Cytopathol. 2019 May-Jun;8(3):117–9. PMID:31097286

711. Saieg M, Pitman MB. Experience and future perspectives on the use of the Papanicolaou Society of Cytopathology Terminology System for reporting pancreaticobiliary cytology. Diagn Cytopathol. 2020 May;48(5):494–8. PMID:32031332

712. Saieg MA, Munson V, Colletti S, et al. The impact of the new proposed Papanicolaou Society of Cytopathology terminology for pancreaticobiliary cytology in endoscopic US-FNA: a single-institutional experience. Cancer Cytopathol. 2015 Aug;123(8):488–94. PMID:25994860

713. Sakhdari A, Moghaddam PA, Pejchal M, et al. Sequential molecular and cytologic analyses provides a complementary approach to the diagnosis of pancreatic cystic lesions: a decade of clinical practice. J Am Soc Cytopathol. 2020 Jan-Feb;9(1):38–44. PMID:31711852

714. Sallinen V, Le Large TY, Galeev S, et al. Surveillance strategy for small asymptomatic non-functional pancreatic neuroendocrine tumors - a systematic review and meta-analysis. HPB (Oxford). 2017 Apr;19(4):310–20. PMID:28254159

715. Salomao M, Gonda TA, Margolskee E, et al. Strategies for improving diagnostic accuracy of biliary strictures. Cancer Cytopathol. 2015 Apr;123(4):244–52. PMID:25564796

716. Salomao M, Remotti H, Allendorf JD, et al. Fine-needle aspirations of pancreatic serous cystadenomas: improving diagnostic yield with cell blocks and α-inhibin immunohistochemistry. Cancer Cytopathol. 2014 Jan;122(1):33–9. PMID:23939868

717. Salvia R, Fernández-del Castillo C, Bassi C, et al. Main-duct intraductal papillary mucinous neoplasms of the pancreas: clinical predictors of malignancy and long-term survival following resection. Ann Surg. 2004 May;239(5):678–85. PMID:15082972

718. Samad A, Shah AA, Stelow EB, et al. Cercariform cells: another cytologic feature distinguishing solid pseudopapillary neoplasms from pancreatic endocrine neoplasms and acinar cell carcinomas in endoscopic ultrasound-guided fine-needle aspirates. Cancer Cytopathol. 2013 Jun;121(6):298–310. PMID:23765692

719. Sandrasegaran K, Tomasian A, Elsayes KM, et al. Hematologic malignancies of the pancreas. Abdom Imaging. 2015 Feb;40(2):411–23. PMID:25120155

720. Sangfelt P, Sundin A, Wanders A, et al. Monitoring dominant strictures in primary sclerosing cholangitis with brush cytology and FDG-PET. J Hepatol. 2014 Dec;61(6):1352–7. PMID:25111173

721. Sangoi AR, Ohgami RS, Pai RK, et al. PAX8 expression reliably distinguishes pancreatic well-differentiated neuroendocrine tumors from ileal and pulmonary well-differentiated neuroendocrine tumors and pancreatic acinar cell carcinoma. Mod Pathol. 2011 Mar;24(3):412–24. PMID:20890270

722. Sano M, Homma T, Hayashi E, et al. Clinicopathological characteristics of anaplastic carcinoma of the pancreas with rhabdoid features. Virchows Arch. 2014 Nov;465(5):531–8. PMID:25031015

723. Sarin H, Manucha V, Verma K. Extramedullary plasmacytoma, a report of five cases diagnosed by FNAC. Cytopathology. 2009 Oct;20(5):328–31. PMID:19416311

724. Sarr MG, Carpenter HA, Prabhakar LP, et al. Clinical and pathologic correlation of 84 mucinous cystic neoplasms of the pancreas: Can one reliably differentiate benign from malignant (or premalignant) neoplasms? Ann Surg. 2000 Feb;231(2):205–12. PMID:10674612

725. Sarr MG, Kendrick ML, Nagorney DM, et al. Cystic neoplasms of the pancreas: benign to malignant epithelial neoplasms. Surg Clin North Am. 2001 Jun;81(3):497–509. PMID:11459267

726. Sato T, Kato S, Watanabe S, et al. Primary leiomyoma of the pancreas diagnosed by endoscopic ultrasound-guided fine-needle aspiration. Dig Endosc. 2012 Sep;24(5):380. PMID:22925296

727. Sato Y, Sasaki M, Harada K, et al. Pathological diagnosis of flat epithelial lesions of the biliary tract with emphasis on biliary intraepithelial neoplasia. J Gastroenterol. 2014 Jan;49(1):64–72. PMID:23616173

728. Savant D, Lee L, Das K. Intraductal tubulopapillary neoplasm of the pancreas masquerading as pancreatic neuroendocrine carcinoma: review of the literature with a case report. Acta Cytol. 2016;60(3):267–74. PMID:27459312

729. Savari O, Al-Duwal Z, Wang Z, et al. Pancreatic lymphoma: a cytologic diagnosis challenge. Diagn Cytopathol. 2020 Apr;48(4):350–5. PMID:31774250

730. Savic S, Bubendorf L. Common fluorescence in situ hybridization applications in cytology. Arch Pathol Lab Med. 2016 Dec;140(12):1323–30. PMID:27479335

731. Saxena P, El Zein M, Stevens T, et al. Stylet slow-pull versus standard suction for endoscopic ultrasound-guided fine-needle aspiration of solid pancreatic lesions: a multicenter randomized trial. Endoscopy. 2018 May;50(5):497–504. PMID:29272906

732. Scarpa A, Chang DK, Nones K, et al. Whole-genome landscape of pancreatic neuroendocrine tumours. Nature. 2017 Mar 2;543(7643):65–71. PMID:28199314

733. Scheid JF, Rosenbaum MW, Przybyszewski EM, et al. Next-generation sequencing in the evaluation of biliary strictures in patients with primary sclerosing cholangitis. Cancer Cytopathol. 2022 Mar;130(3):215–30. PMID:34726838

734. Schizas D, Charalampakis N, Kole C, et al. Immunotherapy for pancreatic cancer: a 2020 update. Cancer Treat Rev. 2020 Jun;86:102016. PMID:32247999

735. Schlitter AM, Born D, Bettstetter M, et al. Intraductal papillary neoplasms of the bile duct: stepwise progression to carcinoma involves common molecular pathways. Mod Pathol. 2014 Jan;27(1):73–86. PMID:23828315

736. Schlitter AM, Jang KT, Klöppel G, et al. Intraductal tubulopapillary neoplasms of the bile ducts: clinicopathologic, immunohistochemical, and molecular analysis of 20 cases. Mod Pathol. 2015 Sep;28(9):1249–64. PMID:26111977

737. Schmidt CM, Matos JM, Bentrem DJ, et al. Acinar cell carcinoma of the pancreas in the United States: prognostic factors and comparison to ductal adenocarcinoma. J Gastrointest Surg. 2008 Dec;12(12):2078–86. PMID:18836784

738. Schmidt MT, Himmelfarb EA, Shafi H, et al. Use of IMP3, S100P, and pVHL immunopanel to aid in the interpretation of bile duct biopsies with atypical histology or suspicious for malignancy. Appl Immunohistochem Mol Morphol. 2012 Oct;20(5):478–87. PMID:22495381

739. Schmidt RL, Witt BL, Lopez-Calderon LE, et al. The influence of rapid onsite evaluation on the adequacy rate of fine-needle aspiration cytology: a systematic review and meta-analysis. Am J Clin Pathol. 2013 Mar;139(3):300–8. PMID:23429365

740. Schmidt RL, Witt BL, Matynia AP, et al. Rapid on-site evaluation increases endoscopic ultrasound-guided fine-needle aspiration adequacy for pancreatic lesions. Dig Dis Sci. 2013 Mar;58(3):872–82. PMID:23053888

741. Schmitt F, editor. Molecular applications in cytology. Cham (Switzerland): Springer; 2018.

742. Schmitz D, Kazdal D, Allgäuer M, et al. KRAS/GNAS-testing by highly sensitive deep targeted next generation sequencing improves the endoscopic ultrasound-guided workup of suspected mucinous neoplasms of the pancreas. Genes Chromosomes Cancer. 2021 Jul;60(7):489–97. PMID:33686791

743. Schnelldorfer T, Sarr MG, Nagorney DM, et al. Experience with 208 resections for intraductal papillary mucinous neoplasm of the pancreas. Arch Surg. 2008 Jul;143(7):639–46. PMID:18645105

744. Schreiner AM, Mansoor A, Faigel DO, et al. Intrapancreatic accessory spleen: mimic of pancreatic endocrine tumor diagnosed by endoscopic ultrasound-guided fine-needle aspiration biopsy. Diagn Cytopathol. 2008 Apr;36(4):262–5. PMID:18335556

745. Schüssler MH, Skoudy A, Ramaekers F, et al. Intermediate filaments as differentiation markers of normal pancreas and pancreas cancer. Am J Pathol. 1992 Mar;140(3):559–68. PMID:1372155

746. Schwartz DA, Unni KK, Levy MJ, et al. The rate of false-positive results with EUS-guided fine-needle aspiration. Gastrointest Endosc. 2002 Dec;56(6):868–72. PMID:12447300

747. Schwenk J, Makovitzky J. Tissue expression of the cancer-associated antigens CA 19-9 and CA-50 in chronic pancreatitis and pancreatic carcinoma. Int J Pancreatol. 1989 Jul;5(1):85–98. PMID:2746048

748. Scourtas A, Dudley JC, Brugge WR, et al. Preoperative characteristics and cytological features of 136 histologically confirmed pancreatic mucinous cystic neoplasms. Cancer Cytopathol. 2017 Mar;125(3):169–77. PMID:27926784

749. Seidel G, Zahurak M, Iacobuzio-Donahue C, et al. Almost all infiltrating colloid carcinomas of the pancreas and periampullary region arise from in situ papillary neoplasms: a study of 39 cases. Am J Surg Pathol. 2002 Jan;26(1):56–63. PMID:11756769

750. Seki M, Ninomiya E, Hayashi K, et al. Widespread and multifocal carcinomas in situ (CISs) through almost the entire pancreas: report of a case with preoperative cytological diagnosis. Langenbecks Arch Surg. 2010 Jun;395(5):589–92. PMID:20013290

751. Sekulic M, Amin K, Mettler T, et al. Pancreatic involvement by metastasizing neoplasms as determined by endoscopic ultrasound-guided fine needle aspiration: a clinicopathologic characterization. Diagn Cytopathol. 2017 May;45(5):418–25. PMID:28205397

752. Selvaggi SM. Bile duct brushing cytology: cytohistologic/fine-needle aspiration correlation and diagnostic pitfalls. J Am Soc Cytopathol. 2016 Sep-Oct;5(5):296–300. PMID:31042506

753. Senoo J, Mikata R, Kishimoto T, et al. Immunohistochemical analysis of IMP3 and p53 expression in endoscopic ultrasound-guided fine needle aspiration and resected specimens of pancreatic diseases. Pancreatology. 2018 Mar;18(2):176–83. PMID:29305088

754. Sessa F, Bonato M, Frigerio B, et al. Ductal cancers of the pancreas frequently express markers of gastrointestinal epithelial cells. Gastroenterology. 1990 Jun;98(6):1655–65. PMID:1692551

755. Shah M, Mcclelland A, Moadel R, et al. Splenule disguised as pancreatic mass: elucidated with SPECT liver-spleen scintigraphy. Clin Nucl Med. 2014 Sep;39(9):e405–6. PMID:24097009

756. Shah MH, Goldner WS, Halfdanarson TR, et al. NCCN guidelines insights: Neuroendocrine and adrenal tumors, Version 2.2018. J Natl Compr Canc Netw. 2018 Jun;16(6):693–702. PMID:29891520

757. Shami VM, Sundaram V, Stelow EB, et al. The level of carcinoembryonic antigen and the presence of mucin as predictors of cystic pancreatic mucinous neoplasia. Pancreas. 2007 May;34(4):466–9. PMID:17446847

758. Sharma A, Mukewar S, Vege SS. Clinical profile of pancreatic cystic lesions in von Hippel-Lindau disease: a series of 48 patients seen at a tertiary institution. Pancreas. 2017 Aug;46(7):948–52. PMID:28697137

759. Sharpe SM, In H, Winchester DJ, et al. Surgical resection provides an overall survival benefit for patients with small pancreatic neuroendocrine tumors. J Gastrointest Surg. 2015 Jan;19(1):117–23. PMID:25155459

760. Shen GQ, Aleassa EM, Walsh RM, et al. Next-generation sequencing in pancreatic cancer. Pancreas. 2019 Jul;48(6):739–48. PMID:31206465

761. Shen J, Brugge WR, Dimaio CJ, et al. Molecular analysis of pancreatic cyst fluid: a comparative analysis with current practice of diagnosis. Cancer. 2009 Jun 25;117(3):217–27. PMID:19415731

762. Shi C, Klein AP, Goggins M, et al. Increased prevalence of precursor lesions in familial pancreatic cancer patients. Clin Cancer Res. 2009 Dec 15;15(24):7737–43. PMID:19996207

763. Shi J, Liu H, Wang HL, et al. Diagnostic utility of von Hippel-Lindau gene product, maspin, IMP3, and S100P in adenocarcinoma of the gallbladder. Hum Pathol. 2013 Apr;44(4):503–11. PMID:23079206

764. Shi Z, Cao D, Zhuang Q, et al. MR imaging features of pancreatic schwannoma: a Chinese case series and a systematic review of 25 cases. Cancer Imaging. 2021 Feb 15;21(1):23. PMID:33588954

765. Shibahara H, Tamada S, Goto M, et al. Pathologic features of mucin-producing bile duct tumors: two histopathologic categories as counterparts of pancreatic intraductal papillary-mucinous neoplasms. Am J Surg Pathol. 2004 Mar;28(3):327–38. PMID:15104295

766. Shidham VB, Chang CC, Rao RN, et al. Immunostaining of cytology smears: a comparative study to identify the most suitable method of smear preparation and fixation with reference to commonly used immunomarkers. Diagn Cytopathol. 2003 Oct;29(4):217–21. PMID:14506675

767. Shimosegawa T, Chari ST, Frulloni L, et al. International consensus diagnostic criteria for autoimmune pancreatitis: guidelines of the International Association of Pancreatology. Pancreas. 2011 Apr;40(3):352–8. PMID:21412117

768. Shin LK, Jeffrey RB, Pai RK, et al. Multidetector CT imaging of the pancreatic groove: differentiating carcinomas from paraduodenal pancreatitis. Clin Imaging. 2016 Nov-Dec;40(6):1246–52. PMID:27636383

769. Shukla VK, Pandey M, Kumar M, et al. Ultrasound-guided fine needle aspiration cytology of malignant gallbladder masses. Acta Cytol. 1997 Nov-Dec;41(6):1654–8. PMID:9390120

770. Siddiqui AA, Kowalski TE, Shahid H, et al. False-positive EUS-guided FNA cytology for solid pancreatic lesions. Gastrointest Endosc. 2011 Sep;74(3):535–40. PMID:21737075

771. Sigel C, Reidy-Lagunes D, Lin O, et al. Cytological features contributing to the misclassification of pancreatic neuroendocrine tumors. J Am Soc Cytopathol. 2016 Sep-Oct;5(5):266–76. PMID:31042503

772. Sigel CS. Advances in the cytologic diagnosis of gastroenteropancreatic neuroendocrine neoplasms. Cancer Cytopathol. 2018 Dec;126(12):980–91. PMID:30485690

773. Sigel CS, Guo H, Sigel KM, et al. Cytology assessment can predict survival for patients with metastatic pancreatic neuroendocrine neoplasms. Cancer Cytopathol. 2017 Mar;125(3):188–96. PMID:28094897

774. Sigel CS, Klimstra DS. Cytomorphologic and immunophenotypical features of acinar cell neoplasms of the pancreas. Cancer Cytopathol. 2013 Aug;121(8):459–70. PMID:23408736

775. Sigel CS, Krauss Silva VW, Reid MD, et al. Well differentiated grade 3 pancreatic neuroendocrine tumors compared with related neoplasms: a morphologic study. Cancer Cytopathol. 2018 May;126(5):326–35. PMID:29451738

776. Silverman JF, Dabbs DJ, Finley JL, et al. Fine-needle aspiration biopsy of pleomorphic (giant cell) carcinoma of the pancreas. Cytologic, immunocytochemical, and ultrastructural findings. Am J Clin Pathol. 1988 Jun;89(6):714–20. PMID:3369361

777. Silverman JF, Holbrook CT, Pories WJ, et al. Fine needle aspiration cytology of pancreatoblastoma with immunocytochemical and ultrastructural studies. Acta Cytol. 1990 Sep-Oct;34(5):632–40. PMID:2220242

778. Simons-Linares CR, Yadav D, Lopez R, et al. The utility of intracystic glucose levels in differentiating mucinous from non mucinous pancreatic cysts. Pancreatology. 2020 Oct;20(7):1386–92. PMID:32919884

779. Singh P, Kumar P, Rohilla M, et al. Fine needle aspiration cytology with the aid of immunocytochemistry on cell-block confirms the diagnosis of solid pseudopapillary neoplasm of the pancreas. Cytopathology. 2021 Jan;32(1):57–64. PMID:32319130

780. Singh R, Basturk O, Klimstra DS, et al. Lipid-rich variant of pancreatic endocrine neoplasms. Am J Surg Pathol. 2006 Feb;30(2):194–200. PMID:16434893

781. Singh VK, Yadav D, Garg PK. Diagnosis and management of chronic pancreatitis: a review. JAMA. 2019 Dec 24;322(24):2422–34. PMID:31860051

782. Singhal RL, Monaco SE, Pantanowitz L. Cytopathology of myeloid sarcoma: a study of 16 cases. J Am Soc Cytopathol. 2015 Mar-Apr;4(2):98–103. PMID:31051716

783. Singhi AD, Ali SM, Lacy J, et al. Identification of targetable ALK rearrangements in pancreatic ductal adenocarcinoma. J Natl Compr Canc Netw. 2017 May;15(5):555–62. PMID:28476735

784. Singhi AD, Klimstra DS. Well-differentiated pancreatic neuroendocrine tumours (PanNETs) and poorly differentiated pancreatic neuroendocrine carcinomas (PanNECs): concepts, issues and a practical diagnostic approach to high-grade (G3) cases. Histopathology. 2018 Jan;72(1):168–77. PMID:29239037

785. Singhi AD, Lilo M, Hruban RH, et al. Overexpression of lymphoid enhancer-binding factor 1 (LEF1) in solid-pseudopapillary neoplasms of the pancreas. Mod Pathol. 2014 Oct;27(10):1355–63. PMID:24658583

786. Singhi AD, Liu TC, Roncaioli JL, et al. Alternative lengthening of telomeres and loss of DAXX/ATRX expression predicts metastatic disease and poor survival in patients with pancreatic neuroendocrine tumors. Clin Cancer Res. 2017 Jan 15;23(2):600–9. PMID:27407094

787. Singhi AD, McGrath K, Brand RE, et al. Preoperative next-generation sequencing of pancreatic cyst fluid is highly accurate in cyst classification and detection of advanced neoplasia. Gut. 2018 Dec;67(12):2131–41. PMID:28970292

788. Singhi AD, Nikiforova MN, Chennat J, et al. Integrating next-generation sequencing to endoscopic retrograde cholangiopancreatography (ERCP)-obtained biliary specimens improves the detection and management of patients with malignant bile duct strictures. Gut. 2020 Jan;69(1):52–61. PMID:30971436

789. Singhi AD, Nikiforova MN, Fasanella KE, et al. Preoperative GNAS and KRAS testing in the diagnosis of pancreatic mucinous cysts. Clin Cancer Res. 2014 Aug 15;20(16):4381–9. PMID:24938521

790. Singhi AD, Wood LD, Parks E, et al. Recurrent rearrangements in PRKACA and PRKACB in intraductal oncocytic papillary neoplasms of the pancreas and bile duct. Gastroenterology. 2020 Feb;158(3):573–582.e2. PMID:31678302

791. Singhi AD, Zeh HJ, Brand RE, et al. American Gastroenterological Association guidelines are inaccurate in detecting pancreatic cysts with advanced neoplasia: a clinicopathologic study of 225 patients with supporting molecular data. Gastrointest Endosc. 2016 Jun;83(6):1107–1117.e2. PMID:26709110

792. Smith AL, Abdul-Karim FW, Goyal A. Cytologic categorization of pancreatic neoplastic mucinous cysts with an assessment of the risk of malignancy: a retrospective study based on the Papanicolaou Society of Cytopathology guidelines. Cancer Cytopathol. 2016 Apr;124(4):285–93. PMID:26618476

793. Smith AL, Odronic SI, Springer BS, et al. Solid tumor metastases to the pancreas diagnosed by FNA: a single-institution experience and review of the literature. Cancer Cytopathol. 2015 Jun;123(6):347–55. PMID:25828394

794. Smith EH, Bartrum RJ Jr, Chang YC. Ultrasonically guided percutaneous aspiration biopsy of the pancreas. Radiology. 1974 Sep;112(3):737–8. PMID:4843311

795. Smith EH, Bartrum RJ Jr, Chang YC, et al. Percutaneous aspiration biopsy of the pancreas under ultrasonic guidance. N Engl J Med. 1975 Apr 17;292(16):825–8. PMID:1113814

796. Smoczynski M, Jablonska A, Matyskiel A, et al. Routine brush cytology and fluorescence in situ hybridization for assessment of pancreatobiliary strictures. Gastrointest Endosc. 2012 Jan;75(1):65–73. PMID:22078103

797. Sohn TA, Yeo CJ, Cameron JL, et al. Intraductal papillary mucinous neoplasms of the pancreas: an increasingly recognized clinicopathologic entity. Ann Surg. 2001 Sep;234(3):313–21. PMID:11524584

798. Sohn TA, Yeo CJ, Cameron JL, et al. Intraductal papillary mucinous neoplasms of the pancreas: an updated experience. Ann Surg. 2004 Jun;239(6):788–97. PMID:15166958

799. Soltani AK, Krishnan K. Current status of newer generation endoscopic ultrasound core needles in the diagnostic evaluation of gastrointestinal lesions. J Am Soc Cytopathol. 2020 Sep-Oct;9(5):389–95. PMID:32680792

800. Sooklal S, Chahal P. Endoscopic ultrasound. Surg Clin North Am. 2020 Dec;100(6):1133–50. PMID:33128884

801. Sopha SC, Gopal P, Merchant NB, et al. Diagnostic and therapeutic implications of a novel immunohistochemical panel detecting duodenal mucosal invasion by pancreatic ductal adenocarcinoma. Int J Clin Exp Pathol. 2013 Oct 15;6(11):2476–86. PMID:24228110

802. Soyer OM, Baran B, Ormeci AC, et al. Role of biochemistry and cytological analysis of cyst fluid for the differential diagnosis of pancreatic cysts: a retrospective cohort study. Medicine (Baltimore). 2017 Jan;96(1):e5513. PMID:28072692

803. Specht K, Zhang L, Sung YS, et al. Novel BCOR-MAML3 and ZC3H7B-BCOR gene fusions in undifferentiated small blue round cell sarcomas. Am J Surg Pathol. 2016 Apr;40(4):433–42. PMID:26752546

804. Speisky D, Villarroel M, Vigovich F, et al. Undifferentiated carcinoma with osteoclast-like giant cells of the pancreas diagnosed by endoscopic ultrasound guided biopsy. Ecancermedicalscience. 2020 Jul 17;14:1072. PMID:32863866

805. Spencer LA, Spizarny DL, Williams TR. Imaging features of intrapancreatic accessory spleen. Br J Radiol. 2010 Aug;83(992):668–73. PMID:19690077

806. Sperti C, Pasquali C, Di Prima F, et al. Percutaneous CT-guided fine needle aspiration cytology in the differential diagnosis of pancreatic lesions. Ital J Gastroenterol. 1994 Apr;26(3):126–31. PMID:8061338

807. Spier BJ, Johnson EA, Gopal DV, et al. Predictors of malignancy and recommended follow-up in patients with negative endoscopic ultrasound-guided fine-needle aspiration of suspected pancreatic lesions. Can J Gastroenterol. 2009 Apr;23(4):279–86. PMID:19373422

808. Springer S, Masica DL, Dal Molin M, et al. A multimodality test to guide the management of patients with a pancreatic cyst. Sci Transl Med. 2019 Jul 17;11(501):eaav4772. PMID:31316009

809. Springer S, Wang Y, Dal Molin M, et al. A combination of molecular markers and clinical features improve the classification of pancreatic cysts. Gastroenterology. 2015 Nov;149(6):1501–10. PMID:26253305

810. Srivastava A, Hornick JL. Immunohistochemical staining for CDX-2, PDX-1, NESP-55, and TTF-1 can help distinguish gastrointestinal carcinoid tumors from pancreatic endocrine and pulmonary carcinoid tumors. Am J Surg Pathol. 2009 Apr;33(4):626–32. PMID:19065104

811. Stelow EB, Bardales RH, Lai R, et al. The cytological spectrum of chronic pancreatitis. Diagn Cytopathol. 2005 Feb;32(2):65–9. PMID:15637684

812. Stelow EB, Bardales RH, Shami VM, et al. Cytology of pancreatic acinar cell carcinoma. Diagn Cytopathol. 2006 May;34(5):367–72. PMID:16604543

813. Stelow EB, Bardales RH, Stanley MW. Pitfalls in endoscopic ultrasound-guided fine-needle aspiration and how to avoid them. Adv Anat Pathol. 2005 Mar;12(2):62–73. PMID:15731574

814. Stelow EB, Pambuccian SE, Bardales RH, et al. The cytology of pancreatic foamy gland adenocarcinoma. Am J Clin Pathol. 2004 Jun;121(6):893–7. PMID:15198363

815. Stelow EB, Shami VM, Abbott TE, et al. The use of fine needle aspiration cytology for the distinction of pancreatic mucinous neoplasia. Am J Clin Pathol. 2008 Jan;129(1):67–74. PMID:18089490

816. Stevens KJ, Lisanti C. Pancreas imaging. 2022 Mar 11. In: StatPearls. Treasure Island (FL): StatPearls Publishing; 2022 Jan–. PMID:31613505

817. Stewart CJ, Mills PR, Carter R, et al. Brush cytology in the assessment of pancreatico-biliary strictures: a review of 406 cases. J Clin Pathol. 2001 Jun;54(6):449–55. PMID:11376018

818. Stewart FW. The diagnosis of tumors by aspiration. Am J Pathol. 1933;9(Suppl):801–812.3. PMID:19970115

819. Stone JH, Khosroshahi A, Deshpande V, et al. Recommendations for the nomenclature of IgG4-related disease and its individual organ system manifestations. Arthritis Rheum. 2012 Oct;64(10):3061–7. PMID:22736240

820. Strobel O, Hartwig W, Bergmann F, et al. Anaplastic pancreatic cancer: presentation, surgical management, and outcome. Surgery. 2011 Feb;149(2):200–8. PMID:20542529

821. Suda K, Hirai S, Matsumoto Y, et al. Variant of intraductal carcinoma (with scant mucin production) is of main pancreatic duct origin: a clinicopathological study of four patients. Am J Gastroenterol. 1996 Apr;91(4):798–800. PMID:8677955

822. Suh YK, Shin HJ. Fine-needle aspiration biopsy of granulocytic sarcoma: a clinicopathologic study of 27 cases. Cancer. 2000 Dec 25;90(6):364–72. PMID:11156520

823. Sundling KE, Kurtycz DFI. Standardized terminology systems in cytopathology. Diagn Cytopathol. 2019 Jan;47(1):53–63. PMID:30499199

824. Sung S, Del Portillo A, Gonda TA, et al. Update on risk stratification in the Papanicolaou Society of Cytopathology System for Reporting Pancreaticobiliary Cytology categories: 3-year, prospective, single-institution experience. Cancer Cytopathol. 2020 Jan;128(1):29–35. PMID:31722125

825. Sung S, Rao R, Sharaiha RZ, et al. Fine-needle aspiration cytology of pancreatic schwannoma. Diagn Cytopathol. 2017 Jul;45(7):668–70. PMID:28217914

826. Suthipintawong C, Leong AS, Vinyuvat S. Immunostaining of cell preparations: a comparative evaluation of common fixatives and protocols. Diagn Cytopathol. 1996 Aug;15(2):167–74. PMID:8872443

827. Suzuki R, Lee JH, Krishna SG, et al. Repeat endoscopic ultrasound-guided fine needle aspiration for solid pancreatic lesions at a tertiary referral center will alter the initial inconclusive result. J Gastrointestin Liver Dis. 2013 Jun;22(2):183–7. PMID:23799217

828. Suzuki S, Kaji S, Koike N, et al. Pancreatic schwannoma: a case report and literature review with special reference to imaging features. JOP. 2010 Jan 8;11(1):31–5. PMID:20065549

829. Sweeney J, Rao R, Margolskee E, et al. Immunohistochemical staining for S100P, SMAD4, and IMP3 on cell block preparations is sensitive and highly specific for pancreatic ductal adenocarcinoma. J Am Soc Cytopathol. 2018 Nov-Dec;7(6):318–23. PMID:31043302

830. Syed A, Babich O, Rao B, et al. Endoscopic ultrasound guided fine-needle aspiration vs core needle biopsy for solid pancreatic lesions: comparison of diagnostic accuracy and procedural efficiency. Diagn Cytopathol. 2019 Nov;47(11):1138–44. PMID:31313531

831. Tajima S. Intraductal tubulopapillary neoplasm of the pancreas suspected by endoscopic ultrasonography-fine-needle aspiration cytology: report of a case confirmed by surgical specimen histology. Diagn Cytopathol. 2015 Dec;43(12):1003–6. PMID:26390029

832. Tajiri T, Tate G, Inagaki T, et al. Intraductal tubular neoplasms of the pancreas: histogenesis and differentiation. Pancreas. 2005 Mar;30(2):115–21. PMID:15714133

833. Tajiri T, Tate G, Kunimura T, et al. Histologic and immunohistochemical comparison of intraductal tubular carcinoma, intraductal papillary-mucinous carcinoma, and ductal adenocarcinoma of the pancreas. Pancreas. 2004 Aug;29(2):116–22. PMID:15257103

834. Takahashi K, Mikata R, Tsuyuguchi T, et al. Granular cell tumor of the pancreas diagnosed by endoscopic ultrasound-guided fine-needle aspiration. Clin J Gastroenterol. 2018 Jun;11(3):193–9. PMID:29380119

835. Takahashi M, Fujinaga Y, Notohara K, et al. Diagnostic imaging guide for autoimmune pancreatitis. Jpn J Radiol. 2020 Jul;38(7):591–612. PMID:32297064

836. Tanaka M, Chari S, Adsay V, et al. International consensus guidelines for management of intraductal papillary mucinous neoplasms and mucinous cystic neoplasms of the pancreas. Pancreatology. 2006;6(1-2):17–32. PMID:16327281

837. Tanaka M, editor. Intraductal papillary mucinous neoplasm of the pancreas. Tokyo (Japan): Springer; 2014.

838. Tanaka M, Fernández-del Castillo C, Adsay V, et al. International consensus guidelines 2012 for the management of IPMN and MCN of the pancreas. Pancreatology. 2012 May-Jun;12(3):183–97. PMID:22687371

839. Tanaka M, Fernández-Del Castillo C, Kamisawa T, et al. Revisions of international consensus Fukuoka guidelines for the management of IPMN of the pancreas. Pancreatology. 2017 Sep-Oct;17(5):738–53. PMID:28735806

840. Tanaka Y, Kato K, Notohara K, et al. Significance of aberrant (cytoplasmic/nuclear) expression of beta-catenin in pancreatoblastoma. J Pathol. 2003 Feb;199(2):185–90. PMID:12533831

841. Tang LH, Basturk O, Sue JJ, et al. A practical approach to the classification of WHO grade 3 (G3) well-differentiated neuroendocrine tumor (WD-NET) and poorly differentiated neuroendocrine carcinoma (PD-NEC) of the pancreas. Am J Surg Pathol. 2016 Sep;40(9):1192–202. PMID:27259015

842. Tang LH, Untch BR, Reidy DL, et al. Well-differentiated neuroendocrine tumors with a morphologically apparent high-grade component: a pathway distinct from poorly differentiated neuroendocrine carcinomas. Clin Cancer Res. 2016 Feb 15;22(4):1011–7. PMID:26482044

843. Tang ZH, Zou SQ, Hao YH, et al. The relationship between loss expression of DPC4/Smad4 gene and carcinogenesis of pancreatobiliary carcinoma. Hepatobiliary Pancreat Dis Int. 2002 Nov;1(4):624–9. PMID:14607700

844. Tatsas AD, Owens CL, Siddiqui MT, et al. Fine-needle aspiration of intrapancreatic accessory spleen: cytomorphologic features and differential diagnosis. Cancer Cytopathol. 2012 Aug 25;120(4):261–8. PMID:22298506

845. Terris B, Cavard C. Diagnosis and molecular aspects of solid-pseudopapillary neoplasms of the pancreas. Semin Diagn Pathol. 2014 Nov;31(6):484–90. PMID:25524568

846. Tewari N, Rollins K, Wu J, et al. Lymphoepithelial cyst of the pancreas and elevated cyst fluid carcinoembryonic antigen: a diagnostic challenge. JOP. 2014 Sep 28;15(5):504–7. PMID:25262722

847. Thoeni RF. The revised Atlanta classification of acute pancreatitis: its importance for the radiologist and its effect on treatment. Radiology. 2012 Mar;262(3):751–64. PMID:22357880

848. Thornton GD, McPhail MJ, Nayagam S, et al. Endoscopic ultrasound guided fine needle aspiration for the diagnosis of pancreatic cystic neoplasms: a meta-analysis. Pancreatology. 2013 Jan-Feb;13(1):48–57. PMID:23395570

849. Tian L, Lv XF, Dong J, et al. Clinical features and CT/MRI findings of pancreatic acinar cell carcinoma. Int J Clin Exp Med. 2015 Sep 15;8(9):14846–54. PMID:26628966

850. Tiemann K, Heitling U, Kosmahl M, et al. Solid pseudopapillary neoplasms of the pancreas show an interruption of the Wnt-signaling pathway and express gene products of 11q. Mod Pathol. 2007 Sep;20(9):955–60. PMID:17632456

851. Tokunaga K, Yamamura A, Ueno S, et al. Isolated pancreatic myeloid sarcoma associated with t(8;21)/RUNX1-RUNX1T1 rearrangement. Intern Med. 2018 Feb 15;57(4):563–8. PMID:29151502

852. Toll AD, Bibbo M. Identification of gastrointestinal contamination in endoscopic ultrasound-guided pancreatic fine needle aspiration. Acta Cytol. 2010 May-Jun;54(3):245–8. PMID:20518405

853. Toll AD, Hruban RH, Ali SZ. Acinar cell carcinoma of the pancreas: clinical and cytomorphologic characteristics. Korean J Pathol. 2013 Apr;47(2):93–9. PMID:23667367

854. Tracht J, Reid MD, Hissong E, et al. Serous cystadenoma of the pancreas with complex florid papillary architecture: a case report and review of the literature. Int J Surg Pathol. 2019 Dec;27(8):907–11. PMID:31187681

855. Traverso LW, Peralta EA, Ryan JA Jr, et al. Intraductal neoplasms of the pancreas. Am J Surg. 1998 May;175(5):426–32. PMID:9600293

856. Trisolini E, Armellini E, Paganotti A, et al. KRAS mutation testing on all non-malignant diagnosis of pancreatic endoscopic ultrasound-guided fine-needle aspiration biopsies improves diagnostic accuracy. Pathology. 2017 Jun;49(4):379–86. PMID:28450086

857. Tseng JF, Warshaw AL, Sahani DV, et al. Serous cystadenoma of the pancreas: tumor growth rates and recommendations for treatment. Ann Surg. 2005 Sep;242(3):413–9. PMID:16135927

858. Tsui WM, Lam PW, Mak CK, et al. Fine-needle aspiration cytologic diagnosis of intrahepatic biliary papillomatosis (intraductal papillary tumor): report of three cases and comparative study with cholangiocarcinoma. Diagn Cytopathol. 2000 May;22(5):293–8. PMID:10790236

859. Tsukada A, Ishizaki Y, Nobukawa B, et al. Paraganglioma of the pancreas: a case report and review of the literature. Pancreas. 2008 Mar;36(2):214–6. PMID:18376320

860. Tummala P, Munigala S, Eloubeidi MA, et al. Patients with obstructive jaundice and biliary stricture ± mass lesion on imaging: prevalence of malignancy and potential role of EUS-FNA. J Clin Gastroenterol. 2013 Jul;47(6):532–7. PMID:23340062

861. Tylén U, Arnesjö B, Lindberg LG, et al. Percutaneous biopsy of carcinoma of the pancreas guided by angiography. Surg Gynecol Obstet. 1976 May;142(5):737–9. PMID:1265615

862. Tyson GL, El-Serag HB. Risk factors for cholangiocarcinoma. Hepatology. 2011 Jul;54(1):173–84. PMID:21488076

863. Ueno S, Muranaka T, Maekawa S, et al. Radiographic features in lymphoepithelial cyst of the pancreas. Abdom Imaging. 1994 May-Jun;19(3):232–4. PMID:8019350

864. Umehara H, Okazaki K, Masaki Y, et al. Comprehensive diagnostic criteria for IgG4-related disease (IgG4-RD), 2011. Mod Rheumatol. 2012 Feb;22(1):21–30. PMID:22218969

865. Unno J, Kanno A, Masamune A, et al. The usefulness of endoscopic ultrasound-guided fine-needle aspiration for the diagnosis of pancreatic neuroendocrine tumors based on the World Health Organization classification. Scand J Gastroenterol. 2014 Nov;49(11):1367–74. PMID:25180490

866. Val-Bernal JF, Yllera E, Moris M, et al. Endoscopic ultrasound-guided fine-needle aspiration cytology in the diagnosis of the gastrointestinal stromal tumor of the stomach. Diagn Cytopathol. 2020 Sep;48(9):833–9. PMID:32400969

867. Vâlsănescu T, Mateescu MA, Schell HD, et al. All-reagent test tablets and method for rapid and selective alpha-amylase iodometric determination. Anal Biochem. 1985 May 1;146(2):299–306. PMID:3875297

868. Valsangkar NP, Morales-Oyarvide V, Thayer SP, et al. 851 resected cystic tumors of the pancreas: a 33-year experience at the Massachusetts General Hospital. Surgery. 2012 Sep;152(3 Suppl 1):S4–12. PMID:22770958

869. van Heek NT, Meeker AK, Kern SE, et al. Telomere shortening is nearly universal in pancreatic intraepithelial neoplasia. Am J Pathol. 2002 Nov;161(5):1541–7. PMID:12414502

870. van Heek T, Rader AE, Offerhaus GJ, et al. K-ras, p53, and DPC4 (MAD4) alterations in fine-needle aspirates of the pancreas: a molecular panel correlates with and supplements cytologic diagnosis. Am J Clin Pathol. 2002 May;117(5):755–65. PMID:12090425

871. van Huijgevoort NCM, Del Chiaro M, Wolfgang CL, et al. Diagnosis and management of pancreatic cystic neoplasms: current evidence and guidelines. Nat Rev Gastroenterol Hepatol. 2019 Nov;16(11):676–89. PMID:31527862

872. van Riet PA, Cahen DL, Poley JW, et al. Mapping international practice patterns in EUS-guided tissue sampling: outcome of a global survey. Endosc Int Open. 2016 Mar;4(3):E360–70. PMID:27227103

873. VandenBussche CJ, Allison DB, Graham MK, et al. Alternative lengthening of telomeres and ATRX/DAXX loss can be reliably detected in FNAs of pancreatic neuroendocrine tumors. Cancer Cytopathol. 2017 Jul;125(7):544–51. PMID:28371511

874. VandenBussche CJ, Maleki Z. Fine-needle aspiration of squamous-lined cysts of the pancreas. Diagn Cytopathol. 2014 Jul;42(7):592–9. PMID:24376211

875. Vandervoort J, Soetikno RM, Montes H, et al. Accuracy and complication rate of brush cytology from bile duct versus pancreatic duct. Gastrointest Endosc. 1999 Mar;49(3 Pt 1):322–7. PMID:10049415

876. van der Waaij LA, van Dullemen HM, Porte RJ. Cyst fluid analysis in the differential diagnosis of pancreatic cystic lesions: a pooled analysis. Gastrointest Endosc. 2005 Sep;62(3):383–9. PMID:16111956

877. Vannas MJ, Boyd S, Färkkilä MA, et al. Value of brush cytology for optimal timing of liver transplantation in primary sclerosing cholangitis. Liver Int. 2017 May;37(5):735–42. PMID:28453918

878. Vege SS, Ziring B, Jain R, et al. American gastroenterological association institute guideline on the diagnosis and management of asymptomatic neoplastic pancreatic cysts. Gastroenterology. 2015 Apr;148(4):819–22. PMID:25805375

879. Vij M, Agrawal V, Pandey R. Malignant extra-gastrointestinal stromal tumor of the pancreas. A case report and review of literature. JOP. 2011 Mar 9;12(2):200–4. PMID:21386653

880. Villa NA, Berzosa M, Wallace MB, et al. Endoscopic ultrasound-guided fine needle aspiration: the wet suction technique. Endosc Ultrasound. 2016 Jan-Feb;5(1):17–20. PMID:26879162

881. Vilmann P, Jacobsen GK, Henriksen FW, et al. Endoscopic ultrasonography with guided fine needle aspiration biopsy in pancreatic disease. Gastrointest Endosc. 1992 Mar-Apr;38(2):172–3. PMID:1568614

882. Virani N, Pang J, Lew M. Cytologic and immunohistochemical evaluation of low-grade spindle cell lesions of the gastrointestinal tract. Arch Pathol Lab Med. 2016 Oct;140(10):1038–44. PMID:27684974

883. Virk RK, Gamez R, Mehrotra S, et al. Variation of cytopathologists' use of the indeterminate diagnostic categories "atypical" and "suspicious for malignancy" in the cytologic diagnosis of solid pancreatic lesions on endoscopic ultrasound-guided fine-needle aspirates. Diagn Cytopathol. 2017 Jan;45(1):3–13. PMID:27873469

884. Viscosi F, Fleres F, Mazzeo C, et al. Cystic lymphangioma of the pancreas: a hard diagnostic challenge between pancreatic cystic lesions-review of recent literature. Gland Surg. 2018 Oct;7(5):487–92. PMID:30505770

885. Vlajnic T, Somaini G, Savic S, et al. Targeted multiprobe fluorescence in situ hybridization analysis for elucidation of inconclusive pancreatobiliary cytology. Cancer Cytopathol. 2014 Aug;122(8):627–34. PMID:24753508

886. Volk N, Lacy B. Anatomy and physiology of the small bowel. Gastrointest Endosc Clin N Am. 2017 Jan;27(1):1–13. PMID:27908510

887. Volkan Adsay N. Cystic lesions of the pancreas. Mod Pathol. 2007 Feb;20 Suppl 1:S71–93. PMID:17486054

888. Volmar KE, Jones CK, Xie HB. Metastases in the pancreas from nonhematologic neoplasms: report of 20 cases evaluated by fine-needle aspiration. Diagn Cytopathol. 2004 Oct;31(4):216–20. PMID:15452907

889. Volmar KE, Routbort MJ, Jones CK, et al. Primary pancreatic lymphoma evaluated by fine-needle aspiration: findings in 14 cases. Am J Clin Pathol. 2004 Jun;121(6):898–903. PMID:15198364

890. Volmar KE, Vollmer RT, Routbort MJ, et al. Pancreatic and bile duct brushing cytology in 1000 cases: review of findings and comparison of preparation methods. Cancer. 2006 Aug 25;108(4):231–8. PMID:16541448

891. Vortmeyer AO, Lubensky IA, Fogt F, et al. Allelic deletion and mutation of the von Hippel-Lindau (VHL) tumor suppressor gene in pancreatic microcystic adenomas. Am J Pathol. 1997 Oct;151(4):951–6. PMID:9327728

892. Vyas M, Hechtman JF, Zhang Y, et al. DNAJB1-PRKACA fusions occur in oncocytic pancreatic and biliary neoplasms and are not specific for fibrolamellar hepatocellular carcinoma. Mod Pathol. 2020 Apr;33(4):648–56. PMID:31676785

893. Waddell N, Pajic M, Patch AM, et al. Whole genomes redefine the mutational landscape of pancreatic cancer. Nature. 2015 Feb 26;518(7540):495–501. PMID:25719666

895. Wallace ZS, Naden RP, Chari S, et al. The 2019 American College of Rheumatology/European League Against Rheumatism classification criteria for IgG4-related disease. Ann Rheum Dis. 2020 Jan;79(1):77–87. PMID:31796497

896. Wallace ZS, Naden RP, Chari S, et al. The 2019 American College of Rheumatology/European League Against Rheumatism classification criteria for IgG4-related disease. Arthritis Rheumatol. 2020 Jan;72(1):7–19. PMID:31793250

897. Walts AE. Osteoclast-type giant-cell tumor of the pancreas. Acta Cytol. 1983 Sep-Oct;27(5):500–4. PMID:6578648

898. Wang L, Basturk O, Wang J, et al. A FISH assay efficiently screens for BRAF gene rearrangements in pancreatic acinar-type neoplasms. Mod Pathol. 2018 Jan;31(1):132–40. PMID:28884748

899. Wang S, Xing C, Wu H, et al. Pancreatic schwannoma mimicking pancreatic cystadenoma: a case report and literature review of the imaging features. Medicine (Baltimore). 2019 Jun;98(24):e16095. PMID:31192973

900. Wang T, Askan G, Adsay V, et al. Intraductal oncocytic papillary neoplasms: clinical-pathologic characterization of 24 cases, with an emphasis on associated invasive carcinomas. Am J Surg Pathol. 2019 May;43(5):656–61. PMID:30986801

901. Wani S. Basic techniques in endoscopic ultrasound-guided fine-needle aspiration: role of a stylet and suction. Endosc Ultrasound. 2014 Jan;3(1):17–21. PMID:24949406

902. Wani S, Early D, Kunkel J, et al. Diagnostic yield of malignancy during EUS-guided FNA of solid lesions with and without a stylet: a prospective, single blind, randomized, controlled trial. Gastrointest Endosc. 2012 Aug;76(2):328–35. PMID:22695205

903. Wani S, Gupta N, Gaddam S, et al. A comparative study of endoscopic ultrasound guided fine needle aspiration with and without a stylet. Dig Dis Sci. 2011 Aug;56(8):2409–14. PMID:21327919

904. Wani S, Muthusamy VR, McGrath CM, et al. AGA white paper: Optimizing endoscopic ultrasound-guided tissue acquisition and future directions. Clin Gastroenterol Hepatol. 2018 Mar;16(3):318–27. PMID:29074447

905. Watanabe T, Araki K, Ishii N, et al. A surgically resected pancreatic schwannoma with obstructive jaundice with special reference to differential diagnosis from other cystic lesions in the pancreas. Case Rep Gastroenterol. 2018 Feb 21;12(1):85–91. PMID:29606941

906. Waters L, Si Q, Caraway N, et al. Secondary tumors of the pancreas diagnosed by endoscopic ultrasound-guided fine-needle aspiration: a 10-year experience. Diagn Cytopathol. 2014 Sep;42(9):738–43. PMID:24554612

907. Waugh MS, Guy CD, Maygarden SJ, et al. Use of the ThinPrep method in bile duct brushings: analysis of morphologic parameters associated with malignancy and determination of interobserver reliability. Diagn Cytopathol. 2008 Sep;36(9):651–6. PMID:18677761

908. Westra WH, Sturm P, Drillenburg P, et al. K-ras oncogene mutations in osteoclast-like giant cell tumors of the pancreas and liver: genetic evidence to support origin from the duct epithelium. Am J Surg Pathol. 1998 Oct;22(10):1247–54. PMID:9777987

909. Whitehair R, Stelow EB. The cytologic and immunohistochemical findings of pancreatic mixed acinar-endocrine carcinoma. Diagn Cytopathol. 2021 Feb;49(2):287–94. PMID:33128511

910. WHO Classification of Tumours Editorial Board. Digestive system tumours. Lyon (France): International Agency for Research on Cancer; 2019. (WHO classification of tumours series, 5th ed.; vol. 1). https://publications.iarc.fr/579.

911. WHO Classification of Tumours Editorial Board. Haematolymphoid tumours. Lyon (France): International Agency for Research on Cancer; forthcoming. (WHO classification of tumours series, 5th ed.). https://publications.iarc.fr/.

912. WHO Classification of Tumours Editorial Board. Soft tissue and bone tumours. Lyon (France): International Agency for Research on Cancer; 2020. (WHO classification of tumours series, 5th ed.; vol. 3). https://publications.iarc.fr/588.

913. Wieczorek TJ, Faquin WC, Rubin BP, et al. Cytologic diagnosis of gastrointestinal stromal tumor with emphasis on the differential diagnosis with leiomyosarcoma. Cancer. 2001 Aug 25;93(4):276–87. PMID:11507702

914. Wiersema MJ, Kochman ML, Cramer HM, et al. Endosonography-guided real-time fine-needle aspiration biopsy. Gastrointest Endosc. 1994 Nov-Dec;40(6):700–7. PMID:7859968

915. Wiersema MJ, Vilmann P, Giovannini M, et al. Endosonography-guided fine-needle aspiration biopsy: diagnostic accuracy and complication assessment. Gastroenterology. 1997 Apr;112(4):1087–95. PMID:9097990

916. Williet N, Kassir R, Cuilleron M, et al. Difficult endoscopic diagnosis of a pancreatic plasmacytoma: case report and review of literature. World J Clin Oncol. 2017 Feb 10;8(1):91–5. PMID:28246589

917. Wisnoski NC, Townsend CM Jr, Nealon WH, et al. 672 patients with acinar cell carcinoma of the pancreas: a population-based comparison to pancreatic adenocarcinoma. Surgery. 2008 Aug;144(2):141–8. PMID:18656619

918. Witt BL, Kristen Hilden RN, Scaife C, et al. Identification of factors predictive of malignancy in patients with atypical biliary brushing results obtained via ERCP. Diagn Cytopathol. 2013 Aug;41(8):682–8. PMID:23008113

919. Wolske KM, Ponnatapura J, Kolokythas O, et al. Chronic pancreatitis or pancreatic tumor? A problem-solving approach. Radiographics. 2019 Nov-Dec;39(7):1965–82. PMID:31584860

920. Wong NACS, Suortamo S, George E, et al. Paraduodenal/pancreatic Ewing sarcoma is very rare and therefore may be mistaken for neuroendocrine carcinoma. J Clin Pathol. 2022 Jan;75(1):71–2. PMID:33619219

921. Wong W, Raufi AG, Safyan RA, et al. BRCA mutations in pancreas cancer: spectrum, current management, challenges and future prospects. Cancer Manag Res. 2020 Apr 23;12:2731–42. PMID:32368150

922. Woo SM, Park JW, Han SS, et al. Isolated pancreatic metastasis of hepatocellular carcinoma after curative resection. World J Gastrointest Oncol. 2010 Apr 15;2(4):209–12. PMID:21160600

923. Wood LD, Hruban RH. Pathology and molecular genetics of pancreatic neoplasms. Cancer J. 2012 Nov-Dec;18(6):492–501. PMID:23187835

924. Wright PK, Shelton DA, Holbrook MR, et al. Outcomes of endoscopic ultrasound-guided pancreatic FNAC diagnosis for solid and cystic lesions at Manchester Royal Infirmary based upon the Papanicolaou Society of Cytopathology pancreaticobiliary terminology classification scheme. Cytopathology. 2018 Feb;29(1):71–9. PMID:29193477

925. Wu J, Jiao Y, Dal Molin M, et al. Whole-exome sequencing of neoplastic cysts of the pancreas reveals recurrent mutations in components of ubiquitin-dependent pathways. Proc Natl Acad Sci U S A. 2011 Dec 27;108(52):21188–93. PMID:22158988

926. Wu J, Matthaei H, Maitra A, et al. Recurrent GNAS mutations define an unexpected pathway for pancreatic cyst development. Sci Transl Med. 2011 Jul 20;3(92):92ra66. PMID:21775669

927. Xiao AY, Tan ML, Wu LM, et al. Global incidence and mortality of pancreatic diseases: a systematic review, meta-analysis, and meta-regression of population-based cohort studies. Lancet Gastroenterol Hepatol. 2016 Sep;1(1):45–55. PMID:28404111

928. Xie C, Aloreidi K, Patel B, et al. Indeterminate biliary strictures: a simplified approach. Expert Rev Gastroenterol Hepatol. 2018 Feb;12(2):189–99. PMID:29034764

929. Xu MM, Sethi A. Diagnosing biliary malignancy. Gastrointest Endosc Clin N Am. 2015 Oct;25(4):677–90. PMID:26431597

931. Xue Y, Reid MD, Pehlivanoglu B, et al. Morphologic variants of pancreatic neuroendocrine tumors: clinicopathologic analysis and prognostic stratification. Endocr Pathol. 2020 Sep;31(3):239–53. PMID:32488621

932. Xue Y, San Luis B, Lane DP. Intratumour heterogeneity of p53 expression; causes and consequences. J Pathol. 2019 Nov;249(3):274–85. PMID:31322742

933. Yachida S, Vakiani E, White CM, et al. Small cell and large cell neuroendocrine carcinomas of the pancreas are genetically similar and distinct from well-differentiated pancreatic neuroendocrine tumors. Am J Surg Pathol. 2012 Feb;36(2):173–84. PMID:22251937

934. Yamaguchi H, Kuboki Y, Hatori T, et al. Somatic mutations in PIK3CA and activation of AKT in intraductal tubulopapillary neoplasms of the pancreas. Am J Surg Pathol. 2011 Dec;35(12):1812–7. PMID:21945955

935. Yamaguchi H, Kuboki Y, Hatori T, et al. The discrete nature and distinguishing molecular features of pancreatic intraductal tubulopapillary neoplasms and intraductal papillary mucinous neoplasms of the gastric type, pyloric gland variant. J Pathol. 2013 Nov;231(3):335–41. PMID:23893889

936. Yamaguchi H, Shimizu M, Ban S, et al. Intraductal tubulopapillary neoplasms of the pancreas distinct from pancreatic intraepithelial neoplasia and intraductal papillary mucinous neoplasms. Am J Surg Pathol. 2009 Aug;33(8):1164–72. PMID:19440145

937. Yamaguchi S, Fujii T, Izumi Y, et al. Identification and characterization of a novel adenomatous polyposis coli mutation in adult pancreatoblastoma. Oncotarget. 2018 Jan 6;9(12):10818–27. PMID:29535845

938. Yamaguchi T, Shirai Y, Nakamura N, et al. Usefulness of brush cytology combined with pancreatic juice cytology in the diagnosis of pancreatic cancer: significance of pancreatic juice cytology after brushing. Pancreas. 2012 Nov;41(8):1225–9. PMID:23086246

939. Yamao K, Takenaka M, Ishikawa R, et al. Partial pancreatic parenchymal atrophy is a new specific finding to diagnose small pancreatic cancer (≤10 mm) including carcinoma in situ: comparison with localized benign main pancreatic duct stenosis patients. Diagnostics (Basel). 2020 Jul 1;10(7):445. PMID:32630180

940. Yamao K, Yanagisawa A, Takahashi K, et al. Clinicopathological features and prognosis of mucinous cystic neoplasm with ovarian-type stroma: a multi-institutional study of the Japan Pancreas Society. Pancreas. 2011 Jan;40(1):67–71. PMID:20924309

941. Yamazaki K, Eyden B. An immunohistochemical and ultrastructural study of pancreatic microcystic serous cyst adenoma with special reference to tumor-associated microvasculature and vascular endothelial growth factor in tumor cells. Ultrastruct Pathol. 2006 Jan-Feb;30(1):119–28. PMID:16517478

942. Yan BM, Pai RK, Van Dam J. Diagnosis of pancreatic gastrointestinal stromal tumor by EUS guided FNA. JOP. 2008 Mar 8;9(2):192–6. PMID:18326928

943. Yang F, Liu E, Sun S. Rapid on-site evaluation (ROSE) with EUS-FNA: the ROSE looks beautiful. Endosc Ultrasound. 2019 Sep-Oct;8(5):283–7. PMID:31603143

944. Yang F, Wu W, Wang X, et al. Grading solid pseudopapillary tumors of the pancreas: the Fudan prognostic index. Ann Surg Oncol. 2021 Jan;28(1):550–9. PMID:32424583

945. Yang MJ, Hwang JC, Yoo BM, et al. A prospective randomized trial of EUS-guided tissue acquisition using a 25-gauge core biopsy needle with and without a stylet. Surg Endosc. 2018 Sep;32(9):3777–82. PMID:29572629

946. Yang W, Sun Y. Promising molecular targets for the targeted therapy of biliary tract cancers: an overview. Onco Targets Ther. 2021 Feb 25;14:1341–66. PMID:33658799

947. Yang X, Guo JF, Sun LQ, et al. Assessment of different modalities for repeated tissue acquisition in diagnosing malignant biliary strictures: a two-center retrospective study. J Dig Dis. 2021 Feb;22(2):102–7. PMID:33247545

948. Yang Z, Gong Y, Ji M, et al. Differential diagnosis of pancreatoblastoma (PB) and solid pseudopapillary neoplasms (SPNs) in children by CT and MR imaging. Eur Radiol. 2021 Apr;31(4):2209–17. PMID:32997172

949. Yang Z, Klimstra DS, Hruban RH, et al. Immunohistochemical characterization of the origins of metastatic well-differentiated neuroendocrine tumors to the liver. Am J Surg Pathol. 2017 Jul;41(7):915–22. PMID:28498280

950. Yasuda H, Takada T, Amano H, et al. Surgery for mucin-producing pancreatic tumor. Hepatogastroenterology. 1998 Nov-Dec;45(24):2009–15. PMID:9951855

951. Yeh MM, Tang LH, Wang S, et al. Inhibin expression in ovarian-type stroma in mucinous cystic neoplasms of the pancreas. Appl Immunohistochem Mol Morphol. 2004 Jun;12(2):148–52. PMID:15354741

952. Yeo MK, Kim KH, Lee YM, et al. The usefulness of adding p53 immunocytochemistry to bile drainage cytology for the diagnosis of malignant biliary strictures. Diagn Cytopathol. 2017 Jul;45(7):592–7. PMID:28411396

953. Yepuri N, Pruekprasert N, Naous R. High-grade malignant pancreatic neoplasm with sarcomatoid features. AME Case Rep. 2018 Aug 22;2:39. PMID:30363708

954. Yin BW, Dnistrian A, Lloyd KO. Ovarian cancer antigen CA125 is encoded by the MUC16 mucin gene. Int J Cancer. 2002 Apr 10;98(5):737–40. PMID:11920644

955. Yip-Schneider MT, Wu H, Dumas RP, et al. Vascular endothelial growth factor, a novel and highly accurate pancreatic fluid biomarker for serous pancreatic cysts. J Am Coll Surg. 2014 Apr;218(4):608–17. PMID:24491241

956. Ylagan LR, Edmundowicz S, Kasal K, et al. Endoscopic ultrasound guided fine-needle aspiration cytology of pancreatic carcinoma: a 3-year experience and review of the literature. Cancer. 2002 Dec 25;96(6):362–9. PMID:12478684

957. Yokode M, Akita M, Fujikura K, et al. High-grade PanIN presenting with localised stricture of the main pancreatic duct: a clinicopathological and molecular study of 10 cases suggests a clue for the early detection of pancreatic cancer. Histopathology. 2018 Aug;73(2):247–58. PMID:29660164

958. Yoon WJ, Daglilar ES, Fernández-del Castillo C, et al. Peritoneal seeding in intraductal papillary mucinous neoplasm of the pancreas patients who underwent endoscopic ultrasound-guided fine-needle aspiration: the PIPE Study. Endoscopy. 2014 May;46(5):382–7. PMID:24619804

959. Yoon WJ, Daglilar ES, Mino-Kenudson M, et al. Characterization of epithelial subtypes of intraductal papillary mucinous neoplasm of the pancreas with endoscopic ultrasound and cyst fluid analysis. Endoscopy. 2014 Dec;46(12):1071–7. PMID:25208034

960. Yoon WJ, Daglilar ES, Pitman MB, et al. Cystic pancreatic neuroendocrine tumors: endoscopic ultrasound and fine-needle aspiration characteristics. Endoscopy. 2013;45(3):189–94. PMID:23296363

961. Yoon WJ, Lee JK, Lee KH, et al. Cystic neoplasms of the exocrine pancreas: an update of a nationwide survey in Korea. Pancreas. 2008 Oct;37(3):254–8. PMID:18815545

962. Yoshida A, Goto K, Kodaira M, et al. CIC-rearranged sarcomas: a study of 20 cases and comparisons with Ewing sarcomas. Am J Surg Pathol. 2016 Mar;40(3):313–23. PMID:26685084

963. Younan G. Pancreas solid tumors. Surg Clin North Am. 2020 Jun;100(3):565–80. PMID:32402301

964. Youngwirth LM, Freischlag K, Nussbaum DP, et al. Primary sarcomas of the pancreas: a review of 253 patients from the National Cancer Data Base. Surg Oncol. 2018 Dec;27(4):676–80. PMID:30449492

965. Youssef Y, Shen R, Tonkovich D, et al. Clinical features, onsite evaluation, and follow-up results in patients with suspicious for adenocarcinoma on EUS-guided FNA of pancreas. J Am Soc Cytopathol. 2018 Jul-Aug;7(4):212–8. PMID:31043279
966. Yu J, Wang Q, Xue P, et al. A model for the impact of FFPE section thickness on gene copy number measurement by FISH. Sci Rep. 2019 May 17;9(1):7518. PMID:31101839
967. Zaheer A, Pokharel SS, Wolfgang C, et al. Incidentally detected cystic lesions of the pancreas on CT: review of literature and management suggestions. Abdom Imaging. 2013 Apr;38(2):331–41. PMID:22534872
968. Zamboni G, Lüttges J, Capelli P, et al. Histopathological features of diagnostic and clinical relevance in autoimmune pancreatitis: a study on 53 resection specimens and 9 biopsy specimens. Virchows Arch. 2004 Dec;445(6):552–63. PMID:15517359
969. Zamboni G, Scarpa A, Bogina G, et al. Mucinous cystic tumors of the pancreas: clinicopathological features, prognosis, and relationship to other mucinous cystic tumors. Am J Surg Pathol. 1999 Apr;23(4):410–22. PMID:10199470
970. Zamboni GA, D'Onofrio M, Idili A, et al. Ultrasound-guided percutaneous fine-needle aspiration of 545 focal pancreatic lesions. AJR Am J Roentgenol. 2009 Dec;193(6):1691–5. PMID:19933666
971. Zen Y, Adsay NV, Bardadin K, et al. Biliary intraepithelial neoplasia: an international interobserver agreement study and proposal for diagnostic criteria. Mod Pathol. 2007 Jun;20(6):701–9. PMID:17431410
972. Zen Y, Fujii T, Itatsu K, et al. Biliary cystic tumors with bile duct communication: a cystic variant of intraductal papillary neoplasm of the bile duct. Mod Pathol. 2006 Sep;19(9):1243–54. PMID:16741522
973. Zen Y, Fujii T, Itatsu K, et al. Biliary papillary tumors share pathological features with intraductal papillary mucinous neoplasm of the pancreas. Hepatology. 2006 Nov;44(5):1333–43. PMID:17058219
974. Zen Y, Harada K, Sasaki M, et al. IgG4-related sclerosing cholangitis with and without hepatic inflammatory pseudotumor, and sclerosing pancreatitis-associated sclerosing cholangitis: Do they belong to a spectrum of sclerosing pancreatitis? Am J Surg Pathol. 2004 Sep;28(9):1193–203. PMID:15316319
975. Zen Y, Ishikawa A, Ogiso S, et al. Follicular cholangitis and pancreatitis - clinicopathological features and differential diagnosis of an under-recognized entity. Histopathology. 2012 Jan;60(2):261–9. PMID:22211284
976. Zen Y, Kawakami H, Kim JH. IgG4-related sclerosing cholangitis: all we need to know. J Gastroenterol. 2016 Apr;51(4):295–312. PMID:26817943
977. Zen Y, Quaglia A, Heaton N, et al. Two distinct pathways of carcinogenesis in primary sclerosing cholangitis. Histopathology. 2011 Dec;59(6):1100–10. PMID:22175890
978. Zen Y, Sasaki M, Fujii T, et al. Different expression patterns of mucin core proteins and cytokeratins during intrahepatic cholangiocarcinogenesis from biliary intraepithelial neoplasia and intraductal papillary neoplasm of the bile duct–an immunohistochemical study of 110 cases of hepatolithiasis. J Hepatol. 2006 Feb;44(2):350–8. PMID:16360234
979. Zhai J. UroVysion multi-target fluorescence in situ hybridization assay for the detection of malignant bile duct brushing specimens: a comparison with routine cytology. Acta Cytol. 2018;62(4):295–301. PMID:29734171
980. Zhang H, Jensen MH, Farnell MB, et al. Primary leiomyosarcoma of the pancreas: study of 9 cases and review of literature. Am J Surg Pathol. 2010 Dec;34(12):1849–56. PMID:21107091
981. Zhang H, Zhu J, Ke F, et al. Radiological imaging for assessing the respectability of hilar cholangiocarcinoma: a systematic review and meta-analysis. Biomed Res Int. 2015;2015:497942. PMID:26448940
982. Zhang ML, Arpin RN, Brugge WR, et al. Moray micro forceps biopsy improves the diagnosis of specific pancreatic cysts. Cancer Cytopathol. 2018 Jun;126(6):414–20. PMID:29660844
983. Zhao L, Hart J, Xiao SY, et al. Cytological features of pancreatic intraductal tubulopapillary neoplasm and an unexpected immunohistochemical profile. Pathology. 2014 Dec;46(7):662–5. PMID:25393265
984. Zhelnin K, Xue Y, Quigley B, et al. Nonmucinous biliary epithelium is a frequent finding and is often the predominant epithelial type in mucinous cystic neoplasms of the pancreas and liver. Am J Surg Pathol. 2017 Jan;41(1):116–20. PMID:27673548
985. Zhong L. Magnetic resonance imaging in the detection of pancreatic neoplasms. J Dig Dis. 2007 Aug;8(3):128–32. PMID:17650223
986. Zhou DK, Gao BQ, Zhang W, et al. Sarcomatoid carcinoma of the pancreas: a case report. World J Clin Cases. 2019 Jan 26;7(2):236–41. PMID:30705901
987. Zhou J, Wu H, Lin J, et al. Fine needle aspiration evaluation of pancreatic lymphoma: a retrospective study of 25 cases in a single institution. Diagn Cytopathol. 2018 Feb;46(2):131–8. PMID:29143491
988. Zhu LC, Sidhu GS, Cassai ND, et al. Fine-needle aspiration cytology of pancreatoblastoma in a young woman: report of a case and review of the literature. Diagn Cytopathol. 2005 Oct;33(4):258–62. PMID:16138370
989. Zikos T, Pham K, Bowen R, et al. Cyst fluid glucose is rapidly feasible and accurate in diagnosing mucinous pancreatic cysts. Am J Gastroenterol. 2015 Jun;110(6):909–14. PMID:25986360
990. Zou C, Yang F, Fu D. Meta-analysis of Ki-67 expression for recurrence in patients with solid pseudopapillary tumor of the pancreas. HPB (Oxford). 2020 Apr;22(4):631–2. PMID:31668755

Subject index

Bold page numbers indicate the main discussion(s) of the topic.

The IAC-IARC-WHO Cytopathology Reporting Systems

Lung

International Academy of Cytology – International Agency for Research on Cancer – World Health Organization Joint Editorial Board. WHO Reporting System for Lung Cytopathology. Lyon (France): International Agency for Research on Cancer; 2022. (IAC-IARC-WHO cytopathology reporting systems series, 1st ed.; vol. 1). https://publications.iarc.fr/620.

Pancreaticobiliary system

International Academy of Cytology – International Agency for Research on Cancer – World Health Organization Joint Editorial Board. WHO Reporting System for Pancreaticobiliary Cytopathology. Lyon (France): International Agency for Research on Cancer; 2022. (IAC-IARC-WHO cytopathology reporting systems series, 1st ed.; vol. 2). https://publications.iarc.fr/621.

WHO Classification of Tumours Online

The content of this new, innovative, and comprehensive cytopathology reporting series is also available in a convenient digital format, at https://tumourclassification.iarc.who.int